Study Guide
Cooper & Gosnell

Foundations and Adult Health Nursing

Seventh Edition

Candice Kumagai

Formerly Instructor in Clinical Nursing
University of Texas at Austin
Austin, Texas

ELSEVIER
MOSBY

ELSEVIER
MOSBY

3251 Riverport Lane
St. Louis, Missouri 63043

STUDY GUIDE FOR FOUNDATIONS AND
ADULT HEALTH NURSING, Seventh edition   ISBN: 978-0-323-11219-2

Content Strategist: Nancy O'Brien
Content Development Specialist: Kelly Skelton
Publishing Services Manager: Jeff Patterson
Project Manager: Mary G. Stueck
Design Direction: Karen Pauls

Printed in the United States of America

Last digit is the print number: 9 8 7 6 5 4 3 2 1

To the Student

Understanding fundamental concepts and principles of nursing will prepare you for patient care experiences. By mastering the content of your *Foundations and Adult Health Nursing* textbook, you will have the necessary knowledge and skills for nursing practice. This Study Guide was created to help you achieve the objectives of each chapter in the textbook, establish a solid base of knowledge in the fundamentals of nursing, and evaluate your understanding of this critical information.

Each Study Guide chapter is organized into sections, each with its own topic and related objectives from the textbook. Different types of learning activities, including short answer, multiple choice, fill-in-the blank, matching, and true/false, assist you in meeting these content objectives. To maximize the benefits of this Study Guide and prepare for the learning activities:

1. Carefully read the chapter in the textbook and highlight, note, or outline important information.
2. Review the Key Points, access the Additional Learning Resources, and complete the Review Questions for the NCLEX® Examination at the end of each textbook chapter.
3. Complete the Study Guide exercises to the best of your ability.
4. Time and pace yourself during the completion of each exercise. You should spend approximately 1 minute for each multiple choice, true/false, and matching question, and approximately 2 minutes for completion activities or short answer questions.
5. After completing an exercise, refer to the textbook page references as needed. You can then repeat any exercises for additional practice and review. A complete Answer Key is provided in your Additional Learning Resources on Evolve.

ADDITIONAL LEARNING RESOURCES

Additional Learning Resources are available on the Evolve website at http://evolve.elsevier.com/Cooper/foundationsadult/.

Evolve

- Review Questions for the NCLEX® Examination (for each chapter)
- Answer Key for all Study Guide questions
- Calculators
- Fluids and Electrolytes Tutorial
- Spanish/English Glossary
- Additional Animations
- Additional Audio Clips
- Additional Video Clips
- Skills Performance Checklists
- Body Spectrum Electronic Anatomy Coloring Book

STUDY HINTS FOR ALL STUDENTS

- *Ask questions!* There are no bad questions. If you do not know something or are not sure, you need to find out. Other people may be wondering the same thing but may be too shy to ask. The answer could mean life or death to your patient, which certainly is more important than feeling embarrassed about asking a question.
- *Make use of chapter objectives.* At the beginning of each chapter in the textbook are objectives that you should have mastered when you finished studying that chapter. Write these objectives in your notebook, leaving a blank space after each. Fill in the answers as you find them while reading the chapter. Review to make sure your answers are correct and complete, and use these answers when

you study for tests. This should also be done for separate course objectives that your instructor has listed in your class syllabus.

- *Locate and understand key terms.* At the beginning of each chapter in the textbook are key terms that you will encounter as you read the chapter. Page numbers are provided for easy reference and review, and the key terms are in bold, blue font the first time they appear in the chapter. Phonetic pronunciations are provided for terms that might be difficult to pronounce.
- *Review Key Points.* Use the Key Points at the end of each chapter in the textbook to help you review for exams.
- *Get the most from your textbook.* When reading each chapter in the textbook, look at the subject headings to learn what each section is about. Read first for the general meaning, then reread parts you did not understand. It may help to read those parts aloud. Carefully read the information given in each table and study each figure and its caption.
- *Follow up on difficult concepts.* While studying, put difficult concepts into your own words to see if you understand them. Check this understanding with another student or the instructor. Write these in your notebook.
- *Take useful notes.* When taking lecture notes in class, leave a large margin on the left side of each notebook page and write only on right-hand pages, leaving all left-hand pages blank. Look over your lecture notes soon after each class, while your memory is fresh. Fill in missing words, complete sentences and ideas, and underline key phrases, definitions, and concepts. At the top of each page, write the topic of that page. In the left margin, write the key word for that part of your notes. On the opposite left-hand page, write a summary or outline that combines material from both the textbook and the lecture. These can be your study notes for review.
- *Join or form a study group.* Form a study group with some other students so you can help one another. Practice speaking and reading aloud, ask questions about material you are not sure about, and work together to find answers.
- *Improve your study skills.* Good study skills are essential for achieving your goals in nursing. Time management, efficient use of study time, and a consistent approach to studying are all beneficial. There are various study methods for reading a textbook and for taking class notes. Some methods that have proven helpful can be found in *Saunders Student Nurse Planner: A Guide to Success in Nursing School* by Susan C. deWit. This book contains helpful information on test-taking and preparing for clinical experiences. It includes an example of a "time map" for planning study time and a blank form that you can use to formulate a personal time map.

ADDITIONAL STUDY HINTS FOR STUDENTS WHO USE ENGLISH AS A SECOND LANGUAGE (ESL)

- *Find a first-language buddy.* ESL students should find a first-language buddy—another student who is a native speaker of English and is willing to answer questions about word meanings, pronunciations, and culture. Maybe your buddy would like to learn about your language and culture. This could help in his or her nursing experience as well.
- *Expand your vocabulary.* If you find a nontechnical word you do not know (e.g., *drowsy*), try to guess its meaning from the sentence (e.g., *With electrolyte imbalance, the patient may feel fatigued and drowsy*). If you are not sure of the meaning, or if it seems particularly important, look it up in the dictionary.
- *Keep a vocabulary notebook.* Keep a small alphabetized notebook or address book in which you can write down new nontechnical words you read or hear along with their meanings and pronunciations. Write each word under its initial letter so you can find it easily, as in a dictionary. For words you do not know or for words that have a different meaning in nursing, write down how they are used and sound. Look up their meanings in a dictionary or ask your instructor or first-language buddy. Then write the different meanings or usages that you have found in your book, including the nursing meaning. Continue to add new words as you discover them. For example:
  - *Primary*—Of most importance; main (e.g., *the primary problem or disease*); The first one; elementary (e.g., *primary school*)
  - *Secondary*—Of less importance; resulting from another problem or disease (e.g., *a secondary symptom*); The second one (e.g., *secondary school* ["high school" in the United States])

Illustration Credits

Chapter 5
P. 27: Maslow A: *Motivation and personality*, ed 2, New York, 1970, Harper & Row.

Chapter 13
P. 75: Maslow A: *Motivation and personality*, ed 2, New York, 1970, Harper & Row.

Chapter 15
P. 86: Potter PA, Perry AG, Stockert P, and Hall A: *Fundamentals of nursing: Concepts, process, and practice*, ed 8, St. Louis, 2013, Mosby.
P. 87: Elkin MK et al: *Nursing interventions and clinical skills*, ed 4, St. Louis, 2008, Mosby.

Chapter 16
P. 96: Sheehy SB & Lombardi J: *Manual of emergency care*, ed 4, St. Louis, 1995, Mosby.

Chapter 21
P. 133: Clayton BD & Stock YN: *Basic pharmacology for nurses*, ed 14, St. Louis, 2007, Mosby.

Chapter 26
P. 169: Lowdermilk DL, et al: *Maternity and women's health care*, ed 10, St. Louis, 2012, Mosby.

Chapter 30
P. 194: Hockenberry MJ: *Wong's essentials of pediatric nursing*, ed 8, St. Louis, 2009, Mosby.

Chapter 31
P. 204: Hockenberry MJ: *Wong's essentials of pediatric nursing*, ed 8, St. Louis, 2009, Mosby.

Chapter 40
P. 261: Harkreader H, Hogan MA, & Thobaben M: *Fundamentals of nursing: caring and clinical judgment*, ed 3, St. Louis, 2007, Saunders.

Chapter 42
P. 275: Thibodeau GA & Patton KT: *Anthony's textbook of anatomy and physiology*, ed 20, St. Louis, 2013, Mosby.

Chapter 43
P. 279: Patton KT & Thibodeau GA: *The human body in health and disease*, ed 6, St. Louis, 2014, Mosby.

Chapter 44
P. 285: Thibodeau GA & Patton KT: *Anatomy and physiology*, ed 8, St. Louis, 2013, Mosby.

Chapter 47
P. 306: Canobbio M: *Mosby's clinical nursing series: Cardiovascular disorders*, St. Louis, 1990, Mosby.

Chapter 50
P. 332: Patton KT & Thibodeau GA: *Anatomy and physiology*, ed 8, St. Louis, 2013, Mosby.

Chapter 51
P. 339: Patton KT & Thibodeau GA: *The human body in health and disease*, ed 6, St. Louis, 2014, Mosby.
P. 342: Seidel HM, et al: *Mosby's guide to physical examination*, ed 7, St. Louis, 2011, Mosby.

Chapter 52
P. 349: Thibodeau GA & Patton KT: *Structure and function of the body*, ed 14, St. Louis, 2012, Mosby.
P. 352: Thibodeau GA & Patton KT: *Anthony's textbook of anatomy and physiology*, ed 20, St. Louis, 2013, Mosby.

Chapter 53

P. 359: Thibodeau GA & Patton KT: Thibodeau GA & Patton KT: *Structure and function of the body*, ed 14, St. Louis, 2012, Mosby.

P. 361: Ignatavicius DD, et al: *Medical-surgical nursing: Patient-centered collaborative care*, ed 6, St. Louis, 2010, Saunders.

Chapter 54

P. 367: Grimes D: *Infectious diseases*, St. Louis, 1991, Mosby.

The Evolution of Nursing

chapter

1

Answer Key: Textbook page references are provided as a guide for answering these questions. A complete Answer Key is provided in your Additional Learning Resources on Evolve.

MATCHING

Directions: Match the nurse on the left with the contribution to nursing on the right.

Nurse		**Contribution to Nursing**
_____	1. Dorothea Dix (1802-1887) *(4)*	a. Credited with the development of our present-day documentation system
_____	2. Clara Barton (1821-1912) *(4)*	b. Pioneer crusader for elevation of standards of care for the mentally ill
_____	3. Mary Ann Ball (1817-1901) *(4)*	c. Worked for acceptance of African-Americans in the nursing profession
_____	4. Linda Richards (1841-1930) *(4)*	d. Developed the American Red Cross in 1881
_____	5. Isabel Hampton Robb (1860-1910) *(4)*	e. Championed the rights and comforts of soldiers; organized diet kitchens, laundries, and ambulance service
_____	6. Lavinia Dock (1858-1956) *(4)*	f. Organized the first graded system of theory and practice in schools of nursing
_____	7. Mary Eliza Mahoney (1845-1926) *(4)*	g. Responsible for the development of public health nursing in the United States through the founding of the Henry Street Settlement in New York City
_____	8. Lillian D. Wald (1867-1940) *(4)*	h. Responsible, with Robb, for the organization of the American Society of Superintendents of Training Schools, which evolved into the National League for Nursing Education
_____	9. Mary Adelaide Nutting (1858-1947) *(4)*	i. Pioneer in nurse-midwifery
_____	10. Mary Breckenridge (1881-1965) *(4)*	j. Developed curriculum concepts and guidelines for student nurses

SHORT ANSWER

Directions: Using your own words, answer each question in the space provided.

11. Identify the role of the National League for Nursing (NLN) in nursing education. *(9, 11)*_____

_____

_____

12. List the purposes of the National Association for Practical Nurse Education and Service (NAPNES) and the National Federation of Licensed Practical Nurses (NFLPN). *(9, 18)*

_____

_____

13. Discuss the role and responsibilities of the practical or vocational nurse in today's health care system. *(18, 19)*

_____

_____

_____

_____

FILL-IN-THE-BLANK SENTENCES

Directions: Complete each sentence by filling in the blank with the correct word or phrase.

14. The duties and responsibilities of the LPN/LVN are determined by the _____. *(1)*

15. The content areas for the NCLEX-PN® are determined by the _____. *(1)*

16. Recognizing patients as individuals and making sure that they receive quality care is ensured by nurses providing care according to the _____. *(15)*

MULTIPLE CHOICE

Directions: Select the best answer(s) for each of the following questions.

17. One of the major problems of hospitals of the early nineteenth century has been addressed by which measure in contemporary health care? *(2)*
    1. Focusing on women's health issues, such as heart disease
    2. Using Standard Precautions to address hygienic practices
    3. Encouraging men to enter the nursing profession
    4. Reducing the nursing shortage during wartime

18. Which patient typifies the demographic changes of the population in the twenty-first century and represents an increased need for nursing care? *(14)*
    1. A 3-month-old infant with developmental disabilities
    2. A 15-year-old homeless adolescent
    3. A 45-year-old man with diabetes
    4. A 78-year-old woman with chronic illness

19. Which nursing action reflects Florence Nightingale's vision of how to improve patient care? *(3)*
    1. Includes the family in the patient education sessions
    2. Considers the patient's cultural and ethnic background
    3. Attends an in-service to learn about a new infusion pump
    4. Safeguards patient's privacy by maintaining confidentiality

20. Which situation includes the four major concepts that are the basis for nursing theories and models? *(17)*
    1. The home health nurse assesses the patient's health and the home setting.
    2. The nurse studies nursing theory in an advanced-practice nursing curriculum.
    3. Nursing programs draw from several psychosocial and nursing theories.
    4. The patient is treated for hypertension, diabetes, and obesity.

21. Which patient is most at risk for being one of the "medically underserved" in the United States? *(8)*
    1. A 30-year-old woman with newly diagnosed breast cancer
    2. An 86-year-old man who resides in a long-term care facility
    3. A 3-year-old whose parents recently emigrated for work
    4. A 65-year-old Vietnam veteran who lives on the street

22. Utilizing Maslow's hierarchy of needs, the nurse gives priority to which problem? *(12)*
    1. Loneliness due to being away from family during hospitalization
    2. Inability to eat because of difficulty with chewing and swallowing
    3. Anxiety due to recent diagnosis of cancer with poor prognosis
    4. Safety related to difficulty with balance during position change

23. A mother tells the nurse that her 17-year-old son, who is wheelchair-bound for one year following an accident, has been depressed because basketball season is starting and he was a star player for his high school team. Utilizing Maslow's hierarchy of needs, which intervention would address the son's priority need? *(12)*
    1. Advise the mother to check the wheelchair access ramps for safe access to the gym.
    2. Explore other interests and activities that would increase his self-esteem.
    3. Initiate a review of body systems to identify the cause of depression.
    4. Suggest the mother and son seek out a wheelchair basketball team.

24. The nurse has identified that a 56-year-old woman has an increased risk for heart problems because of family history. Which modifiable factor(s) should be included in the teaching plan to promote health and self-help practices for wellness for this patient? (Select all that apply.) *(15)*
    1. Smoking cessation and stress reduction
    2. Use of advanced technology and new medications
    3. Weight reduction and decreased alcohol consumption
    4. Cost of health insurance and specialist care
    5. Control over decision-making that affects own body and health

25. Which set of tasks should be assigned to a UAP who has been cross-trained as a unit secretary? *(15)*
    1. Direct visitors and give out patient information
    2. Take vital signs and restock medications
    3. Validate transcriptions and interpret vital signs
    4. Ambulate patients and order unit supplies

26. Which action best demonstrates the nurse's consistent effort to contribute to cost-containment? *(14)*
    1. Obtains malpractice insurance
    2. Uses time and materials economically
    3. Questions excessive diagnostic testing
    4. Refers patients with no insurance to a sliding-scale clinic

27. The nurse is caring for a patient with immobility related to a chronic musculoskeletal disorder. Using Orem's theory of nursing, the nurse would: *(17)*
    1. monitor the patient's self-care deficits.
    2. arrange the patient's pillows to provide joint protection.
    3. support patient's existing coping mechanisms.
    4. encourage the patient to walk down the hallway.

28. The nurse is caring for several patients on the medical-surgical unit. Which action(s) indicate(s) that the nurse is providing care that adheres to the Patient's Bill of Rights? (Select all that apply.) *(15)*
    1. Ensures that the housekeeping staff empties the trash receptacles in a timely fashion
    2. Assists the patient to make a list of questions to ask about a surgical procedure
    3. Identifies a problem with a broken side rail and contacts the maintenance department
    4. Keeps up to date with the latest information on medication and side effects
    5. Ensures that every patient gets a private room with a window and private bathroom
    6. Contacts the hospital's financial counselor if a patient has questions about the bill

29. An intoxicated patient comes to the walk-in clinic and verbally threatens a nurse with bodily harm. The nurse refuses to care for the patient and informs the supervisor about the threats. Which document/concept supports the nurse's right to refuse to care for this patient? *(16)*
    1. Patient's Bill of Rights
    2. Position Paper of the American Nurses Association
    3. Health Care Providers' Rights
    4. NFLPN standards for nursing practice

30. Which action is outside the scope of practice for the LPN/LVN? *(11, 19)*
    1. Offers suggestions to improve the patient's fluid intake
    2. Collects data on the patient while giving medication
    3. Makes independent decision about nursing diagnosis
    4. Uses therapeutic communication with a patient's family

CRITICAL THINKING ACTIVITIES

31. The nurse is interviewing a 65-year-old woman who has hypertension, which is well-controlled by blood pressure medication. She is retired, but recently started volunteering at her church. She describes herself as having some problems, but happily coping and looking forward to spending time with her grandchildren. Describe this woman's state of health by placing an X on the Wellness-Illness continuum and give a rationale for the placement of the X. *(12)*

Wellness ⟷ Illness

Highest level of optimal health   Diminished or impaired state of health

_____

_____

_____

_____

32. a. Compare and contrast the historical significance of the white pleated cap and the apron that were originally part of the nurse's uniform with contemporary mandatory dress codes for nursing students and nurses. *(7)*

_____

_____

_____

_____

   b. Compare and contrast your personal point of view about uniforms with patients' and families' points of view. *(7)*

_____

_____

_____

_____

_____

33. The patient is admitted to the medical-surgical unit for exacerbation of a chronic respiratory disease. While in the hospital he requires medication, oxygen therapy, and diagnostic testing. In addition, the nurse notes that he smokes. He is overweight and making very poor food choices for between-meal snacks. He is unsteady when he ambulates and requires some assistance for activities that require bending and lifting, such as tying his shoelaces or picking up his suitcase. On further assessment, the nurse finds out that the patient lives by himself in a second-story apartment and his primary source of income is from a small pension.

   a. Identify all of the participants in the health care delivery system who will be involved in this patient's care and briefly describe their roles and responsibilities. *(13)*

_____

_____

_____

_____

_____

   b. How could the nurse apply the concepts of health promotion and illness prevention to assist this patient? *(15)*

_____

_____

_____

_____

_____

Legal and Ethical Aspects of Nursing

chapter

2

Answer Key: Textbook page references are provided as a guide for answering these questions. A complete Answer Key is provided in your Additional Learning Resources on Evolve.

MATCHING

Directions: Match the terms on the left to the correct definition on the right.

	Terms		**Definitions**
_____ 1.	abandonment of care (24)	a.	Injury that gives basis for a legal action against the person who caused the damage
_____ 2.	accountability (24)	b.	Failure to perform the duty in a reasonable, prudent manner
_____ 3.	breach of duty (23)	c.	Professional negligence
_____ 4.	proximate cause (23)	d.	Being responsible for one's own actions
_____ 5.	competency (24)	e.	Wrongful termination of providing patient care
		f.	Legal presumption that a person can make decisions for him- or herself unless proven otherwise
_____ 6.	harm (24)	g.	Defines acts whose performance is required, permitted, or prohibited
_____ 7.	malpractice (24)	h.	Occurrence of harm depended directly on the occurrence of the breach
_____ 8.	negligence (24)	i.	Legal responsibility
_____ 9.	standards of care (25)	j.	Absence of due care
_____ 10.	liability (24)		

TRUE OR FALSE

Directions: Write T for true or F for false in the blanks provided.

_____ 11. The purpose of civil law is to make the aggrieved person whole again, to restore the person to where he or she was. *(22)*

_____ 12. The purpose of criminal law is to punish for the crime and deter and prevent further crimes. *(22)*

_____ 13. The duty to care for the patient exists when the nurse accepts a position at a facility. *(24)*

_____ 14. The nurse who uses unnecessary restraints on a patient may be charged with assault. *(24)*

_____ 15. When providing first aid in an emergency situation outside a medical facility, it is important for the nurse to have knowledge of the Good Samaritan Act. *(30)*

MULTIPLE CHOICE

Directions: Select the best answer(s) for each of the following questions.

16. The nursing student needs to obtain patient information to prepare for the clinical experience and decides to stop and say hello the patient. While they are talking, the patient suddenly stops breathing and becomes unresponsive. What should the student do first? *(23)*
    1. Call the nursing instructor and write an incident report.
    2. Call the primary nurse and apply oxygen.
    3. Call the Rapid Response Team and get the crash cart.
    4. Call for help and initiate CPR.

17. In which case is the nurse most likely to be charged with malpractice? *(23)*
    1. The nurse explains the restraint policy to the family and later the elderly patient climbs over the side rail and sustains a hip fracture.
    2. The patient becomes very angry when the nurse refuses to give an additional dose of pain medication before the ordered time.
    3. The family wants the health care provider called at 3:00 AM because "something is wrong;" the nurse waits until 7:00 AM, but the patient is unharmed.
    4. The patient is very demanding and unpleasant, so the nurse ignores the call bell; the patient sustains tissue injury at the IV site.

18. The patient asked the UAP to apply a heating pad to her back, despite the fact that the home health nurse had instructed both to avoid using the device. The patient sustained a burn and decided to sue the UAP and the nurse. Which document(s) is/are likely to be used in this case? (Select all that apply.) *(23)*
    1. Policies and procedures
    2. Standards of care
    3. Equipment maintenance records
    4. Patient's medical records
    5. UAP's personal health records
    6. Personnel files for UAP and nurse

19. The nurse recognizes that in today's health care climate there is an increased likelihood to be involved in litigation. What action could the nurse take to improve the overall situation in the work setting? *(24)*
    1. Agree to take a limited number of high-acuity patients.
    2. Work on a committee to improve discharge teaching.
    3. Work at a facility that covers nurses with malpractice insurance.
    4. Ensure that others are accountable for their own actions.

20. A new UAP is assigned to do a task that was reviewed and demonstrated in orientation and practiced on a manikin. The UAP tells the nurse that she does not know how to do the task. What should the nurse do first? *(25)*
    1. Ask the UAP to recite the steps of the task and assess readiness to perform.
    2. Go with the UAP and perform the task while she observes.
    3. Instruct the UAP to try to perform the task to the best of her ability.
    4. Pull the UAP's orientation file and see if competency was established.

21. The LPN/LVN is instructed by a health care provider to start a unit of blood on a patient, but the institution's policy indicates that LPN/LVNs can monitor blood transfusions, but RNs must initiate blood transfusions. What should the LPN/LVN do? *(26)*
    1. Start the blood transfusion as ordered, because the health care provider is supervising.
    2. Locate the RN in charge so that he/she can start the blood transfusion.
    3. Tell the health care provider that hospital policy prohibits blood transfusion by LPN/LVNs.
    4. Obtain the unit of blood and assist the health care provider as he/she initiates the transfusion.

22. A nursing student must write a clinical report about the care that was given to a patient in the hospital. What should the student do to prevent a HIPAA violation? (Select all that apply.) *(26, 29)*
    1. Do not use the patient's name in any section of the paper.
    2. If laboratory data are used, make sure no identification numbers are included.
    3. Avoid including the health care provider's name in the report.
    4. Do not refer to the room number or the specific unit.
    5. Do not include the patient's vital signs.
    6. Avoid using specific details of the patient's medical condition.

23. Which unaccompanied minor requires parental consent prior to treatment? *(28)*
    1. A 17-year-old who wants a prescription for insulin
    2. An 18-year-old who needs sutures for a laceration to the hand
    3. A 14-year-old who was sexually assaulted by a family member
    4. A 16-year-old who is independent and self-supporting and wants birth control

24. The nurse is working on the medical-surgical unit and answers the telephone. The caller wants to know, "How is Mr. Smith doing?" What is the most important factor that affects the nurse's response? *(28)*
    1. The identity of the caller
    2. The stability of Mr. Smith's condition
    3. The hospital's policy for releasing information
    4. The nurse's knowledge of HIPAA

25. A mother brings her 8-year-old son to the clinic for a broken arm. There are no other apparent injuries and the child and mother appear to have a supportive relationship; however, review of the chart indicates that this child has frequently been treated for other fractures and injuries. What should the nurse do first? *(29)*
    1. Ask the social worker to consult for possible child abuse.
    2. Call child protective services and make a report.
    3. Point out the history of injuries to the health care provider.
    4. Take the child aside and assess his true feelings.

26. The nurse is working in the emergency department. There is a gunshot sound from the waiting room, followed by sounds of yelling and screaming. What should the nurse do first? *(29)*
    1. Grab the crash cart and run to the waiting room.
    2. Reassure all of the patients in the immediate area.
    3. Call 911 and the hospital's security personnel.
    4. Lock the entrance to patient care areas.

27. Which action by the nurse is the best step to avoid a lawsuit? *(30)*
    1. Remain current on practice developments
    2. Know the legal definition of terms, such as *negligence*
    3. Obtain professional malpractice insurance
    4. Validate nursing actions with a supervisor

28. The nurse performs a dressing change on a surgical wound. The procedure is routine and there are no signs of infection or excessive drainage. What should the nurse do about documentation? *(30)*
    1. If using charting by exception, "dressing changed" is adequate.
    2. Document appearance of wound site and type of dressing used.
    3. There is no need to document, because there are no problems with the wound.
    4. Read the previous entry about the wound and document "unchanged as above."

29. The nurse has to go before the state board of nursing because there is a question about her nursing license. Which type of insurance will provide a qualified nurse attorney to represent the nurse? *(30)*
    1. Claims-made policy
    2. Occurrence basis policy
    3. "Tail" agreement for extended coverage
    4. Disciplinary defense insurance

30. The state board of nursing is reviewing a case against the nurse. Rank the severity of the possible sanctions: 1 being the least severe to 5 being the most severe. *(30)*

    _____ a. Suspension with stipulations
    _____ b. Probation with stipulations
    _____ c. Letter of reprimand
    _____ d. Revocation of license
    _____ e. Dismissed charges

31. An elderly patient begins to cry during the review of the advance directive information and refuses to sign. What should the nurse do first? *(31)*
    1. Encourage the patient to express his feelings about the advance directives.
    2. Reassure the patient that his wishes will be respected above all else.
    3. Alert the family to support the patient in the decision.
    4. Document in the patient's record that the information was given and declined.

32. A patient is in very critical condition and unable to make decisions about ongoing treatment. There is conflict among family members on what should be done. Which source, if followed, is the most likely to protect the health care team from liability? *(32)*
    1. Agency's policy and procedure manual
    2. Patient's living will
    3. Patient Self-Determination Act
    4. Accreditation criteria of the Joint Commission

33. A mother and her pregnant 13-year-old daughter are arguing; the mother wants her to keep the baby and the girl wants to have an abortion. The nurse feels very angry toward the mother and very protective toward the girl. What should the nurse do first? *(34)*
    1. Take the girl aside and assess her feelings and wishes regarding the pregnancy.
    2. Ask another nurse to assess the mother's rationale for opposing her daughter.
    3. Seek advice from a supervisor about who can legally make decisions about the pregnancy.
    4. Reflect on own feelings and ability to be supportive and caring toward this family.

34. Which action(s) indicate(s) that the nurse is acting within the code of ethics as developed by the National Federation of Licensed Practical/Vocational Nurses? (Select all that apply.) *(34, 35)*
    1. Collects data about the patient's skin and reports it to the RN
    2. Gives change-of-shift report to the oncoming nurse and the nursing student
    3. Wears professional attire and adheres to the facility's dress code
    4. Observes another nurse being rude and demeaning toward a patient
    5. Cares for a patient with an infectious disease and follows isolation precautions
    6. Uses cell phone to text messages about another nurse's behavior toward coworkers

35. Nurse A knows that Nurse B is stealing small items from elderly residents in the long-term care facility, but Nurse A hesitates to report Nurse B, because they are friends and Nurse B gives good care to the residents. Who should Nurse A talk to first? *(35)*
    1. Ask the residents if they have any complaints about the nurse.
    2. Speak to the families of residents to see if the thefts can be substantiated.
    3. Speak to the supervisor and give facts only; do not offer suspicions.
    4. Talk to an objective third party about personal values clarification.

CRITICAL THINKING ACTIVITIES

36. A new nurse has just started his first job after graduating from nursing school. The nurse sees a health care provider's order to "get surgical consent form," but he is unsure what the order means, so he calls the health care provider for clarification. The provider is a little terse on the phone and says, "just get the consent form signed." The nurse is unsure what to do, so he consults the charge nurse who says, "Oh, the doctors here are too lazy to get their own consent forms signed, so we always do it for them." *(28)*

   a. Discuss the nurse's responsibilities when obtaining an informed consent from a patient before a procedure.

   _____

   _____

   _____

   _____

   b. The nurse is new to the city and this is his first job, so he has limited experience, but he clearly remembers what was taught in school about informed consent. What should he do?

   _____

   _____

   _____

   _____

37. Nurse A is assigned to care for an AIDS patient, but asks Nurse B to switch patients. Nurse B readily agrees, because Nurse A always helps other nurses and members of the health care team. Together, they inform the charge nurse, who gives the okay for the switch of assignments. At the end of the day, Nurse A thanks Nurse B for taking the AIDS patient, because "those kinds of people really bother me." Nurse B feels a little confused by the comment, but shrugs it off. *(35)*

   a. Discuss the behavior of Nurse A and Nurse B, as related to the National Federation of Licensed Practical/Vocational Nurses (NFLPN) code of ethics.

   _____

   _____

   _____

   _____

   b. Nurse B goes home and thinks about the day and about Nurse A's comment. Nurse B realizes that the situation has created some uncomfortable feelings and a potential problem if Nurse A makes a future request to change patient assignments or makes additional comments. What should Nurse B do?

   _____

   _____

   _____

   _____

38. The nurse is caring for a patient who has been quadriplegic for 3 years following a diving accident. One morning the nurse notes that the patient has redness on the sacral area and informs the patient that there is a risk for a pressure ulcer and that very careful turning and scheduled assessment will need to be started. The patient politely thanks the nurse, but informs her that he intends to refuse any treatment for pressure ulcers and is likely to start refusing other nursing measures as well. The nurse is stunned and upset because the patient has always been cooperative and generally very satisfied with the care. *(33, 34)*

   a. What should the nurse do? _____

   _____

   _____

   _____

   _____

   b. How can the nurse continue to interact with this patient if he continues to refuse therapies? _____

   _____

   _____

   _____

   _____

   c. How would you feel if a patient refused to allow you to meet basic needs, such as food, hygiene, or preventive care like turning or receiving immunizations?

   _____

   _____

   _____

   _____

39. The nurse has been working for several years in the hospital. The patient assignments are always very heavy and there has been a continuous nursing shortage. Two patients have died within the past year and although there have been no legal actions taken against the hospital or the staff, the general feeling among the nursing staff is that working conditions are going to result in more harm to the patients. The nurse has talked to her supervisor about her concerns for the patients' safety and the morale of the staff. The supervisor has assured her that everything that can be done has been done. Discuss the legal and ethical implications of these working conditions and the actions that the nurse could take. *(24)*

   _____

   _____

   _____

   _____

   _____

Documentation

chapter

3

Answer Key: Textbook page references are provided as a guide for answering these questions. A complete Answer Key is provided in your Additional Learning Resources on Evolve.

MATCHING

Directions: Match the abbreviations on the left to the correct terminology on the right.

	Abbreviation		Terminology
_____ 1.	CBE *(46)*	a.	Plan, intervention, evaluation
_____ 2.	DRGs *(39)*	b.	Data, action, response, education
_____ 3.	EHR *(38)*	c.	Situation, background, assessment, recommendation, read back
_____ 4.	HIPAA *(54)*	d.	Charting by exception
_____ 5.	PHR *(41)*	e.	Subjective, objective, assessment, plan, evaluation
		f.	Electronic health record
_____ 6.	POC *(40)*	g.	Minimum data sets
_____ 7.	DARE *(45)*	h.	Point-of-care
_____ 8.	SBARR *(41)*	i.	Problem-oriented medical record
_____ 9.	PIE *(46)*	j.	Personal health record
_____ 10.	SOAPE *(44)*	k.	Diagnosis-related groups
_____ 11.	MDS *(53)*	l.	Health Insurance Portability and Accountability Act
_____ 12.	POMR *(44)*		

SHORT ANSWER

Directions: Using your own words, answer each question in the space provided.

13. The five basic purposes of written patient records are: *(39)*_____

_____

_____

14. Compare and contrast focused charting, charting by exception, and narrative charting. *(43, 45, 46)* _____

_____

_____

15. Briefly identify how long-term care and home health care documentation are different from acute care (hospital) documentation. *(53)*

_____

_____

TABLE ACTIVITY

16. In the right-hand column of the table, indicate all of the potential places where the examples of documentation could be recorded. *(39)*

Nursing Process	Where to Document
Assessment	
Alert and oriented to person, place, and time.	
Ambulates independently to bathroom.	
Family assessed for knowledge of wound care.	
Diagnosis	
Risk for infection related to surgical wound	
Knowledge deficit related to wound care at home	
Outcomes Identification/Planning	
Patient will participate in wound care prior to discharge.	
Family will demonstrate ability to perform wound irrigation.	
Implementation	
Wound care procedure demonstrated to patient and family.	
List of supplies and how to obtain reviewed with family.	
Referral made to home health agency.	
Evaluation	
Patient and family participated in wound care. They had questions about asepsis in the home setting; principles of hand hygiene and asepsis were reviewed. They acknowledged understanding of written and verbal information and agreed to follow up with the home health nurse.	

MULTIPLE CHOICE

Directions: Select the best answer(s) for each of the following questions.

17. In using the hospital's computer information system, where would the nurse most likely find documentation about the patient's response to the last dose of pain medication? *(43, 44)*
    1. Individualized care plan
    2. Medication administration record (MAR)
    3. Automated Kardex form
    4. Narrative notes

18. An auditor is randomly reviewing the nurses' charts and the nurse manager has agreed that the auditor can ask questions and give feedback as necessary. Which documentation is the auditor mostly likely to query? *(39)*
    1. Ambulated independently with steady gait to bathroom.
    2. Instructed on method of clean midstream urine collection.
    3. Discharged to home accompanied by spouse.
    4. Placed side rails up x3 with call bell in place.

19. The nurse is working on a medical-surgical unit in a large hospital and observes an unfamiliar person looking at a patient's chart. What should the nurse do? *(54)*
    1. Call hospital security and report the person's behavior and description.
    2. Ask for identification and determine if the person can look at the chart.
    3. Allow the person to continue unless there is suspicious behavior.
    4. Request that the chart be returned and contact the charge nurse.

20. The nursing student attempts to document AM hygienic care, but several computers are broken and the remaining functional computers are being used. What should the student do? *(42)*
    1. Make a note to self of time and relevant details and document at the end of the shift.
    2. Report to the instructor and ask for advice about what to do.
    3. Document the care on a hardcopy form and add it to the patient's chart.
    4. Jot down the time that care was given and document when a computer is available.

21. It is 10:00 AM, and the nurse needs to give a patient a blood pressure medication, but would like to know what the morning vital signs were before administering the medication. The nurse looks at the flow sheet, but the vital signs are not there. Which action should the nurse take first? *(39, 42)*
    1. Give the blood pressure medication now and then check the blood pressure in 30 minutes.
    2. Find the UAP and ask why the morning vital signs have not been documented.
    3. Check the blood pressure, give the medication as appropriate, and then document both.
    4. Check in the nurses' narrative notes to see if the vital signs were documented there.

22. The nurse phones the health care provider to report a change in the patient's condition and uses the SBARR method of communication; however, the health care provider declines to listen to the "read back" and then hangs up. What should the nurse do first? *(41)*
    1. Call the provider back and insist on "read back."
    2. Carry out the orders if they are clear.
    3. Consult a supervisor about the incident.
    4. Document the health care provider's exact words in the patient's chart.

23. The LPN/LVN is reading the documentation that was written by a newly graduated RN. There are numerous spelling mistakes and the grammar is terrible. What should the nurse do? *(41)*
    1. Do nothing; an RN is not accountable to an LPN/LVN.
    2. Offer to teach the new nurse how to document.
    3. Ask the charge nurse to review the documentation.
    4. Correct the spelling errors and initial the changes.

24. The student nurse sees that it is time to give medication to a patient, but the patient is currently in x-ray. The student is aware that there is a 30-minute time window to administer the medication, otherwise it will be considered late. What should the student do? *(42)*
    1. Document that the medication was given at the correct time and then give it as soon as the patient returns from x-ray.
    2. Call the pharmacy and inquire if a delay in administering the medication or holding it until the next dose is harmful to the patient.
    3. Document that the patient is in x-ray, advise the charge nurse, and administer the medication when the patient returns to the unit.
    4. Hold the medication and fill out an incident report that explains the circumstances and details of why the medication was not administered.

25. A patient is admitted to the hospital for a total hip replacement. Care and documentation are performed according to the facility's clinical (critical) pathway for this condition. What information is likely to appear in this documentation tool? *(51)*
    1. Level of activity on a day-to day basis following surgery
    2. Unusual events that have a potential for injury
    3. Nursing care plan with diagnosis and detailed interventions
    4. The LPN/LVN's role in monitoring the patient's progress

26. A patient comes to the nurses' station and demands to have his chart because he has decided to leave the hospital and seek care from a different facility. What is the best response? *(53, 54)*
    1. "Sir, all of the patient records are the property of the hospital."
    2. "Sir, let me contact your health care provider so you can talk to him before leaving."
    3. "Sir, please wait and I will call the nurse manager right now."
    4. "Sir, please return to your room and I will make a copy of the chart."

27. The nursing student leaves a copy of a patient's Kardex on a bedside table. A visitor finds the copy and reads it. What should the student do? *(54)*
    1. Take the Kardex out of the patient's room and immediately shred it.
    2. Apologize to the visitor and patient and explain the information on the Kardex.
    3. Obtain the copy of the Kardex and check for patient identifiers.
    4. Retrieve the Kardex, contact instructor, and complete an incident report.

28. The nurse is documenting with a black pen on the hardcopy nurses' notes about a patient's response to pain medication. The nurse suddenly realizes that she is writing the note in the wrong chart. What is the best action to take? *(43)*
    1. Draw a line through the error and initial it.
    2. Report the error to the charge nurse.
    3. Use white correction fluid to cover the error.
    4. Discard the page that contains the error.

29. The nurse is being advised by an auditor about possible inadequate or inappropriate documentation that could be involved in a malpractice suit. What type(s) of documentation is/are likely to cause problems in malpractice cases? (Select all that apply.) *(43)*
    1. Failed to document latex allergy.
    2. Documented patient's complaint about care by using patient's remarks in quotes.
    3. Charted medication that patient claims he did not receive.
    4. Documented amount of IV fluid, but no assessment of IV site.
    5. Clustered information obtained from physical assessment.
    6. Recorded verbal order using brand-name medication.

30. Which nursing action/behavior would be considered a potential HIPAA violation? *(54)*
    1. Faxes a patient's medical records to a consulting specialist
    2. Leaves the computer monitor display open for easy access
    3. Discusses a patient problem during handover with oncoming staff
    4. Documents contents of an SBARR report for the risk manager

CRITICAL THINKING ACTIVITIES

31. Review the documentation samples below and then refer to Box 3-2, Basic Rules for Documentation and Table 3-2, Legal Guidelines for Documentation to identify errors and examples of poor documentation. *(42)*

Sample #1

Sept, 2014   Patient had a good night. Status was escendially unchanged. Family in to visit and asked about storage of patient's belongings. Reassured that diamond ring and gold watch were in the bedside table. Patient went with family to cafeteria. S. Smith, LPN.

_____

_____

_____

_____

Sample # 2

Sept. 24, 2014 2100   J. Jones RN gave a 500-mL SSE; patient assisted to CC for a return of 600 mL with brown formed stool noted. Procedure well tolerated. J. Jones said that patient had relief of adominal distencion and discomfort. S. Smith, LPN

_____

_____

_____

_____

Sample # 3

Sept 24, 2014   Patient reported pain. Noted in chart that physician made an error and ordered MS. Consulted charge nurse who advised to give morphine sulfate according to the dose written in orders. Patient was angry because he didn't get the pain medication as soon as he asked for it; called me a "stupid lazy fool." Pain medication given later in the shift.

_____

_____

_____

_____

32. Review the material in the textbook and interview nurses during your clinical assignment and then compare and contrast electronic health record (EHR) systems to hardcopy (paper) record systems. *(40)*

_____

_____

_____

_____

Communication

Answer Key: Textbook page references are provided as a guide for answering these questions. A complete Answer Key is provided in your Additional Learning Resources on Evolve.

FILL-IN-THE-BLANK SENTENCES

Directions: Complete each sentence by filling in the blank with the correct word or phrase.

1. A therapeutic nurse-patient interaction is one in which the nurse demonstrates _____, _____, _____, and _____. *(62)*

2. The nurse must first gain the patient's _____ before expecting to have a meaningful or therapeutic interaction. *(69)*

3. While experiencing increased stress, the patient may respond to the nurse with _____, _____, or _____. *(72)*

4. The nursing diagnosis of _____ is used to describe "decreased, delayed, or absent ability to receive, process, transmit, and use a system of symbols." *(72)*

5. Patients who receive mechanical ventilation via endotracheal tube or tracheostomy will experience a(n) _____ because the trachea is obstructed by the tube. *(72)*

MULTIPLE CHOICE

Directions: Select the best answer(s) for each of the following questions.

6. The night nurse is giving report during shift change. A visitor passing by inadvertently is an unintended receiver. What is the best method to prevent this type of occurrence? *(59)*
   1. Ask visitors to leave the unit during shift change.
   2. Give report in a private room with the door closed.
   3. Eliminate negative connotations during report.
   4. Make written notes that are passed only to staff members.

7. The nurse is attempting to elicit the patient's feelings about an upcoming surgery. Which approach is likely to be the most effective? *(65)*
   1. "Are you afraid of having the procedure?"
   2. "Let me give you information about the procedure."
   3. "Look at this series of pictures about the procedure."
   4. "What do you understand about the procedure?"

8. A patient is grimacing while trying to change position himself in bed. He tells the nurse that he is feeling great and is ready to get up and go home. Which response best indicates that the nurse recognizes that the patient's communication is incongruent? *(61)*
   1. "Going home is the goal, but let me help you get up and you can walk around for a while."
   2. "Let me help you sit up and then you can get dressed and pack up your belongings."
   3. "Would you like a dose of pain medication before you go home?"
   4. "That sounds great! I'll call your health care provider and inform her that you are ready to go home."

9. The nurse is about to begin teaching a small group of adolescents about healthy eating habits. Which nonverbal behavior best indicates potential interest in listening to the nurse? *(59-61)*
   1. Talking on a cell phone and smiling at the nurse
   2. Staring at the blackboard with a bored expression
   3. Using the Internet to search for topics of interest
   4. Removing a notebook and pen from a backpack

10. The patient tells the nurse, "I'm supposed to check my blood sugar at least three times each day, but I can't always find the test sticks and they're very expensive." The nurse uses which specific therapeutic technique of clarification when responding? *(65, 66)*
    1. "When did you last check your blood sugar?"
    2. "I'll speak with the health care provider about your situation."
    3. "I see that you know how important it is to check your blood sugar."
    4. "Let me make sure I understand what your concern is with the blood sugar testing."

11. The patient states, "I am worried and don't know what to expect after my biopsy." Which question best encourages the patient to explain the problem to the nurse? *(65, 66)*
    1. "Would you like to talk to your health care provider before the procedure?"
    2. "Are you feeling anxious about the results of your biopsy?"
    3. "What are you worried about?"
    4. "How can I make you feel better?

12. The nurse is trying to take a patient's history, but the patient makes frequent references to her aunt's health, a neighbor's illness, and events that happened many years ago to himself or others. Which therapeutic communication technique is the nurse likely to use with this patient? *(66)*
    1. Clarifying
    2. Paraphrasing
    3. Restating
    4. Closed questioning

13. When communicating with a patient who has expressive aphasia, which communication strategy is the nurse most likely to use? *(74)*
    1. Encourage the patient to speak as much as possible.
    2. Use eye blinks, one for "yes" and two for "no."
    3. Ask family members for information.
    4. Speak loudly and slowly with good enunciation.

14. When communicating with a patient of an unfamiliar culture, the nurse knows that: (Select all that apply.) *(71)*
    1. formal names are used until preference is assessed.
    2. interpretation of social time versus clock time can differ.
    3. touch varies according to gender and relationship.
    4. smiling and handshake are universal greetings.
    5. tone of voice should be soft and deferential.
    6. eye contact has different meaning among cultures.

15. When communicating with an older adult, the nurse is aware that it is important to: *(71)*
    1. speak loudly and at a very slow pace.
    2. allow time for processing information.
    3. provide a dark, quiet environment.
    4. discourage anecdotal or tangential replies.

16. Which nurse behavior/response indicates to the patient that the nurse is actively listening to what he or she is trying to say? *(63)*
    1. Says "Uh-huh"
    2. Smiles and nods at patient
    3. Says "So in other words, you are..."
    4. Looks at patient and leans forward

17. The patient will be discharged from the hospital tomorrow. During the discharge teaching, the patient states, "I don't know how I will be able to care for myself after I leave the hospital." What is the most therapeutic response? *(65)*
    1. "You don't know how you will take care of yourself when you leave the hospital?"
    2. "It sounds like you have some concerns. What do you think is going to happen?"
    3. "Would you like me to review the instructions so the information is clear?"
    4. "Could you get someone to stay with you until you are feeling better?"

18. The nurse is working with a patient from a different culture. Which action by the nurse is most likely to cause offense if patient's sense of intimate space differs from the nurse's? *(69)*
    1. Assists the patient to transfer from bed to chair
    2. Sits in a chair and speaks with the patient
    3. Speaks to the family in the presence of the patient
    4. Hangs the patient's clothes in the closet

19. The nurse is completing the patient's history. Which question encourages the patient to provide a specific answer with relevant detail? *(66)*
    1. "What type of surgeries have you had in the past?"
    2. "What kinds of problems do you have?"
    3. "Are you having any pain?"
    4. "How do you feel about your current health status?"

20. The patient tells the nurse that the UAP is always making jokes. What is the best response? *(68)*
    1. "Laughter is the best medicine."
    2. "What do you think about the UAP's jokes?"
    3. "Yes, the UAP really is a funny person."
    4. "Would you tell me a joke?"

21. The nurse is explaining a change in a patient's condition to a health care provider. The provider rudely and sarcastically replies, "Well, what do you want me to do about that?" What is the best response? *(61, 62)*
    1. "Well, mostly I just wanted you to know about the situation."
    2. "That's really your decision. I'm merely reporting the patient's condition."
    3. "Please come and examine the patient, because the condition has changed."
    4. "Sorry to bother you. I'll just keep monitoring the patient's condition."

22. The patient has just died. The wife and daughter are holding each other and crying at the bedside, while the little boy is standing apart staring out the window. Which communication approach would be the best to support everyone in the family? *(63)*
    1. Talk to the little boy about what he is feeling and what he sees out the window.
    2. Stand beside the wife and daughter and direct the little boy to join the group.
    3. Use therapeutic touch with the wife and daughter and allow the little boy to have his space.
    4. Stand beside the little boy and keep an open body position toward the mother and daughter.

23. The nurse is present when the health care provider informs a 17-year-old that she is pregnant. The adolescent shrugs, appears bored and says, "That's no big deal to me." The nurse, who has been trying to get pregnant for several years, feels angry and hostile toward the patient. What should the nurse do first? *(64, 65)*
    1. Care for the patient and talk about the situation later with a friend.
    2. Perform a self-assessment of ability to convey acceptance.
    3. Be honest with the patient and express concern about her attitude.
    4. Ask another nurse to take over care of the patient.

24. An experienced UAP gives excellent care and is well-liked by all of the residents in the long-term care facility. She calls the female residents "Sweetie" and the male residents "Honey-bunch." The nurse is newly graduated, but recognizes that the UAP is using "elderspeak." What should the nurse do? *(71)*

    1. Let a good thing continue because everyone seems happy and the care is good.
    2. Gain more experience and mimic the UAP's behavior and communication style.
    3. Report to the RN in charge about concerns for the UAP's disrespect of residents.
    4. Praise the UAP for giving excellent care and role-model use of Mr., Mrs., or Ms.

25. A nursing diagnosis of Social isolation is part of the care plan for a resident with a hearing impairment in a long-term care facility. The nurse goes to the patient's room and finds that he is cheerful, conversant, and happy to engage. What should the nurse do? *(72)*

    1. Suggest to the RN that the nursing diagnosis is an error or no longer a problem.
    2. Assess the patient to determine his social skills and the extent of his social network.
    3. Spend more time with the patient, because trust and rapport are established.
    4. Suggest that the patient go into the common room and talk with other residents.

CRITICAL THINKING ACTIVITIES

26. A 58-year-old man is admitted to the medical-surgical unit with a diagnosis of left-sided CVA (stroke). During the admission process, the nurse observes that the patient's speech is unclear and his words are slurred. The nurse also observes that when the patient is asked a question that can be answered with a "yes" or "no" response, he answers the question by moving his head to indicate "yes" or "no." Apply the nursing process to the given situation. *(72, 74)*

    a. Identify communication problems observed by the nurse during the admission process. _____

    _____

    b. Write a realistic goal for the nursing diagnosis Impaired verbal communication. _____

    _____

    _____

    c. Identify at least five nursing actions that can be implemented. _____

    _____

    _____

    d. Write a statement that reflects evaluation of the outcome. _____

    _____

    _____

    e. What would the nurse do if the goal is not being met? _____

    _____

    _____

    _____

27. The nurse is having a very rough day. Another nurse called in sick; a health care provider was very rude; several patients have extremely complex care needs; and Mrs. M., who is an elderly widow, has repeatedly used the call bell all morning. The nurse goes to Mrs. M.'s room and stands in the doorway with her arms across her chest, saying nothing, but looking directly at the patient. Mrs. M. says, "I'm sorry to bother you dear, but I thought I heard my husband in the hallway. Could you check and see if he is here?" The nurse shakes her head and walks out. Analyze this situation and the factors that are influencing the communication between the nurse and the patient. *(72, 73)*

_____

_____

_____

28. Recall a conversation you recently had with a family member, friend, coworker, instructor, or patient in which you used responses that blocked communication. Such responses include false reassurance, giving advice, making false assumptions, giving approval or disapproval, automatic responses, defensive responses, arguing, asking for explanation, or changing the subject. (See Table 4-4 for examples.) Record two or three responses that you used and describe how the other person responded to you. *(73)*

_____

_____

_____

_____

_____

Rephrase your responses listed above so communication remains open. _____

_____

_____

_____

Nursing Process and Critical Thinking

chapter

5

Answer Key: Textbook page references are provided as a guide for answering these questions. A complete Answer Key is provided in your Additional Learning Resources on Evolve.

CROSSWORD PUZZLE

1. Directions: Use the clues for descriptors of taxonomy (see Table 5-3) to complete the crossword puzzle. *(82)*

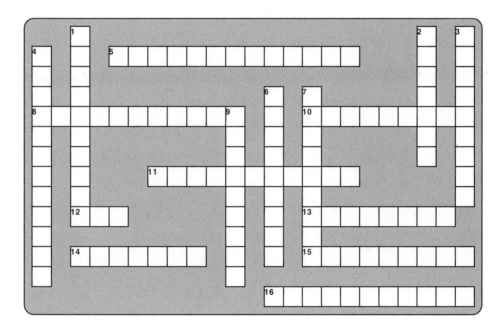

Across

5. Abnormal, incomplete functioning
8. Break in continuity or uniformity
10. Producing the intended or expected effect
11. Related to particular circumstance(s)
12. Containing less than the norm
13. Made worse, weakened, damaged, reduced, or deteriorated
14. Postponed, impeded, or retarded
15. Greater than necessary, desirable, or useful
16. Not producing the desired effect

Down

1. Normal complete functioning
2. Power or capacity to perform actions
3. Awareness by means of the senses with assignment of meaning
4. To realize beforehand; to foresee
6. Incapacity to do or act
7. Used or intended to protect from a perceived threat
9. Making unable or unfit; incapacitating

TRUE OR FALSE

Directions: Write T for true or F for false in the blanks provided.

_____ 2. The nursing process is a systematic problem-solving approach that enables the nurse to identify patient problems and potential problems. *(78)*

_____ 3. The planning phase of the nursing process is the phase where the nurse identifies the health problems. *(81)*

_____ 4. A nursing intervention is created to provide information for the formulation of a care plan. *(85)*

_____ 5. Advising a patient on the type of medication that he could take for his condition is an example of a nursing intervention. *(85)*

_____ 6. *Perceived constipation* is defined as "decrease in normal frequency of defecation accompanied by difficult or incomplete passage of stool and/or passage of excessively hard, dry stool." *(82)*

SHORT ANSWER

Directions: Using your own words, answer each question in the space provided.

7. Write a possible nursing diagnosis and patient-centered outcome for a 52-year-old patient admitted after episodes of severe vomiting and diarrhea. *(83, 84)*

_____

_____

_____

_____

8. Write a possible nursing diagnosis and patient-centered outcome for a 75-year-old patient with right-sided hemiparesis that resulted from a cerebrovascular accident (stroke). *(83, 84)*

_____

_____

9. Provide examples of possible nursing actions that may be implemented for a patient with a nursing diagnosis of Risk for impaired skin integrity due to loss of mobility on right side. *(85)*

_____

_____

10. Using the nursing diagnosis of Constipation related to low intake of dietary fiber as evidenced by straining at stool and patient goal of "patient will pass formed, brown stool without discomfort or straining within 3 days," write possible evaluation statements for a) goal met, b) goal partially met, and c) goal unmet. *(88)*

a. _____

b. _____

c. _____

11. Provide specific examples of how critical thinking is applied in clinical nursing situations. *(91)* _____

_____

_____

12. On the figure below, use a-f to indicate where the following nursing diagnoses would be according to Maslow's Hierarchy. *(85)*

   a. Acute pain
   b. Decreased cardiac output
   c. Situational low self-esteem
   d. Risk for injury
   e. Ineffective relationship
   f. Hopelessness

SELF-ACTUALIZATION
full use of individual talents

ESTEEM
self-respect, self-confidence, feelings of self-worth

LOVE AND BELONGINGNESS
affection, acceptance by peers and community

SAFETY AND SECURITY
stability, protection, security, freedom from fear and anxiety

PHYSIOLOGIC
nutrition, elimination, oxygenation, sexuality

MULTIPLE CHOICE

Directions: Select the best answer(s) for each of the following questions.

13. Place the nursing actions in correct order according to the six steps of the nursing process. *(79)*

  _____ 1. Identifies outcome of "patient will demonstrate respiratory rate of 12-20 breaths/min after being positioned in high Fowler's."

  _____ 2. Assists RN to develop a plan of care that will improve the patient's ability to breathe and expand lungs.

  _____ 3. Collaborates with RN to make diagnosis of Ineffective breathing pattern related to positioning that prevents lung expansion.

  _____ 4. Counts respiratory rate and observes respiratory effort; auscultates lung fields.

  _____ 5. Assists to high Fowler's position or assists to sit in the bedside chair.

  _____ 6. Checks oxygen saturation and asks patient about subjective feelings of relief after being repositioned.

14. The nurse is performing the assessment phase of the nursing process. Which nursing action would be done during this phase? *(78, 79)*
  1. Observe a patient's ability to independently perform AM hygienic care.
  2. Adjust a standardized care plan to meet the needs of the individual patient.
  3. Take blood pressure 30 minutes after giving an antihypertensive medication.
  4. Assist the patient to make a list of questions to ask the health care provider.

15. The nurse observes that the patient is pale; diaphoretic; slightly hunched over; and demonstrates deep, rapid breathing. Based on this objective data, which question will the nurse use to elicit the most relevant subjective data? *(79)*
  1. Do feel chilled or feverish?
  2. Do you need some help to sit up?
  3. Are you having any pain?
  4. When did you start feeling like this?

16. The nurse has identified six relevant nursing diagnoses that would apply to the patient's care. Which nursing action is the most important? *(85)*
    1. Determine how the nursing diagnoses relate to the medical diagnoses.
    2. Plan interventions that will address the six problems that were identified.
    3. Prioritize the nursing diagnoses from most urgent to least urgent.
    4. Ask the patient if the identified problems are consistent with his/her view.

17. The nurse sees on the care plan that there is a new nursing diagnosis of Ineffective breathing pattern related to narrowing of airways, with an intervention of "use inhaler PRN for asthma attacks." How does the nurse implement this intervention? *(79)*
    1. Consult the charge nurse to clarify the specific parameters of the nursing order.
    2. Ask the patient how often he has asthma attacks and what triggers them.
    3. Keep the inhaler at the bedside and tell the patient to use it whenever he needs it.
    4. Observe baseline respiratory effort and repeat at least every 4 hours or as needed.

18. Which data would be included in a cluster relevant to the nursing diagnosis of Constipation? (Select all that apply.) *(80)*
    1. Abdomen firm and nontender to touch
    2. Decreased bowel sounds
    3. Flat, brown, 1-cm lesion noted near umbilicus
    4. Takes opioid pain medications as needed
    5. Passed a small, hard stool yesterday
    6. Prefers to eat meat and potatoes, but lacks appetite

19. The nurse will perform a focused assessment on which patient(s)? (Select all that apply.) *(79)*
    1. Newly admitted to a long-term care facility
    2. Has a head injury that was sustained during a fall
    3. Suddenly becomes confused and does not recognize family
    4. Comes to the clinic for a physical examination for a job
    5. Reports pain in the left leg that worsens with walking
    6. Reports back pain, painful urination, and low-grade fever

20. What is the best rationale for collecting a patient's biographical data, such as age, weight, and place of employment? *(80)*
    1. Creates a complete and comprehensive legal document about the patient
    2. Is required by insurance companies and other third parties for reimbursement
    3. Helps the health care team identify potential risk factors for health problems
    4. Allows patient to participate more fully and have a say in his/her own care

21. What is the major advantage of using the nursing process to identify nursing diagnoses? *(80)*
    1. Helps nurses identify a disease or illness that creates problems for the patient
    2. Allows nurses to use clinical judgment about actual or potential health problems
    3. Permits nurses to use standardized care plans for common patient problems
    4. Limits the type of problems that nurses are responsible for treating

22. The nurse has completed the assessment and reviewed the patient's record. The nursing diagnosis Risk for impaired skin integrity is identified for this patient. Which data would support the choice of this diagnosis? *(82)*
    1. A deep decubitus ulcer is noted over the sacral area.
    2. Documentation includes descriptions of many skin lesions.
    3. Patient reports a painful, open sore on the left ankle.
    4. Patient is underweight and has trouble changing position.

23. Based on the definition, which would be an example of a *collaborative problem*? *(83)*
    1. Edema
    2. Anxiety
    3. Coping
    4. Cancer

24. The home health nurse needs the patient's complete medication history, but the patient tells the nurse that many changes were made in the hospital and at discharge, so he is not really sure what to tell her. What would be the best secondary source for this information? *(79, 80)*
    1. Patient's family
    2. Discharging health care provider
    3. Medication reconciliation form
    4. Local pharmacist

25. The postsurgical patient reports that he is having lower abdominal pain. What would the nurse include in the focused physical assessment? *(79)*
    1. Check peripheral pulses and sensation.
    2. Check for rigidity and rebound tenderness.
    3. Assess the patient's mental status.
    4. Auscultate the lung sounds.

26. The caregiver of a patient with Alzheimer's disease reports that the patient is unsteady and easily loses his balance, leaves the house, and needs coaching to accomplish tasks. Which nursing diagnosis(es) will apply to this patient? (Select all that apply.) *(80-83)*
    1. Acute confusion
    2. Self-care deficit for activities of daily living
    3. Wandering
    4. Risk for caregiver role strain
    5. Risk for falls

27. An elderly patient is wetting the bed because he is unable to independently get up and go to the bathroom. For this particular patient, which phase of the nursing process is most critical to address the patient's needs? *(85)*
    1. Assessment
    2. Diagnosis
    3. Planning
    4. Evaluation

28. The home health nurse has been visiting a patient for several months. One of the nursing diagnoses is "Social isolation related to reluctance to leave the house. The goal of "patient will attend a social function two times per month" has not been met. What should the nurse do first? *(88)*
    1. Document the results obtained after interventions have been performed.
    2. Rewrite the goal and replace "two times per month" with "one time per month."
    3. Agree to visit the patient more frequently to decrease sense of isolation.
    4. Evaluate the factors that are affecting or interfering with the patient's response.

29. Which nursing action demonstrates that the nurse believes that evidence-based practice is important for quality patient care? *(88)*
    1. Routinely reads research articles and applies research to patient care
    2. Works on a committee to update policy and procedure manuals
    3. Looks on the Internet to find clinically relevant data
    4. Asks a clinical nurse specialist to validate nursing care decisions

30. A patient comes to the clinic for a broken toe. The nurse checks the patient's pulse and then attaches him to the cardiac monitor, which reveals an irregular heart rhythm. What is the best rationale for the nurse's action? *(91)*
    1. The nurse saw that the patient had obvious risk factors for cardiac problems.
    2. Standard of care is a complete evaluation when patients first seek health care.
    3. A head-to-toe assessment is implemented when the patient is not distressed.
    4. Palpation of the pulse revealed irregularities, so the nurse considered pathophysiology.

31. The nursing student has diligently read all assignments, attended all lectures and skills practice sessions, but lacks clinical experience to improve critical thinking skills. What should the student do to improve critical thinking as it applies to patient care? (Select all that apply.) *(91)*
    1. Mentally rehearse clinical scenarios: "What would I do if…"
    2. Develop the habit of formulating relevant questions when listening or reading.
    3. Ask the instructor or nurse preceptor to "think out loud."
    4. Discuss with classmates how they reached a certain decision.
    5. Advocate for more clinical time with patients.
    6. Scan for nursing information from a wide variety of sources.

CRITICAL THINKING ACTIVITIES

32. Ms. M., aged 48 years, is admitted to the medical-surgical unit after an abdominal hysterectomy. Her vital signs are stable. The IV in her left forearm is patent, without swelling or tenderness. The dressings are dry and intact. Ms. M. has a Foley catheter in place that is draining clear, yellow urine. She was just transferred from the surgical recovery unit and is expressing severe pain. Select the priority problem for this patient and write a nursing care plan that addresses the problem. *(87)*

_____

_____

_____

_____

_____

_____

_____

_____

_____

_____

33. a. Discuss the LPN/LVN's role in the nursing process. *(89, 90)* _____

_____

_____

_____

_____

_____

b. If the LPN/LVN disagrees with the RN about the choice or priority of a nursing diagnosis, what should the LPN/LVN do? *(89, 90)*

_____

_____

_____

_____

_____

Cultural and Ethnic Considerations

chapter

6

Answer Key: Textbook page references are provided as a guide for answering these questions. A complete Answer Key is provided in your Additional Learning Resources on Evolve.

CROSSWORD PUZZLE

1. Directions: Use the clues to complete the crossword puzzle.

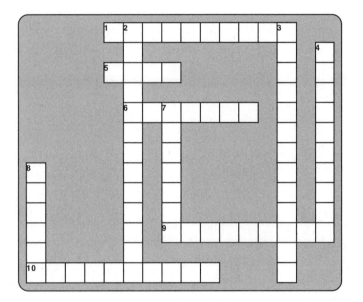

Across

1. Generalized expectation about behavior by members of a particular group *(95)*
5. Shares biologic physical characteristics *(96)*
6. Nation, community, or broad group of people who establish particular aims, beliefs, or standards of living and conduct *(94)*
9. Common social and cultural heritage based on shared traditions, national origin, and physical and biologic characteristics *(96)*
10. Shares characteristics with primary culture, but behaviors and ideals distinguish it from the rest of a cultural group *(94)*

Down

2. Understanding cultural variables and integrating that understanding during interaction *(96)*
3. Belief that own beliefs and cultural practices are the best *(95)*
4. Implies that future activities are possible to recover but not present ones *(100)*
7. Learned beliefs, customs, and practices shared by a group and passed to another generation *(94)*
8. Accepted traditional customs, moral attitudes, or manners of a particular social group *(95)*

FILL-IN-THE-BLANK SENTENCES

Directions: Complete each sentence by filling in the blank with the correct word or phrase.

2. _____ means that the nurse is aware of his or her own cultural beliefs and practices and how they relate to those of others, which may be different. *(95)*

3. A(n) _____ is a fixed concept of how all members of an ethnic group act or think. *(95)*

4. In the United States, the largest increase has occurred in the _____ population, which rose from 12.5% to 16.3% between 2000 and 2010. *(97)*

5. Nursing diagnoses are based on the _____ and may have limitations when used to develop a plan of care for culturally diverse patients with different health beliefs. *(107)*

6. In a culture that is matriarchal, the women probably make the decisions about _____, provide the _____, and _____. *(100)*

MULTIPLE CHOICE

Directions: Select the best answer(s) for each of the following questions.

7. When communicating with a patient who has limited understanding of English, the nurse should: *(97)*
   1. speak loudly to emphasize key information.
   2. keep questions brief and simple.
   3. use sign language and get an interpreter.
   4. provide detailed directions.

8. What cultural difference(s) does the nurse need to be aware of when caring for an older adult? (Select all that apply.) *(96)*
   1. They are more tolerant of other cultures.
   2. They may say hurtful things if cognitive impairment is present.
   3. They are more likely to be rigid in their practices.
   4. They are less likely to use home remedies.
   5. They rely more on traditional religious practices.
   6. They are less likely to be well-educated.

9. The health care provider informs the patient that there is a risk of blood loss during the planned surgical procedure, but the patient is a Jehovah's Witness, so she refuses to sign the consent form. Which nursing action is in the best interest of the patient? *(103)*
   1. Support the patient's decision to refuse the procedure.
   2. Discuss realistic alternatives to blood transfusion with the health care provider.
   3. Document the patient's decision in the medical record.
   4. Contact the risk manager for advice about convincing the patient.

10. A patient who is a Muslim American dies during the night. What action should the nurse perform in order to respect the patient's religious beliefs? *(101)*
    1. Contact the family before giving any post-mortem care.
    2. Stay with the deceased until a family member arrives.
    3. Wait at least 30 minutes before giving post-mortem care.
    4. Contact the organ transplant team because donation is likely.

11. The nurse is from a small town in the southern United States and is starting a new job in a large urban area with a diverse population. What strategy(ies) can the nurse use to develop cultural competence? (Select all that apply.) *(95)*
    1. Perform a self-assessment of beliefs and practices.
    2. Adapt personal beliefs to match those of individual patients.
    3. Keep an open mind about cultural differences.
    4. Treat everyone as equal and act the same toward all patients.
    5. Ignore the differences and focus on exhibiting kindness and care.
    6. Understand own values, preferences, and cultural heritage.

12. The nurse is caring for a patient who is dying. Evidence-based practice about cultural beliefs and rituals that surround death indicates that: *(96)*
    1. the family should be encouraged to pray at the bedside.
    2. respect and protection of the dying person's soul are important.
    3. lack of religious preference increases problems with coping.
    4. rituals and ceremonies to delay or ward off death should be discouraged.

13. The patient who is in no apparent distress is accompanied to the clinic by several family members who cluster around and are all attempting to talk to each other and the nurse at the same time. The nurse can hear a mixture of English and another language being spoken. What should the nurse do first? *(98)*
    1. Try to determine who speaks the best English.
    2. Take only the patient to an examination room and shut the door.
    3. Project calm energy and try to identify the leader of the family.
    4. Physically assess the patient and take vital signs to ascertain stability.

14. A male patient says to the nurse, "That young Asian woman (UAP) who helped me with my bath was really nice, but she seemed scared, never looked up; just kept her head down. Did I do something to scare or offend her?" What should the nurse do first? *(98)*
    1. Find the UAP and ask her to explain her behavior to the patient.
    2. Reassure that he did nothing wrong and that the UAP's behavior is cultural.
    3. Tell the patient that you will check with the UAP and then get back to him.
    4. Apologize to the patient and give then give feedback to the UAP.

15. The nurse is a happy and outgoing person, and comes from a family where hugging, touching, patting, or playfully punching are part of normal everyday interaction. What is the best strategy for the nurse to combine her personal style with giving culturally appropriate care? *(98, 99)*
    1. Assess her own behaviors and try to understand the origin of personal style.
    2. Consider different patient care settings and observe interactions.
    3. Learn which cultures can accept touch by health care personnel.
    4. Request to care for patients who are from her own culture.

16. The nurse is working in an assisted-living facility and most residents take their meals in a common dining area. What is the best method for seating the residents? *(99)*
    1. Assign seating so that everyone has a consistent place at mealtimes.
    2. Encourage the residents to continuously sit with someone new for stimulation.
    3. Observe how ambulatory residents seat and group themselves.
    4. Ask each resident where he/she would like to sit for each meal.

17. The nurse is trying to give all of his patients the 9:00 AM medications. An elderly Hispanic woman needs 15 medications every morning, but is consistently preoccupied whenever the nurse enters the room. What should the nurse do? *(99, 100)*
    1. Administer the medications to other patients first and then help this patient.
    2. Give the patient a 15-minute warning and then stick to the promised time.
    3. Try to find out why the woman is so consistently preoccupied.
    4. Start giving this patient the medications at 8:00 AM so there is extra time.

18. The nursing student is trying to explain the importance of taking blood pressure medication every day to an older patient who is on a fixed income. Which question from the patient suggests that his perception of time tends to be present-oriented? *(99, 100)*
    1. "Can I save the medication on the days when I feel okay?"
    2. "What should I do if I am running out of medication and have no money?"
    3. "My wife takes blood pressure medication too. Can I share her pills?"
    4. "Would you take this medication if you were in my position?"

19. The nurse is discussing the parents' beliefs and use of folk medicine, which they would like to use in the treatment of their child's respiratory infection. Which health care practice is the cause of greatest concern? *(105, 106)*
    1. Placing a religious medal on the bedside table
    2. Having a folk healer come to heal with touch and faith
    3. Giving the child an herbal tea that gives strength and health
    4. Bathing at night instead of in the morning

20. On visiting the patient at home, the nurse finds that the patient is not following the dietary instructions. The nurse discovers that the wife who shops and cooks believes that her husband needs "nutritious home-cooked meals from his native country." What should the nurse do first? *(107)*
    1. Change the dietary plan to meet the patient's and family's cultural preferences.
    2. Consult a nutritionist for ways to adapt the wife's cooking to the dietary plan.
    3. Revise the patient's nutritional goal to incorporate the cultural dietary patterns.
    4. Ask the wife to describe a typical 24-hour day of meal preparation and snacks.

21. The nurse is assessing a patient who reports, "It feels like there is something inside me that wants to come out." Which question(s) would the nurse ask in order to assess the patient's belief system? (Select all that apply.) *(95)*
    1. When did you first notice the feeling?
    2. Why do you think that has happened at this time?
    3. What do you think is causing the problem?
    4. Why do you think this is happening to you?
    5. What do you think will help to clear up the problem?
    6. How long does the feeling last?

CRITICAL THINKING ACTIVITIES

22. The nurse is caring for an older patient who has recently emigrated from another country. The patient's family is at the bedside and the nurse overhears them speaking in English and Spanish. The nurse's first language is English and she understands and speaks a little Spanish.

    a. Identify nursing interventions that may be used to communicate with a non–English-speaking patient. *(95, 98)*

    _____

    _____

    b. Discuss the advantages and disadvantages of using a family member to translate and communicate with the patient. *(98)*

    _____

    _____

    _____

    _____

    _____

    _____

    _____

    c. How should the nurse ask the patient about the following? *(95, 98)*

        i.   Language: _____

        ii. Health: _____

        iii. Family structure:_____

        iv. Dietary practices: _____

        v.   Use of folk medicine: _____

23. Every morning the same day-shift nurse is late for work, so giving handover report is always delayed. The night-shift nurses have mentioned this to the nurse manager, who has promised to take care of the problem, but the late behavior continues. One of the night nurses tries to talk to the day-shift nurse about her behavior, but the nurse says, "Oh you Americans are always so worried about time. Just relax. You know I will always be here." Analyze this situation and make suggestions about how the problem can be addressed. Ask your clinical instructor if you can discuss this topic in a postconference. *(99, 100)*

    _____

    _____

    _____

    _____

    _____

24. Nursing students who grow up and work in the United States sometimes have difficulty describing their own culture and identifying how "American" culture is viewed by people who have not grown up in the United States. *(95, 99)*

    a. If you are an American who grew up in the United States, describe the how "American" culture affects your values and belief system.

    _____

    _____

    _____

    _____

    _____

    _____

    _____

    b. If you are not originally from the United States, discuss how you view "American" culture and how being in that culture is currently affecting you.

    _____

    _____

    _____

    _____

    _____

    _____

    _____

Asepsis and Infection Control

Answer Key: Textbook page references are provided as a guide for answering these questions. A complete Answer Key is provided in your Additional Learning Resources on Evolve.

TRUE OR FALSE

Directions: Write T for true or F for false in the blanks provided.

_____ 1. Following isolation precautions is the most important method of reducing the spread of microorganisms. *(126)*

_____ 2. Immunocompromised patients admitted to health care facilities have an increased risk of being exposed to strains of *Staphylococcus aureus* that are multidrug-resistant (MRSA) and therefore more difficult to treat. *(118)*

_____ 3. One exception to the self-limiting nature of viral infection is acquired immunodeficiency syndrome (AIDS). *(120)*

_____ 4. Protozoa are responsible for valley fever and histoplasmosis, a systemic fungal respiratory disease. *(121)*

_____ 5. An accidental needlestick is an example of portal of exit in the chain of infection. *(122)*

_____ 6. Microorganisms are present only in susceptible hosts. *(122)*

_____ 7. Healthcare-associated infections (HAIs) are most commonly transmitted by direct contact between health care workers and patients or from patient to patient. *(124)*

_____ 8. HIV is the most commonly transmitted infection by contaminated needles. *(125)*

_____ 9. The prodromal stage is often the period in which the individual is most contagious. *(124)*

_____ 10. The intact multilayered mucosa is the body's first line of defense against infection. *(122)*

SHORT ANSWER

Directions: Using your own words, answer each question in the space provided.

11. Identify four major classifications of pathogens and one example of a microorganism for each. *(120)*

_____

_____

12. Discuss disinfection and nursing implications for using disinfectants. *(152)* _____

_____

_____

13. Identify at least five miscellaneous guidelines for Standard Precautions. *(127)* _____

_____

_____

14. What is the proper method for disposal of sharps? *(134, 136)* _____

_____

15. Describe the procedure for gowning for contact isolation. *(133)* _____

_____

_____

16. Review the following nursing tasks and identify whether medical asepsis (MA) or surgical asepsis (SA) is necessary to prevent the spread of infection. Label each task as MA or SA. *(117)*

_____ a. Assisting patient with meal tray

_____ b. Helping patient to brush teeth

_____ c. Obtaining a urine specimen from an existing catheter

_____ d. Obtaining a throat swab for a culture

_____ e. Inserting a urinary catheter

_____ f. Changing the bed linens

_____ g. Replacing a colostomy bag

_____ h. Drawing up medication in a syringe

_____ i. Removing medication from a bubble pack

_____ j. Dressing change of a new surgical incision

_____ k. Suctioning the lower airway

_____ l. Suctioning the oral cavity

17. Place the steps of opening a wrapped sterile package in the correct order. *(145)*

_____ Grasp the outer surface of the last and innermost flap; pull the flap back, allowing it to fall flat.

_____ Place the wrapped sterile package flat in the center of the work surface.

_____ Grasp the outside surface of the first side flap; open the side flap, allow it to lie flat on the table surface.

_____ Grasp the outer surface of the tip of the outermost flap; open the outer flap away from your body.

_____ Grasp the outside surface of the second side flap and allow it to lie flat on the table surface.

_____ Remove the tape or seal indicating the sterilization date.

_____ Perform hand hygiene.

MULTIPLE CHOICE

Directions: Select the best answer(s) for each of the following questions.

18. The patient has a large midline abdominal incision. With the specific purpose of reducing a possible reservoir of infection, the nurse: *(121)*
    1. wears gloves and mask at all times.
    2. isolates the patient's personal articles.
    3. has the patient cover mouth and nose when coughing.
    4. changes the dressing when it becomes soiled.

19. The nurse is preparing a room for a patient with herpes simplex virus. In particular, this type of precaution means that the care should include: *(136, 139)*
    1. a private room with negative air flow.
    2. hand hygiene after filtration masks are removed.
    3. use of gloves and gown upon entering the room.
    4. use of a surgical mask on the patient during transfers.

20. A patient with rubella needs to be transported to the x-ray department. What should the nurse do to prepare the patient for transport? *(135, 138)*
    1. Advise the patient to immediately wash hands after returning from procedure.
    2. Call the x-ray department and inform them to wear gloves at all times.
    3. Dress the patient in an isolation gown and then apply a mask.
    4. Instruct the patient to wear a mask and follow cough etiquette.

21. The nurse is supervising a nursing student. Which action by the student requires correction because it contributes to the potential transmission of pathogens? *(122)*
    1. Uses a dampened cloth to wipe off the overbed table
    2. Shakes linens to remove debris and then places them in laundry bag
    3. Holds soiled linens at a distance to prevent touching uniform
    4. Washes hands with soap and water after emptying and cleaning a bedpan

22. When caring for a patient with tuberculosis who is on airborne precautions, the nurse should routinely use: *(135)*
    1. regular mask and eyewear.
    2. gown and gloves.
    3. surgical handwashing and gloves.
    4. particulate respirator masks.

23. The nurse is observing the new staff member who is preparing to do a sterile dressing change. The nurse determines that the staff member requires correction and additional instruction when he observes: *(145)*
    1. opening the closest flap of the sterile wrapped package first.
    2. placing the cap of the sterile solution inside up on a clean surface.
    3. opening sterile items and dropping them directly onto the sterile field.
    4. maintaining a 1-inch border around the sterile drape.

24. The nurse is aware that the body has normal defenses against infection. Which medication can affect the acidic environment, which is one defense mechanism? *(123)*
    1. ciprofloxacin (Cipro)
    2. aluminum/magnesium antacid (Mylanta)
    3. doxycycline (Vibramycin)
    4. chlorhexidine gluconate (Hibiclens)

25. The patient has been receiving antibiotic therapy. Which laboratory result indicates a need to contact the health care provider for a reevaluation of prescribed therapy? *(154)*
    1. Sensitivity results are positive.
    2. Blood titer is positive for antibodies.
    3. White blood cell count is elevated.
    4. Blood cultures are negative for growth.

26. For what circumstance would it be appropriate to contact the infection-control nurse for assistance? *(125)*
    1. Results of a blood culture are needed to validate antibiotic therapy.
    2. Contaminated waste material needs to be properly disposed.
    3. An unusual cluster of infection is seen in the emergency department.
    4. A newly admitted patient requires droplet and isolation precautions.

27. What is the best rationale for the consistent use of Standard Precautions? *(126)*
    1. CDC recommends that health care workers use "universal blood and body fluid precautions."
    2. It is difficult to accurately identify all patients infected with blood-borne pathogens.
    3. Studies show that infection rates are unaffected by use of protective measures.
    4. Hand hygiene, gloves, masks, eye protection, and gowns are appropriate for patient contact.

28. The patient has tuberculosis and has been placed in a negative-pressure isolation room with airborne precautions. Despite repeated attempts to educate the patient, he keeps sneaking out of his room and going outside to smoke cigarettes. What should the nurse do first? *(135, 137)*
    1. Obtain an order for an around-the-clock sitter.
    2. Report the patient's behavior to the infection-control nurse.
    3. Ask the health care provider to prescribe a nicotine patch.
    4. Discuss the behavior with the patient.

29. Which patient needs to be placed into contact precautions? *(136, 139)*
    1. Has a draining wound colonized with multidrug-resistant bacteria
    2. Has cancer and is currently leukopenic
    3. Has meningitis caused by invasive *Neisseria meningitidis*
    4. Has tuberculosis caused by *Mycobacterium tuberculosis*

30. A patient comes into the clinic and tells the nurse that he has a sore throat and would like to see a doctor. For which task(s) does the nurse need to wear gloves? (Select all that apply.) *(131)*
    1. Interview and taking a history
    2. Taking the blood pressure
    3. Measuring an oral temperature
    4. Taking a throat swab for culture
    5. Reviewing the patient's home medications
    6. Using a tongue blade to look at the throat

31. Immediately after donning a pair of gloves, a family member develops red, watery eyes, and contact dermatitis with itching on the hands. What should the nurse do first? *(131, 132)*
    1. Inform the person that these are the signs/symptoms of latex allergy.
    2. Instruct the person to remove the gloves and wash thoroughly with soap and water.
    3. Contact the health care provider and observe for additional signs of anaphylaxis.
    4. Assess for a personal or family history of latex allergy or other allergies.

32. The nurse sees the UAP trying to take an overly full laundry bag from the patient's room to the dirty utility room. The UAP is struggling to manage the bag and is partially dragging it on the floor. What should the nurse do? *(127)*
    1. Allow the UAP to continue because she is completing her duties.
    2. Report the UAP for creating a situation where proper handling is impossible.
    3. Assist the UAP to carry the bag and then find out how it got so overfilled.
    4. Remind the UAP that overfilling the bag creates a problem for proper disposal.

33. The nurse is assigned to care for patients who are in isolation and patients who are not in isolation. What should the nurse do to try to meet the needs of all of the patients? *(135)*
    1. Provide care for patients who are not in isolation first.
    2. Ask the charge nurse to reassign at least one of the isolation cases to another nurse.
    3. See if patients with same type of isolation can be rearranged to be roommates.
    4. Organize and cluster care of isolation patients to minimize gowning and ungowning.

34. Which patient is the most challenging regarding maintaining sterile technique throughout the procedure? *(140, 141)*
    1. 4-month-old infant who is crying and upset, but needs routine immunization
    2. 30-year-old woman who is obese and confused needs a Foley catheter inserted
    3. 50-year-old man is continuously coughing and needs a dressing change on upper chest
    4. 15-year-old cheerful patient with Down syndrome "wants to help" insert the IV

35. The nurse is assisting a health care provider by setting up a sterile tray for a procedure at the bedside. When the nurse opens the tray, there is moisture on a piece of equipment. What should the nurse do? *(142)*
    1. Continue to set up the tray, because everything inside the kit is considered sterile.
    2. Return the entire tray to the supply area for resterilization and obtain a new tray.
    3. Put on a sterile glove and remove the moist piece of equipment and set it aside.
    4. Inform the health care provider about the problem and obtain a new order for additional equipment.

36. The nurse is supervising a nursing student who is setting up a sterile tray to suction a patient. The nurse would intervene if the student: *(145)*
    1. sets up the field on a clean overbed table that is at waist-level.
    2. touches the outside of the sterile wrapper when handling the package.
    3. picks up a sterile drape by the corner and lets it unfold by itself without touching any object.
    4. puts on sterile gloves, opens the bottle, and sets the cap on the sterile field.

37. A patient who is HIV-positive and ready for discharge expresses fears about exposure of other family members, particularly young children, to the disease. What is the best response to help decrease the patient's fears and concerns? *(121, 122)*
    1. Review general principles of infection control in the home setting.
    2. Review principles of mode of transmission for HIV.
    3. Encourage expression of fears and concerns and validate feelings.
    4. Suggest that the patient maintain contact with family using phone calls, email, or video conferencing.

38. The new nurse observes a health care provider who routinely comes out of a patient's room, goes to the sink, quickly soaps her hands, rinses, and then shakes water from her hands so that it splashes on the floor, sink, and her uniform. What should the new nurse do? *(126, 127)*
    1. Contact the infection-control nurse for advice.
    2. Do nothing because the health care provider is not accountable to the nurse.
    3. Check on the patient's status and then write up an incident report.
    4. Offer the health care provider a paper towel and assess understanding of hand hygiene.

39. Which patient is most likely to be susceptible to infection because of factors affecting immunologic defense mechanisms? *(122)*
    1. A 5-year-old child who is not up to date on school immunizations
    2. A 35-year-old woman who has recently returned from Japan
    3. A 73-year-old man who recently had chemotherapy and radiation treatments
    4. A 55-year-old man who has a high-stress job and is overweight

40. The nursing student has been diagnosed with "strep throat." Under what circumstances can the student go to the clinical unit and care for patients and complete the clinical objectives? *(127)*
    1. Has been taking prescribed antibiotics for at least 24 hours
    2. Agrees to wear a mask whenever caring for patients
    3. Cares only for patients who are not susceptible to infection
    4. Can return to clinical if the instructor is aware of the condition

CRITICAL THINKING ACTIVITIES

41. The nurse is caring for several patients. The patients include a frail 87-year-old woman with a hip fracture; a 78-year-old woman with advanced Alzheimer's who is being treated for dehydration secondary to incontinence of watery diarrhea, and a 60-year-old man who sustained a small perforation during a routine colonoscopy, which was recommended as part of his annual physical examination.

a. Explain conditions that promote the onset of HAIs for these patients. *(124, 125)* _____

_____

_____

b. What measures can be used to prevent HAIs? *(124, 125)*

_____

_____

_____

_____

_____

c. Although the health care provider has not currently ordered isolation precautions for any of these patients, the nurse should consider initiating isolation precautions for which patient? Identify the type of isolation that the nurse would choose and give the rationale that supports the decision. *(124, 125)*

_____

_____

_____

42. The nurse is caring for a 35-year-old patient who sustained a penetrating abdominal wound and multiple bruises and contusions in a farming accident. The abdominal wound was very contaminated, but cleaned before and during surgery. The wound-care specialist has been consulted and has taught the nursing staff how to do the dressing changes. The patient has a peripheral IV and is receiving IV antibiotics and pain medication. The nurse identifies that the patient is at risk for infection.

a. Give examples of questions that the nurse could use to collect data about factors that would affect the patient's immunologic defense mechanisms. *(122, 124)*

_____

_____

_____

_____

_____

b. Explain why this patient is likely to have an inflammatory response and describe the physiologic process that will occur. *(122)*

_____

_____

_____

c. Describe the signs and symptoms that would occur if the patient developed a localized infection at the abdominal wound site or at the IV site. *(123, 124)*

_____

_____

d. Describe the signs and symptoms that the nurse would be alert for that would signal a systemic infection. *(123, 124)*

_____

_____

_____

_____

_____

Body Mechanics and Patient Mobility

chapter

8

Answer Key: Textbook page references are provided as a guide for answering these questions. A complete Answer Key is provided in your Additional Learning Resources on Evolve.

WORD SCRAMBLE

Directions: Unscramble the words that describe different joint movements and then match the term to the correct definition.

Scrambled Term	Unscrambled Term	Definition
1. nfexloi *(170)*		
2. xteennsoi *(170)*		
3. ynsperoexhtein *(170)*		
4. bounctdia *(170)*		
5. dodctianu *(170)*		
6. nupsintioa *(170)*		
7. raopntoni *(170)*		
8. oorsidlexfin *(172)*		
9. uiirccmuctdon *(170)*		

Definition of joint movements

a. Movement of limb away from body
b. Movement of certain joints that decreases angle between two adjoining bones
c. Kind of rotation that allows palm of hand to turn downward
d. To bend or flex backward
e. Movement of certain joints that increases angle between two adjoining bones
f. Movement of limb toward axis of body
g. Kind of rotation that allows palm of hand to turn upwards
h. Extreme or abnormal extension
i. Movement in a circular pattern

MULTIPLE CHOICE

Directions: Select the best answer(s) for each of the following questions.

10. A nurse walks into the patient's room and notices that the patient is having trouble breathing. Which position will the nurse immediately use to help relieve the patient's respiratory distress? *(163)*
    1. Lower the head of the bed and place the patient in a supine anatomical position.
    2. Position the patient on the side with knee and thigh drawn up toward the chest
    3. Lower the patient's head and place the body and legs on a slightly inclined plane.
    4. Raise the head of the bed to 45-60 degrees and with the head in an anatomical position.

11. Which position would be most comfortable for the patient and provide the best access for the nurse to insert a rectal suppository? *(164)*
    1. Sims
    2. Lithotomy
    3. Trendelenberg
    4. Orthopneic

12. Which medications are most likely to contribute to orthostatic hypotension? *(160)*
    1. Medications used to treat osteoporosis
    2. Medications to prevent thrombophlebitis
    3. Medications to reduce high blood pressure
    4. Medications used to treat arthritis pain

13. The nurse is working with a patient who has poor balance to move from the bed to the chair. What is included in the correct technique for assisting the patient to stand and pivot to the chair? *(161)*
    1. Keep the legs slightly bent.
    2. Maintain a narrow base with the feet.
    3. Keep the stomach muscles loose.
    4. Stand at arm's length from the patient.

14. The patient has had a surgical procedure and is getting up to ambulate for the first time. While ambulating down the hallway, the patient says, "I'm going to faint." What should the nurse do first? *(167)*
    1. Call out for someone to obtain a wheelchair.
    2. Pull the patient close and lower him gently to the floor.
    3. Lean the patient against the wall until the episode passes.
    4. Support the patient and move quickly back to the room.

15. The patient will be immobilized for an extended period due to extensive injuries. Which intervention will the nurse use to prevent respiratory complications? *(167)*
    1. Suction the airway every hour.
    2. Change the patient's position every 4-8 hours.
    3. Use oxygen and nebulizer treatments regularly.
    4. Encourage deep-breathing and coughing every hour.

16. Patients who are immobilized in health care facilities require that their psychosocial needs be met along with their physiologic needs. Which statement by the nurse acknowledges these needs? *(166)*
    1. "Visiting hours will be limited so you can rest."
    2. "We will help you do everything so you don't have to worry."
    3. "Let's talk about what you used to do at home during the day."
    4. "A private room can be arranged for you."

17. The patient experienced a cerebrovascular accident (CVA) that left her with severe left-sided paralysis and very limited mobility. Which device would prevent plantar flexion? *(168)*
    1. Footboard
    2. Bed board
    3. Trapeze bar
    4. Trochanter roll

18. When assessing the neurovascular status of a patient, what is an expected finding? *(169)*
    1. Capillary refill after 8 seconds
    2. Pulses strong and easily palpated
    3. Loss of sensation to an affected area
    4. Mild localized discomfort

19. The range of motion (ROM) that can be safely performed on the neck includes: (Select all that apply.) *(170)*
    1. flexion.
    2. supination.
    3. lateral flexion.
    4. rotation.
    5. hyperextension.

20. Which patient has a contracture? *(173)*
    1. Patient has abnormal extension of a finger joint.
    2. Patient's wrist is abnormally flexed and joint is fixed.
    3. Patient's knee is hyperextended.
    4. Patient has abnormal lateral movements of ankle joint.

21. What is the most likely complication if an elderly patient gets pulled across the bed when changing wet linens? *(160)*
    1. Dislocation of a joint.
    2. Increased stress to the joints.
    3. Abnormal hyperextension of a joint.
    4. Shearing or tearing of the skin.

22. For an older female patient who is at risk for osteoporosis, which associated complication can be minimized by participating in a regular exercise program as prescribed by the health care provider? *(160)*
    1. Bone loss that results in fractures
    2. Immobility secondary to joint degeneration
    3. Tissue ischemia and pressure ulcers
    4. Thrombophlebitis secondary to blood clots

23. The nurse is preparing to assist the patient to transfer from the bed to the chair. Which action demonstrates the proper use of body mechanics? *(177)*
    1. Stands by the chair and reaches out to guide the patient toward the chair
    2. Stands by the side of the patient and pulls up on the stronger arm
    3. Stands directly in front of the patient and places hands at the patient's waist level
    4. Stands to the side of patient and assists as the patient pivots

24. The nurse weighs 106 pounds. According to the National Institute for Occupational Safety and Health (NIOSH) Division of Safety Research, what is the maximum amount of weight that she should safely lift? *(182)*
    a. Depends on nurse's health and personal strength
    b. No more than 35 pounds of the patient's weight
    c. No more than 35% of her own 106 pounds
    d. Maximum of 50 pounds regardless of patient's or nurse's weight

25. Which patient behavior should be corrected to reduce the risk of thrombophlebitis? *(162)*
    1. Patient gets out of bed and forgets to put on slippers.
    2. Patient sits in chair and crosses legs while reading a book.
    3. Patient forgets to rise slowly when getting out of bed.
    4. Patient sits in a slouched position on a soft couch.

26. The patient has a cast on the left lower leg. When should assessment be performed to prevent compartment syndrome? *(166)*
    1. Every 3-4 hours as ordered
    2. At the beginning of the shift
    3. When the patient reports pain
    4. Immediately after cast application

27. What is an important consideration for an older patient who is using a continuous passive motion (CPM) machine after knee arthroplasty? *(172)*
    1. CPM is a potential fire hazard, so care must be taken to avoid flammable materials.
    2. CPM creates a risk for skin impairment so pressure points must be frequently assessed.
    3. CPM is preferred for home-bound seniors because it is easy to use.
    4. Many older patients prefer CPM because it is less strenuous than physical therapy.

CRITICAL THINKING ACTIVITIES

28. The nurse is caring for a patient who has had a CVA with right-sided impairment. The identified nursing diagnosis is Impaired physical mobility related to right-sided paresis manifested by difficulty moving right arm and leg and interference with ADLs.

    a. Before turning or transferring this patient, what patient assessment and preparations should be made? *(179)*

    _____

    _____

    b. Identify the appropriate nursing action to assist the patient to move from the bed to a chair. *(176)*

    _____

    _____

    c. While transferring the patient from the bed to a chair, the patient starts to fall. What should the nurse do? *(167)*

    _____

    _____

    d. The patient is unable to perform ROM of the right extremities. What can the nurse do to help the patient accomplish the ROM exercises? *(169)*

    _____

    _____

29. The nurse is caring for a patient who is in a comatose state after sustaining a severe head injury several months ago. He is breathing on his own and his vital signs are stable but he shows no purposeful movements.

    a. What are the complications of immobility for this patient? *(166)* _____

    _____

    b. What nursing interventions may be implemented to prevent the occurrence of complications of immobility? *(166)*

    _____

    _____

    _____

    c. During morning hygiene, the nurse notes a reddened area on the patient's sacrum. What nursing interventions can be used to address this finding? *(166)*

    _____

    _____

    _____

Hygiene and Care of the Patient's Environment

chapter

9

Answer Key: Textbook page references are provided as a guide for answering these questions. A complete Answer Key is provided in your Additional Learning Resources on Evolve.

TRUE OR FALSE

Directions: Write T for true or F for false in the blanks provided.

_____ 1. Although the rules of touch are typically unspoken and unwritten, they are usually visible to the observer. *(186)*

_____ 2. Urinary incontinence is expected among very elderly adults. *(188)*

_____ 3. Medicare and Medicaid will cover the costs of treating pressure ulcers that developed during the patient's hospitalization if the condition is well-documented. *(200)*

_____ 4. When the external pressure against the skin is greater than the pressure in the capillary bed, blood flow increases to the adjacent tissues. *(200)*

_____ 5. Routine hygiene would include trimming or shaving an unsightly beard, mustache, or sideburns for surgical procedures or to maintain personal cleanliness. *(207)*

FILL-IN-THE-BLANK SENTENCES

Directions: Complete each sentence by filling in the blank with the correct word or phrase.

6. Assisting a patient with hygiene gives the nurse an opportunity to perform a complete and thorough _____. *(185)*

7. The recommended room temperature for most adult patients is _____. *(186)*

8. If external pressure on the skin or tissues continues without relief for more than _____ hours, cells in the involved layers of skin tend to undergo necrosis. *(200)*

9. Inserting objects into the internal auditory canal can damage the _____ or cause _____ to become impacted in the canal. *(214)*

10. Patients who are immobilized, poorly nourished, and have reduced sensation are at risk for impaired _____. *(225)*

MULTIPLE CHOICE

Directions: Select the best answer(s) for each of the following questions.

11. The nurse is teaching a patient who has diabetes about foot care. What should be included in the self-care instructions? *(223)*
    1. Carefully cut corns and apply moleskin.
    2. Inspect feet daily for breaks in the skin.
    3. Wear loose shoes or sandals to air the feet.
    4. Use alcohol to increase dryness between the toes.

12. An older adult patient wears dentures, and the nurse will delegate the denture care to the UAP. What instructions should the nurse give to the UAP about the patient's dentures? *(204)*
    1. Use hot water and a mild soap.
    2. Let the patient wear them at night.
    3. Brush dentures with a soft toothbrush.
    4. Wrap them in a soft towel when not worn.

13. In delegating the early morning care that should occur before breakfast, what does the nurse remind the UAP to do for the patient? *(187)*
    1. Shampoo the patient's hair and comb it.
    2. Assist the patient with a bath and clean gown.
    3. Offer the patient a backrub with warmed lotion.
    4. Help the patient wash hands and face.

14. A patient who is paralyzed from the waist down is at risk for developing a pressure ulcer on the sacral area. Which intervention would the nurse use for this patient? *(202)*
    1. Frequently check and change the bed linens.
    2. Teach to shift weight every 15 minutes.
    3. Obtain an order for a donut cushion for sitting.
    4. Keep skin moist and frequently reapply lotion.

15. While completing the bath, the nurse notices a reddened area on the patient's sacrum. What should the nurse do first? *(200)*
    1. Cleanse the skin with alcohol.
    2. Wash the area with hot water and soap.
    3. Massage the area vigorously.
    4. Assess for other areas of erythema.

16. The nurse is assessing the oral cavity of an unconscious patient and sees tenacious, dried exudate on the tongue, teeth, and gums. What instructions should be given to the UAP? *(205, 206)*
    1. Use a moistened sponge applicator and gently clean crusts several times per shift.
    2. Spray the mouth with a bulb syringe and use oral suction to remove the fluid.
    3. Use a toothbrush with paste and scrub the area until the crusts are removed.
    4. Wrap a gauze sponge around a tongue blade and apply hydrogen peroxide.

17. The nurse is evaluating the eye care that has been delegated to and is being provided by a new staff member. Which action is appropriate? *(213)*
    1. Removing dried secretions with moist gauze
    2. Using soap and water on a washcloth
    3. Cleansing the eyes from the outer to the inner canthus
    4. Wiping plastic eyeglasses with a clean paper towel

18. The nurse observes the patient performing ear care. Identify which behavior indicates a need for additional teaching? *(214)*
    1. Cleans the pinna with a cotton-tipped swab
    2. Turns the hearing aid off when not in use
    3. Leaves the hearing aid by a sunny window
    4. Rotates a clean washcloth to clean ear canal

19. The nurse is caring for a postpartum patient. Which assessment should the nurse perform first before starting perineal care? *(211)*
    1. Note presence of accumulated secretions.
    2. Evaluate the appearance of episiotomy.
    3. Assess ability to perform own care.
    4. Ask about burning with urination.

20. The nurse is caring for an elderly patient who requires assistance with elimination. He can walk very slowly, but is frequently incontinent of urine before he can get to the toilet. What should the nurse do to help the patient with elimination? (Select all that apply.) *(220, 221)*
    1. Instruct the UAP to be alert for the call signal and answer promptly.
    2. Obtain an order for an indwelling catheter until bladder training is achieved.
    3. Show the patient how to use a urinal and place it within his reach.
    4. Obtain an order for a commode chair and place it close to the bed.
    5. Restrict fluids to exact intervals to establish a voiding pattern.
    6. Make a plan with the patient to call sooner, rather than delaying.

21. The nursing student is told to observe the bowel movements of an adult patient and report any abnormalities to the nurse. What should the student report as an unexpected finding? *(219)*
    1. Stool was a dull clay color.
    2. Stool had soft, formed consistency.
    3. Patient had two bowel movements.
    4. Stool had the shape of the rectum.

22. The nurse is caring for a new patient who needs assessment of skin and self-care abilities; perineal care; partial bath; and the bed linen changed. The patient is very obese. What is the best strategy to meet the needs of the patient? *(185, 190)*
    1. Instruct the UAP to perform all tasks except the skin assessment.
    2. Ask the UAP to call when the patient's back is positioned for assessment.
    3. Assess skin and self-care abilities while working with the UAP to complete care.
    4. Assess skin and self-care abilities, then allow the patient to perform her own care.

23. Which patient is most likely to request that the room temperature be turned down? *(186, 187)*
    1. Has chronic pulmonary disease
    2. Has alternating chills and fever
    3. Has peripheral vascular disease
    4. Has end-stage pancreatic cancer

24. The nurse is caring for elderly residents in an assisted-living facility. What is the best strategy to prevent skin breakdown among this vulnerable group? *(188)*
    1. Make daily rounds and assess skin condition.
    2. Instruct UAPs to help residents out of bed as much as possible.
    3. Plan a toileting schedule for the residents at greatest risk.
    4. Ask the dietary department to serve high-quality protein foods.

25. A family member tells the nurse that the staff is spending too much time laughing and chatting at the nurses' station and it is disturbing the patient's rest and comfort. What should the nurse do first? *(187)*
    1. Instruct the staff to be more discreet and move conversation to the breakroom.
    2. Assess other environmental factors that are interfering with patient's comfort.
    3. Apologize to the family member and assure that the situation will be corrected.
    4. Assess the patient's discomfort and ask what other things are interfering with rest.

26. The nurse is supervising a nursing student who is giving a patient a bed bath. The nurse would intervene if the student performed which action? *(189)*
    1. Lowers the side rail to perform care
    2. Raises the head of the bed to a semi-Fowler's position
    3. Bathes arms using long, firm strokes
    4. Puts up all four side rails after completing the bath

27. The nurse instructed the UAP to encourage the patient's independence in accomplishing ADLs. Which behavior best indicates that the UAP understood what to do? *(190)*
    1. The UAP waits until the patient uses the call light for assistance.
    2. The nurse sees that the commode chair is close to the bed.
    3. The nurse observes that the patient is brushing his own teeth.
    4. The UAP tells the nurse that the patient is independent for ADLs.

28. An unconscious patient needs oral care. What instructions should the nurse give to the UAP to ensure the safety of the patient? (Select all that apply.) *(205, 206)*
    1. Position the patient upright; use pillows for support as needed.
    2. Report bleeding, sores in the mouth, or obvious problems with teeth or gums.
    3. Check for gag reflex by gently inserting a tongue blade into the throat.
    4. Use a soft toothbrush and brush teeth as for any other patient.
    5. Have an oral suction device ready and check function prior to starting.
    6. Perform hand hygiene before donning clean gloves.

29. A neighbor tells the nurse that he has muscle soreness and stiffness after performing a new exercise program. What would the nurse recommend? *(191)*
    1. A tub bath with the proper temperature of 113° to 115° F (45° to 46° C).
    2. A bath with the water temperature at a tepid 98.6° F (37° C).
    3. A sitz bath that lasts 20-30 minutes for soaking and relaxing.
    4. A shower with a recommended water temperature of 109.4° F (43° C).

30. A patient with dementia needs assistance with bathing. What strategy(ies) is/are best to use to help the patient accomplish this task? (Select all that apply.) *(192)*
    1. Maintain a relaxed demeanor, smile frequently, and use a calm tone of voice.
    2. Demonstrate and explain the desired behavior, such as turning on the water.
    3. Reassure frequently and say things such as, "You are doing well. We are almost done."
    4. Try to repeat the same hygiene pattern every day and wash the same body parts.
    5. Use distraction rather than trying to negotiate or making demands.
    6. Attempt to have the same caregivers as often as possible for hygienic care.

CRITICAL THINKING ACTIVITIES

31. For the following patients, identify how bathing may be affected or altered.

    a. The patient is extremely fatigued. *(215)* _____

    _____

    b. The patient is on complete bedrest. *(202, 204, 207)* _____

    _____

    c. The patient has right-sided paralysis following a CVA. *(199)* _____

    _____

    d. There is inflammation of the perianal tissue. *(191)* _____

    _____

    e. The patient is an East Indian Hindu. *(186)* _____

    _____

    f. The patient is an older adult who is incontinent. *(220, 221)* _____

    _____

32. A 30-year-old female patient has quadriplegia secondary to a diving accident that occurred five years ago. She was very healthy and athletic prior to the accident, but within the last several months she has been hospitalized several times for recurrent urinary tract infections and significant weight loss. She currently has a poor appetite.

   a. Identify possible risk factors that will contribute to development of pressure ulcers for this patient. *(200)*

   _____

   _____

   b. The nurse observes a stage I pressure ulcer on the patient's sacral area. Describe the criteria for a stage I pressure ulcer. *(201)*

   _____

   _____

   _____

   c. The nurse observes suspected deep tissue injury on the patient's right heel. Describe the criteria for suspected deep tissue injury. *(202)*

   _____

   _____

   d. How can the nurse prevent the development of pressure ulcers? *(200, 201)* _____

   _____

   _____

   e. Identify general guidelines for care of pressure ulcers. *(202)* _____

   _____

   _____

   _____

   _____

Safety

Answer Key: Textbook page references are provided as a guide for answering these questions. A complete Answer Key is provided in your Additional Learning Resources on Evolve.

ABBREVIATIONS

Directions: For each abbreviation, write out the full term or phrase.

1. RACE: _____ *(241)*

2. CDC: _____ *(239)*

3. OSHA:_____ *(239)*

4. PASS:_____ *(241)*

5. SRD: _____ *(231)*

TRUE OR FALSE

Directions: Write T for true or F for false in the blanks provided.

_____ 6. It is acceptable to delegate monitoring patient behavior for risk for injury and promoting a safe environment as a responsibility of the UAP, in addition to the nursing staff. *(229)*

_____ 7. Growth and the acquisition of new motor skills place children at increased risk for injury. *(230)*

_____ 8. Safety reminder devices (SRDs) are primarily used in long-term care facilities. *(231, 232)*

_____ 9. There is a 5% chance of a health care worker becoming infected with HIV from a sharps injury. *(239)*

_____ 10. Electrical accidents are often prevented by reporting frayed or broken electrical cords or any shocks felt when using equipment. *(251)*

MULTIPLE CHOICE

Directions: Select the best answer(s) for each of the following questions.

11. The patient is using an older thermometer at home that contains mercury. The thermometer is dropped and breaks, releasing mercury onto the floor. What is the priority nursing action? (238, 239)
    1. Evacuate everyone from the room.
    2. Close the interior doors and open windows.
    3. Vacuum the mercury and the glass shards.
    4. Mop the floor with hot water and soap.

12. The nurse is caring for a patient who relies on mechanical ventilation. The nurse hears a fire alarm and flames are visible in a back corridor. What should the nurse do first? (241)
    1. Seek assistance to move the patient and the ventilator to safety.
    2. Turn off the oxygen supply and provide manual respiratory support.
    3. Close the patient's door, call 911, and fight the fire in the corridor.
    4. Delegate the UAP to move ambulatory patients toward the exit.

13. The nurse is planning to teach a community group about fire safety in the home. What information should be included in the presentation? (Select all that apply.) (239-241)
    1. No smoking by the patient, family, or visitors in areas where oxygen is used.
    2. Use safety matches to light candles or fireplaces.
    3. Install fire alarms, smoke detectors, and carbon monoxide detectors.
    4. Practice fire escape routes from each room and practice exit drills.
    5. Use one electrical circuit to facilitate monitoring of cords and appliances.
    6. Cover electrical cords with a secure carpet to prevent falls.

14. An older adult patient in a long-term care facility has been wandering around outside of the room during the late evening hours. The patient has a history of falls. The nurse intervenes by: (232)
    1. obtaining an order for a bed and chair alarm.
    2. keeping the light on and the television playing all night.
    3. putting up the side rails and frequently checking on the patient.
    4. having the family come to check on the patient at night.

15. A male patient of average build requires assistance to ambulate down the hall. He has some weakness on the left side. The nurse assists this patient to ambulate by applying a gait belt and standing at his: (230)
    1. left side and holding the weak left arm.
    2. right side and holding the front of the gait belt.
    3. left side and holding the back of the gait belt.
    4. right side and holding one arm around his waist.

16. The nurse is considering the use of an SRD to prevent a patient from self-injury. When using an SRD, the nurse should: (Select all that apply.) (231, 232)
    1. obtain a health care provider's order for the SRD.
    2. explain the purpose of the SRD to the patient.
    3. explain the purpose of the SRD to the family.
    4. obtain consensus of nursing staff for type of SRD.
    5. exhaust all alternatives before using an SRD.

17. The nurse notices smoke coming from the wastebasket in a patient's room. Upon entering the room, the nurse sees a fire that is starting to flare up. What should the nurse do first? (242, 243)
    1. Extinguish the fire.
    2. Remove the patient from the room.
    3. Close the door to the room.
    4. Turn off all electrical equipment.

18. Which occurrence is mostly likely to be investigated as a "sentinel event"? *(229)*
    1. Patient leaves the hospital against medical advice because she gets angry with the nurse.
    2. An older patient sustains a broken arm related to the use of an SRD.
    3. A nurse is 2 hours late administering routine scheduled medications.
    4. During a follow-up phone call, a patient reports that care in the hospital was poor.

19. The nurse is conducting a fall risk assessment on an elderly patient who is moving into an assisted-living center. Which question(s) would the nurse ask? (Select all that apply.) *(230)*
    1. Have you had any falls in the past year?
    2. Are you able to independently get up after a fall?
    3. Do you feel unsteady when you stand up?
    4. Are you able to independently walk from room to room?
    5. Have you ever lost consciousness after a fall?
    6. Do you use a cane or other assistive device?

20. The nurse is giving instructions to the UAP about patient safety and fall prevention. What should the nurse tell the UAP about helping the patient go to the bathroom? *(233)*
    1. Help the patient whenever she needs help.
    2. Ask her if she wants to walk or use the bedpan.
    3. Have her sit up slowly and dangle her legs before standing.
    4. Help her to the commode chair if she seems weak.

21. For the care of a patient who has an SRD in place, which task can be delegated to a UAP? *(229)*
    1. Observe for circulation distal to the SRD.
    2. Check for respiratory effort and breathing.
    3. Change position every 2 hours.
    4. Determine when the SRD can be removed.

22. Which instructions should be given to the UAP who is assigned to assist in the care of a patient who is being treated with internal radiation? *(229)*
    1. Do not go into the room unless the patient uses the call bell.
    2. Help children to don a lead shield apron before entering the room.
    3. Wear a mask, eye shield, and isolation gown when entering the room.
    4. Wear your dosimeter during patient care or when handling patient items.

23. A patient begins to have a grand mal seizure. Which action should be delegated to the UAP? *(229)*
    1. Ensure that the tongue is not occluding the airway.
    2. Place pillows or other soft materials on side rails.
    3. Suction the mouth for frothy secretions to prevent aspiration.
    4. Gently insert an oral airway between the teeth.

24. The nurse is talking to a young mother who has an infant who has just started to crawl. Based on knowledge of growth and development, which safety issue is currently the most important to discuss with the mother? *(230)*
    1. What to do when using pots and pans on the stove
    2. How to ensure backyard pool safety measures
    3. How to manage electrical sockets and cords
    4. Where to obtain safety labels for cleaning products

25. Which new equipment creates the greatest risk for falls for an older adult? *(230, 231)*
    1. Wheelchair
    2. Prescription lenses
    3. Safety bar in shower
    4. Walker

26. The postoperative patient demonstrates some mild dizziness and mild shortness of breath when moving from sitting to standing position. Which laboratory value would the nurse check first? *(231)*
    1. Red blood cell count
    2. White blood cell count
    3. Blood urea nitrogen
    4. Creatinine level

27. The patient reports dizziness when standing up too fast. Which over-the-counter medication is most likely to be contributing to the patient's orthostatic hypotension? *(231)*
    1. Nonaspirin pain reliever
    2. Antihistamine
    3. Vitamin supplement
    4. Medicated cough drop

28. An infant has a wound with a dressing on the left upper arm. He repeatedly attempts to remove the dressing. Which SRD would the nurse select? *(235)*
    1. Mummy wrap
    2. Wrap jacket
    3. Bilateral wrist SRDs
    4. Right elbow SRD

29. A mother brings her alert and playful child to the clinic because she "found him playing with this empty bottle of baby aspirin." Which question is the most important to ask the mother?" *(244)*
    1. "Has he ever done anything like this before?"
    2. "How many times has he vomited since the ingestion?"
    3. "How many pills do you think were in the container?"
    4. "Did you contact poison control before you drove to the clinic?"

30. A patient with a latex allergy is exposed to latex. Which sign or symptom is cause for the greatest concern? *(238)*
    1. Hives
    2. Laryngeal edema
    3. Runny eyes and nose
    4. Localized swelling

31. Before the nurse can intervene, a UAP pushes contaminated material into an overfilled sharps container and sustains a puncture wound. What should the nurse do first? *(239)*
    1. Tell the UAP to immediately report to the infection-control nurse.
    2. Assist the UAP to scrub the wound with copious amounts of soap and water.
    3. Report the UAP for improper handling of hazardous material.
    4. Dispose of the sharps container to prevent any additional injuries to others.

32. The nurse started a new job in a small long-term care facility in a rural area. The back exit hallway is being used as a storage area and "a new storage area is being planned." What should the nurse do first? *(239, 241)*
    1. Report the facility for unsafe conditions.
    2. Express unwillingness to work in unsafe conditions.
    3. Review the facility's policies/procedures for emergencies.
    4. Check the building for other safety issues.

33. In the event of a bioterrorist attack, what is the first role that the nurse must perform? *(246, 247)*
    1. Isolate suspected cases.
    2. Advocate for public safety.
    3. Liaison with the public health department.
    4. Recognize high-risk syndromes.

34. It is suspected that a patient has been exposed to cyanide gas. The nurse is alert for which symptom? *(249)*
    1. Erratic behavior
    2. Nausea and vomiting
    3. Respiratory distress
    4. Vesicle formation

35. The nurse is reviewing the disaster preparedness plan for a small nursing home. What should be included in the plan? (Select all that apply.) *(244-246)*
    1. Emergency treatment for the most critically injured
    2. Possible admission to a hospital or transfer to a temporary shelter
    3. Log to document residents' names and locations
    4. System to notify families and health care providers
    5. Designation of an area for decontamination
    6. Method of patient identification, such as a bracelet or picture ID

36. The nurse working in a local health department knows that a bioterrorist attack that can occur via the food-borne route is: *(247)*
    1. anthrax.
    2. botulism.
    3. plague.
    4. smallpox.

CRITICAL THINKING ACTIVITIES

37. The nurse is caring for a patient in a long-term care facility. The patient has a history of falls in the home.

    a. For the nursing diagnosis Risk for injury/falls, identify a patient outcome and three nursing interventions. *(229)*

    _____

    _____

    _____

    _____

    b. Describe how the nurse can promote safe ambulation for the patient in a health care facility. *(229)*

    _____

    _____

    _____

    _____

    c. Identify three additional factors that influence the safety of the older adult in the home or health care environment. *(229)*

    _____

    _____

38. The nurse is working in a small urban outpatient clinic. The nurse manager has just informed the staff that the disaster plan may have to be activated because the emergency department of a nearby hospital has identified a possible bioterrorism-related event.

    a. What is the role of the nurse in a disaster event? *(244, 246)* _____

    _____

    _____

    b. What indications would alert the nurse to a possible bioterrorism-related event? *(246, 247)* _____

    _____

    _____

39. List your personal fears or concerns about safety for family, friends, and self that might occur during a bioterrorism event. Discuss these fears and concerns with a classmate or your instructor.

    _____

    _____

    _____

    _____

    _____

Vital Signs

Answer Key: Textbook page references are provided as a guide for answering these questions. A complete Answer Key is provided in your Additional Learning Resources on Evolve.

WORD SCRAMBLE

Directions: Unscramble the words that are related to taking and interpreting vital signs and then match the term to the correct definition or characteristic listed below.

Scrambled Term	Unscrambled Term	Definition or Characteristic
1. cardiaydarb *(265)*		
2. dysaenp *(271)*		
3. pertherhymia *(258)*		
4. pneabrady *(270)*		
5. eeafbril *(257)*		
6. achypneat *(270)*		
7. yyhhdrstmia *(265)*		
8. pohymiather *(258)*		
9. diacartachy *(265)*		
10. sionpertenhy *(273)*		

Definition or characteristic of terms related to taking and interpreting vital signs

a. Irregularity in the normal rhythm of the heart
b. Normal finding for well-conditioned athlete
c. No elevation in temperature
d. Expected respiratory pattern while exercising
e. Laboring with difficulty to get enough oxygen
f. Slow respiratory rate, below 10 per minute
g. Above-normal body temperature
h. Expected heart rate if very frightened or angry
i. The silent killer
j. Occurs more frequently in cold weather

FIGURE LABELING

11. Directions: Label the figure below with the names and sites for assessment of peripheral pulses. *(266)*

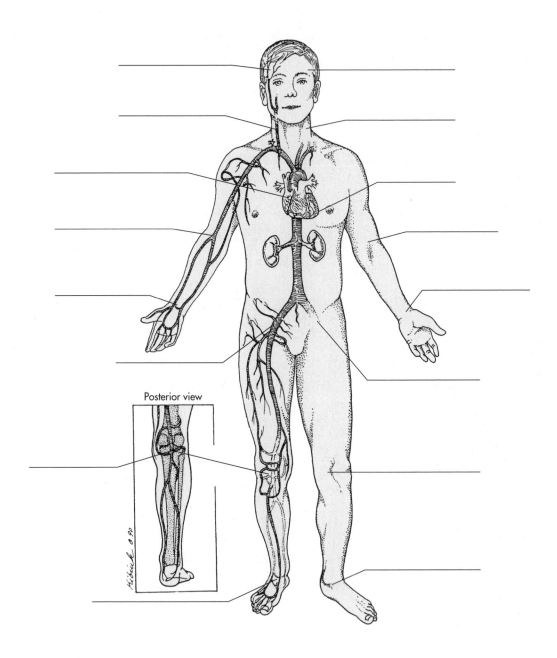

Posterior view

FILL-IN-THE-BLANK SENTENCES

Directions: Complete each sentence by filling in the blank with the correct word or phrase.

12. Normal body cells are at risk for damage when the temperature exceeds _____. *(258)*

13. The normal body temperature can range from _____. *(257)*

14. When obtaining a rectal temperature from an adult, the nurse inserts the electronic thermometer probe into the rectum approximately _____. *(261)*

15. The patient's pulse is difficult to assess and disappears with slight pressure. The pulse strength is described as _____. *(266)*

16. Respiratory rate is controlled by the _____. *(270)*

17. Occasional sighing is normal and allows for all _____ to be aerated. *(270)*

18. Blood pressure reflects _____ output, the quality of the _____, the blood volume, and blood viscosity. *(273)*

FIGURE LABELING

19. Directions: Identify on the aneroid gauge where the Korotkoff's sounds were heard for a blood pressure of 136/78 mm Hg. *(275)*

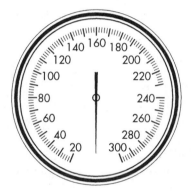

TABLE ACTIVITY

20. Directions: Complete the table below with the expected vital signs for different age groups. *(256)*

Age Group	Heart Rate (per Minute)	Respiratory Rate (per Minute)	Blood Pressure (mm Hg)
Neonate			Systolic:
Infant			Systolic:
Toddler			Systolic:
School-age (6-10 years)			Systolic: Diastolic:
Adolescent (10-18 years)			Systolic: Diastolic:
Adult			Systolic: Diastolic:
Older adult			Systolic: Diastolic:

MULTIPLE CHOICE

Directions: Select the best answer(s) for each of the following questions.

21. An experienced UAP reports that the patient is alert and asking for breakfast. Vital signs have been completed and recorded as follows: axillary temperature of 100.6° F, pulse of 80/min, respirations 16/min and blood pressure 120/70. What is the nurse's first action? *(263)*
    1. Instruct the UAP to obtain a breakfast tray for the patient.
    2. Ask the UAP to repeat the temperature using the oral or tympanic method.
    3. Direct the UAP to repeat all of the vital signs and observe technique.
    4. Ask the UAP to explain the choice of axillary method to measure the temperature.

22. A new nurse has taken a job on a medical-surgical unit. According to the shift report, the four assigned patients are stable and should have a predictable clinical stay. How often does the nurse plan to take the vital signs? *(283)*
    1. Every hour until stability is validated
    2. Every 2 hours and before medication
    3. Every 4 hours, unless status changes
    4. At the beginning and end of the shift

23. The nursing student takes a blood pressure on a patient who has been in a coma for several months. The student reports to the nurse that the blood pressure seems too low. What would the nurse do first? *(282)*
    1. Direct the student to retake the blood pressure on the opposite extremity.
    2. Go with the student and assess the patient for other signs/symptoms.
    3. Instruct the student to check the chart to see what is baseline for the patient.
    4. Remind the student that a prolonged coma will cause changes in vital signs.

24. A patient who is brought to the emergency department was discovered lying in an alley. He is cold and wet and demonstrates slurred speech. His temperature is 94° F. How does his condition affect his pulse rate? *(265)*
    1. Tachycardia is likely due to the stress of cold exposure.
    2. Since he is conscious, there should be no effects on pulse.
    3. A decreased heart rate reflects lowered metabolism.
    4. Palpating pulses will be impossible because of vasoconstriction.

25. The UAP takes vital signs at 3:00 AM and reports to the nurse that the patient's temperature is 97.6° F (36.4° C). The nurse sees that the patient's temperature at 6:00 PM was 99.6° F (37.5° C) and at 11:00 PM was 98.2° F (36.8° C). What should the nurse do? *(258)*
    1. Thank the UAP and explain that lower temperatures occur between 1 AM and 4 AM
    2. Repeat the temperature, but use a different method than what the UAP used
    3. Tell the UAP to document the temperature and not to worry about it
    4. Ask the UAP to get the patient a warm blanket and increase the room temperature

26. Two nurses simultaneously assess to determine if a patient has a pulse deficit. One nurse counts the apical pulse at 105 beats/min. The other nurse takes the radial pulse and counts 96 beats/min. What is the pulse deficit? _____ *(266, 267)*

27. When assessing the apical pulse, the nurse counts the pulse rate for: *(270)*
    1. 20 seconds and multiplies by 3.
    2. 60 seconds and does not multiply.
    3. 30 seconds and multiplies by 2.
    4. 15 seconds and multiplies by 4.

28. The nurse is supervising a first-year nursing student who is checking the patient's peripheral pulses. The nurse would intervene if the student performed which action? *(266)*
    1. Palpated all of the pulses, including carotids and femorals bilaterally
    2. Positioned the patient in the prone position to assess the popliteal artery
    3. Palpated the point of maximal impulse and assessed the apical pulse for 60 seconds
    4. Palpated the radial pulse with the pads of the index and third fingers

29. The nurse is aware that a patient's respiratory rate may be increased by: (271)
    1. opioids.
    2. acute pain.
    3. hypothermia.
    4. brainstem injury.

30. The nurse counts respirations immediately following measurement of the radial pulse while the fingers are still in place over the artery. What is the best rationale for this technique? (272)
    1. Rapport has been established so the patient is likely to be less anxious.
    2. Therapeutic touch of the nurse's fingers on the patient's wrist is soothing.
    3. Patients can voluntarily alter respiratory rate if they know they are being monitored.
    4. Counting respirations immediately after pulse check is an efficient time-saver.

31. A nursing student is preparing to take the blood pressure on a patient who has excessive adipose tissue on the upper arm. If the student uses a normal-sized cuff, what is likely to occur? (277)
    1. The blood pressure will be falsely elevated.
    2. The patient will be uncomfortable during the procedure.
    3. The systolic pressure will be artificially lower.
    4. The blood pressure is likely to be very close to baseline.

32. The nurse receives the end-of-shift report from the off-going nurse. Based on the vital sign information for the assigned adult patients, which patient should the nurse check on first? (270)
    1. BP 120/80, P 68, R 16
    2. BP 110/74, P 72, R 14
    3. BP 130/90, P 80, R 18
    4. BP 120/90, P 62, R 9

33. The nurse sees in the patient's documentation that the patient has a radial pulse of 4+. What assessment would the nurse plan to make for this patient? (266)
    1. Doppler assessment of pulses for hands and feet
    2. Observe for pallor or cyanosis in the hands
    3. Assess blood pressure for hypertension
    4. Assess apical and radial pulse for a pulse deficit

34. The patient's pulse oximetry reading appears to be lower than expected. The patient is breathing easily, the lungs are clear, the oxygen is delivered as ordered and the patient reports, "feeling fine." What would the nurse do first? (257)
    1. Check the position of the pulse oximeter.
    2. Feel the patient's fingers for coolness or warmth.
    3. Apply the pulse oximeter to own finger to test function.
    4. Ask the patient if he has any circulation problems.

35. The nurse needs to take the temperature of a baby who was brought to the clinic for his 6 month well-baby visit. Which method of measuring the temperature is the best choice for this patient? (263)
    1. Oral
    2. Axillary
    3. Rectal
    4. Temporal arterial

36. The nurse received a new stethoscope as a graduation present. What will he/she do to care for and appropriately use the stethoscope? (265)
    1. Drape the stethoscope around the neck to have it readily available.
    2. Clean the tubing with alcohol swabs after every patient contact.
    3. Remove the earpieces regularly and clean off cerumen, dust, and oils.
    4. Frequently rub the tubing between the palms to keep it soft.

37. The nurse is caring for a patient who is several days postoperative for major abdominal surgery. The UAP reports that the pulse is 120/min. The nurse rechecks the pulse and gets 122/min. The nurse will assess for: (Select all that apply.) (265)
    1. pain.
    2. infection.
    3. anxiety.
    4. hemorrhage.
    5. substance abuse.
    6. hypothermia.

38. The patient has a sudden deterioration in condition with confusion; diaphoresis; pallor; and cold, clammy skin. Which peripheral pulse site is the best to quickly determine the pulse rate? *(266)*
    1. Radial
    2. Femoral
    3. Carotid
    4. Brachial

39. The nurse hears in report that the patient has bilateral dorsalis pedis pulses 3+. How does the nurse use this information in planning care? *(266)*
    1. Allots time to check circulation and sensation on both feet every 2 hours
    2. Plans to follow up and ensure that the health care provider is aware of the finding
    3. Instructs the UAP to do full range of motion to hands and wrists every 3 hours
    4. Plans to do routine change-of-shift assessment and observe as needed

40. The UAP tells the nurse that the patient has a respiratory rate of 32/min and "is having trouble breathing." What additional sign(s) and symptom(s) is the nurse most likely to observe? (Select all that apply.) *(271)*
    1. Pursed-lip breathing
    2. Flared nostrils
    3. Epistaxis
    4. Costal retractions
    5. Fatigue
    6. Shortness of breath

41. The nurse checks the patient's blood pressure and obtains a reading of 160/90 mm Hg. What is the pulse pressure? _____ *(273)*

42. The nurse hears in report that the patient has an auscultatory gap. The nurse plans to adapt the technique for measuring which vital sign? *(276)*
    1. Temperature
    2. Pulse
    3. Respiratory rate
    4. Blood pressure

MATH AND CONVERSION

43. Convert the following temperature readings. *(257)*
    a. 37° C   =   _____ ° F
    b. 101.2° F   =   _____ ° C
    c. 39.2° C   =   _____ ° F
    d. 97.8° F   =   _____ ° C

44. Convert weight in pounds to the equivalent in kilograms. *(281)*
    a. A patient who weighs 44 lbs weighs _____ kg.
    b. A patient who weighs 210 lbs weighs _____ kg.

45. Convert weight in kilograms to the equivalent in pounds. *(281)*
    a. A patient who weighs 6 kilograms weighs _____ lbs.
    b. A patient who weighs 16 kilograms weighs _____ lbs.

46. Convert height in feet and inches to the equivalent in centimeters. *(559, Chapter 21)*
    a. A patient who is 5 feet 9 inches tall is _____ centimeters.
    b. A patient who is 2 feet 3 inches tall is _____ centimeters.

47. Fluid balance may be assessed by weighing the patient. If the patient weighs 2 kg less today than yesterday, how much fluid was lost? _____ mL *(281)*

CRITICAL THINKING ACTIVITIES

48. A 58-year-old female patient was admitted with pneumonia 2 days ago. The nurse recognizes that the patient must be monitored for signs of worsening infection. The patient's temperature taken at 7:00 AM is 101.2° F.

a. Discuss factors that may be affecting the body temperature of this patient. *(257, 258)* _____

_____

_____

b. What systemic signs and symptoms are associated with an elevated temperature? *(258)* _____

_____

_____

c. What should the nurse do if the patient's temperature is above normal? *(258)* _____

_____

_____

49. The nurse is caring for a patient who was admitted for a chronic respiratory problem. Upon entering the room, the nurse observes that the patient is struggling to move from a supine position to a sitting position and breathing is rapid and labored. The nurse notes tension in neck and shoulder muscles with each inspiration. The patient is anxious and repeatedly apologizes for "being a bother" while trying to explain why he came to the hospital and how his disease is affecting his life and his family.

a. For this patient, what factors may be contributing to the increased respiratory rate? *(271)* _____

_____

_____

_____

b. What should the nurse do if the patient's respirations are rapid and labored? *(271)* _____

_____

_____

_____

c. Write a response that the nurse could use to help this patient deal with the immediate respiratory problem. *(271)*

_____

_____

_____

50. Discuss how the nurse uses clinical judgment to determine the frequency, method, and interpretation of vital signs. *(254, 255)*

_____

_____

_____

_____

_____

_____

_____

_____

_____

Physical Assessment

Answer Key: Textbook page references are provided as a guide for answering these questions. A complete Answer Key is provided in your Additional Learning Resources on Evolve.

TABLE ACTIVITY

1. Directions: Complete the table by supplying the correct terms that you would use to document the physical assessment findings described on the right. Aim for correct spelling! *(289)*

Term	Description
	Lack of appetite resulting in the inability to eat
	Difficulty passing stools or infrequent passage of hard stools
	Bluish discoloration of the skin and mucous membranes
	Profuse sweating
	Frequent passage of loose, liquid stools
	Shortness of breath or difficulty breathing
	Extravasation of blood into the subcutaneous tissues
	Abnormal accumulation of fluid in interstitial spaces
	Redness or inflammation of the skin or mucous membranes
	Pertaining to something that has a foul, putrid, or offensive odor
	The protective response of the tissues of the body to irritation or injury
	Yellow tinge to the skin
	State or quality of being indifferent, apathetic, or sluggish
	Sensation often leading to the urge to vomit
	Must sit upright or stand in order to breathe comfortably
	Unnatural paleness or absence of color in the skin
	Itching and an uncomfortable sensation leading to an urge to scratch
	Creamy, viscous, pale yellow, or yellow-green exudate; liquefied necrosis of tissues
	Unhealthy yellow color; usually said of a complexion or skin
	Yellow color of the sclera
	Heart contractions at a rate greater than 100 beats per minute
	Abnormally rapid rate of breathing
	Expel the contents of the stomach out of the mouth

FILL-IN-THE-BLANK SENTENCES

Directions: Complete each sentence by filling in the blank with the correct word or phrase.

2. Congenital diseases appear at _____. *(287)*

3. Deficiency diseases are a result of _____. *(287)*

4. The most frequently used skill in the physical nursing assessment is _____. *(293)*

5. The first step in initiating the nurse-patient relationship is to _____. *(293)*

6. More than _____ of all health problems are the result of behavior and lifestyle. *(298)*

MULTIPLE CHOICE

Directions: Select the best answer(s) for each of the following questions.

7. The patient is diagnosed with sickle cell anemia. Based on the nurse's knowledge of the origin of disease, which intervention is most likely to be recommended for the patient? *(287)*
    1. Review of allergens in the home environment
    2. Referral for genetic counseling
    3. Dietary evaluation to identify deficiencies
    4. Prescription for broad-spectrum antibiotics

8. The nurse recognizes that an example of a metabolic disease is: *(287)*
    1. ulcerative colitis.
    2. diabetes mellitus.
    3. cystic fibrosis.
    4. heart failure.

9. The risk factor that can lead to the development of coronary artery disease is: *(288)*
    1. protein deficiency.
    2. asbestos exposure.
    3. trauma to the chest cavity.
    4. high cholesterol level.

10. To decrease the risk for lung disease, which lifestyle modification is the most important to recommend to patients? *(288)*
    1. Seek cancer screening
    2. Exercise regularly
    3. Stop smoking
    4. Limit dietary fats

11. While obtaining the vital signs of an adult, the nurse observes that the patient is diaphoretic and flushed. Which change in vital signs would the nurse expect to accompany this observation? *(288, 289)*
    1. Respiratory rate of 10/min
    2. Pulse of 65/min
    3. Blood pressure of 100/60
    4. Temperature of 101° F (38.3° C)

12. The nurse hears in report that the patient has had occasional episodes of cyanosis and dyspnea. Which physical assessment does the nurse plan to frequently perform during the shift? *(297)*
    1. Check for abdominal pain
    2. Assess respiratory effort
    3. Monitor urinary output
    4. Assess for headache

13. While assessing the patient, the nurse observes that the patient experiences orthopnea. What instruction will the nurse give the UAP about assisting the patient? *(289)*
    1. The patient is too weak to walk to the bathroom.
    2. Dizziness will occur if the patient stands up too quickly.
    3. Keep the head of the bed elevated at all times.
    4. The dominant hand is not functioning properly.

14. The patient's oral temperature is 101.2° F. The patient tells the nurse that he doesn't feel well, but has no known health conditions. What question would the nurse ask first to try to localize the source of infection? *(289)*
    1. What other symptoms are you having?
    2. Do you have any known allergies?
    3. Have you ever felt like this before?
    4. When did you first notice the fever?

15. The nurse hears in report that a patient who has cancer is experiencing anorexia. Which assessment does the nurse plan to conduct during the shift? *(208)*
    1. Assess need for supplemental oxygen
    2. Evaluate ability to independently ambulate
    3. Review efficacy of PRN pain medication
    4. Assess need for supplemental nutrition

16. The nurse is interviewing an older patient and notices that the patient is slumping and irritable and frequently sighs. Which question would the nurse ask to validate the most likely interpretation of the patient's behavior? *(299)*
    1. "Are you short of breath?"
    2. "Are you feeling tired?"
    3. "Would you like some water?"
    4. "Are you having pain?"

17. A patient tells the nurse that she is afraid of the doctor. How could this affect the objective data? *(291)*
    1. Description of pain will be exaggerated.
    2. Patient is likely to experience nausea.
    3. Blood pressure could be higher than expected.
    4. Pupils will be constricted and nonreactive.

18. The health care provider tells the nurse that the patient has pruritus. Which objective finding is the nurse most likely to observe? *(290)*
    1. Scratch marks on skin
    2. Abdominal distention
    3. Abnormal breath sounds
    4. Low-grade temperature

19. The nurse uses the OPQRSTUV method for obtaining the most information about the patient's pain. Which question addresses the P in the OPQRSTUV? *(295)*
    1. On a scale of 1 to 10, what number is the pain?
    2. What causes the pain to increase or decrease?
    3. When did you first notice the pain?
    4. Is the pain spreading out to other areas?

20. The nurse reads in the patient's chart that the patient has crackles in the posterior lower lobes. What does the nurse expect to hear during auscultation if the patient's condition is unchanged? *(304)*
    1. Short, discrete, bubbling sounds on inspiration
    2. High-pitched, musical sounds on inspiration
    3. Grating sounds on expiration
    4. Coarse gurgling on expiration

21. Which evaluation statement indicates that the antibiotic therapy has successfully resolved the patient's leg infection? *(289)*
    1. Patient reports that pain is decreased compared to previously.
    2. Patient is observed independently ambulating in hallway.
    3. Wound site shows no signs of erythema; white cell count is normal.
    4. Wound site shows edema, redness, and white cell count is elevated.

22. Which method would be the best to assess an elderly patient's ability to accomplish activities of daily living (ADLs)? *(296)*
    1. Accompany the patient during ambulation to the bathroom.
    2. Ask the patient what he normally eats during the day.
    3. Take a full set of vital signs and include pain assessment.
    4. Observe the patient's level of consciousness and orientation.

23. The nurse is assessing an older patient. Which explanation should the nurse use? *(299)*
    1. "I am going to auscultate the posterior lung fields."
    2. "I will be checking your motor function."
    3. "I would like to check your perineal area."
    4. "I am going to listen to your heartbeat."

24. The nurse is most likely to use the Glasgow Coma Scale (GCS) for which patient? *(302)*
    1. Recently had a myocardial infarction
    2. Sustained a serious head injury
    3. Shows some signs of septic shock
    4. Has risk for respiratory failure

25. The nurse observes jugular venous distention on a patient who is sitting in the interview chair. What other signs/symptoms would the nurse check to validate suspicion of right-sided heart failure? *(303)*
    1. Low heart rate
    2. Decreased urinary output
    3. Dependent edema in legs
    4. Jaundice of sclera

26. A new nurse documents PERRLA in the patient's chart. When the preceptor nurse asks her to describe the findings, the new nurse is unable to explain. What should the preceptor nurse do first? *(304)*
    1. Show the new nurse how to perform the assessment.
    2. Ask the new nurse how she knew to document PERRLA.
    3. Instruct the new nurse to seek out the nurse educator.
    4. Report the new nurse for falsifying the documentation.

27. The nurse is assessing the patency of the nostrils. What is the best method to use? *(304)*
    1. Use a penlight and observe for blockage or excess mucus.
    2. Press against one nostril and ask the patient to breathe.
    3. Give the patient a tissue and instruct to blow the nose.
    4. Ask the patient to breathe quietly and listen for air movement.

28. What is the UAP's role in assessing the respiratory system? *(304)*
    1. Observe and report changes in rate and depth.
    2. Determine a position that accommodates orthopnea.
    3. Auscultate the lung sounds every 4 hours or as needed.
    4. Monitor and interpret the pulse oximeter readings.

29. What would be considered a normal finding when assessing the patient's spine? *(305)*
    1. A gentle inward curvature of the lumbosacral curve
    2. A large posterior curvature of the thoracic spine
    3. An increased curvature of the lumbar spine
    4. A right or left lateral spinal curvature

30. The nurse is unable to palpate the popliteal pulse. What assessment would the nurse perform before informing the health care provider? Check the: *(306, 308)*
    1. femoral pulse.
    2. dorsalis pedis pulse.
    3. brachial pulse.
    4. apical pulse.

CRITICAL THINKING ACTIVITIES

31. A 40-year-old man comes to the clinic. He desires a general physical check-up and reports, "not feeling quite 100%." This is the patient's first visit to the clinic, so there are no medical records available for comparison. Provide examples of questions that the nurse could ask to obtain information during a review of systems. *(297)*

    a. Respiratory: _____

        _____

    b. Endocrine: _____

        _____

    c. Gastrointestinal: _____

        _____

    d. Cardiac: _____

        _____

    e. Neurologic: _____

        _____

    f. Genitourinary: _____

        _____

32. A 30-year-old woman comes to the emergency department. Her chief complaint is pain in the lower abdomen. She appears very uncomfortable and is walking in a slightly bent-over position. Her hands are supporting her lower abdomen as she moves toward the examination room.

    a. Use the OPQRSTUV method to elicit information about the chief complaint. *(295)* _____

        _____

        _____

        _____

        _____

        _____

        _____

    b. Describe how the nurse performs the physical assessment of the abdomen. *(308, 309)* _____

        _____

        _____

        _____

        _____

33. How does the nurse use the concept of "chief complaint" to generate subjective and objective data when the patient's chief complaint is "I have a really bad headache"? *(295)*

_____

_____

_____

_____

_____

34. The nurse is conducting an interview with a patient who was just admitted to the medical-surgical unit. The nurse stands at the bedside and initially smiles at the patient, but as the nurse is asking the questions, she frequently glances out the window and shifts restlessly back and forth. She diligently fills out the admission form while reading the questions from the form. When the patient tries to explain a point, she cuts him off and moves on to the next question. She checks the equipment that is necessary for the patient's care while the patient is trying to explain his symptoms. Discuss this nurse-patient interaction from the patient's point of view. *(293-296)*

_____

_____

_____

_____

_____

_____

_____

_____

_____

_____

_____

_____

Admission, Transfer, and Discharge

chapter **13**

Answer Key: Textbook page references are provided as a guide for answering these questions. A complete Answer Key is provided in your Additional Learning Resources on Evolve.

IDENTIFYING PATIENTS' REACTIONS TO HOSPITALIZATION

1. Directions: Identify and record the patient's reaction to hospitalization in the blanks provided; then on the figure below (use a, b, c, or d), indicate where each patient would be according to Maslow's Hierarchy. The first item is completed for you as an example.

    a. Patient appears anxious as he enters his hospital room for the first time. He nervously begins to ask the nurse a series of questions about what will happen to him. Reaction: Fear of the unknown

    b. A preschooler who is admitted to the hospital is happily engaged in playing with the toys that the nurse has provided, but when her parents prepare to leave, she begins to cry and clings to them. Reaction: _____ *(313)*

    c. An elderly woman who has just moved into an assisted-living facility seems to need a lot of social interaction. She becomes very talkative when the nurse tries to leave the room. Reaction: _____ *(314)*

    d. An adolescent is admitted to the hospital, but refuses to take off his clothes and put on a hospital gown. Reaction: _____ *(314)*

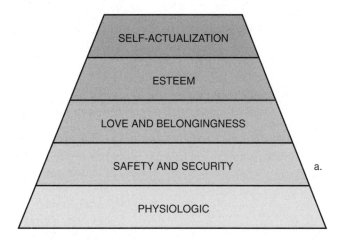

FILL-IN-THE-BLANK SENTENCES

Directions: Complete each sentence by filling in the blank with the correct word or phrase.

2. _____ addresses the patient's right to refuse or accept medical treatment as well as information regarding advance directives. *(315)*

3. The _____, _____, and _____ require that all hospitals and other health care facilities present a Patient's Bill of Rights to the patient or the patient's legal guardian at the time of admission. *(315)*

4. An interagency transfer requires documentation from the _____ and the health care provider as well as a(n) _____ from the patient indicating that he or she understands the risks and benefits associated with the transfer. *(322)*

5. The Joint Commission (TJC) requires each hospitalized patient to have an admission assessment prepared by a registered nurse within _____ hour(s) of admission. *(318)*

MULTIPLE CHOICE

Directions: Select the best answer(s) for each of the following questions.

6. A rational patient wishes to leave the hospital against medical advice (AMA), despite the nurse's best attempt at therapeutic communication. What is the nurse's first responsibility? *(328)*
   1. Notify the health care provider.
   2. Document the incident.
   3. Detain the patient.
   4. Obtain an AMA form.

7. The patient has an old head injury and demonstrates intermittent periods of belligerence and confusion interspersed with appropriate behavior. He is currently angry and wants to leave AMA. The nurse is unable to reach the health care provider. What should the nurse do first? *(327)*
   1. Explain the AMA form and consequences to the patient.
   2. Notify the RN, because the patient now has acute needs.
   3. Contact the family and ask them to take responsibility.
   4. Call the risk manager and ask for permission to detain.

8. During the admission of a patient to a health care facility, the responsibilities of the admission department representative include: (Select all that apply.) *(314, 315)*
   1. obtaining identifying information.
   2. giving information on Health Insurance Portability and Accountability Act.
   3. placing the correct ID band on the patient's wrist.
   4. obtaining a list of current medications.
   5. obtaining emergency contact information.
   6. gathering insurance information.

9. Which newly admitted patient is mostly likely to need and benefit from an individualized explanation of the bathroom facilities? *(316)*
   1. A 75-year-old woman with advanced Alzheimer's disease
   2. A 20-month-old child who has just started toilet training
   3. A 65-year-old man who is from a rural farming region of China
   4. A 50-year-old woman who has stress incontinence

10. The nurse is placing an ID band on a patient who was admitted through the emergency department. What is the best thing to say as the band is applied? *(314)*
   1. "This is your assigned hospital identification number."
   2. "The primary purpose of the band is to maintain safety."
   3. "All the patients have to wear these; it's standard procedure."
   4. "We don't want to lose you while you are in the hospital."

11. The patient is newly admitted and seems anxious, but also appears very tentative about asking questions. Which statement by the nurse best demonstrates empathy? *(314)*
    1. "Call me if you need anything; I'll be happy to help you."
    2. "There's nothing to worry about; we'll take good care of you."
    3. "I know you must have a lot of questions; I know I would."
    4. "You seem a little uncertain; do you have some questions?"

12. The nurse is trying to explain the bed controls and the call button and other items related to hospitalization, but the elderly patient keeps telling the nurse to "wait for my son to get here." What should the nurse do first? *(314)*
    1. Go find the son or other available family members.
    2. Leave written information at the bedside.
    3. Give brief information using very simple language.
    4. Offer comfort measures and ensure patient safety.

13. Which task(s) related to admitting a new patient can be delegated to the UAP? (Select all that apply.) *(315, 316)*
    1. Obtain personal care items, such as water pitcher or packaged cleansing cloths.
    2. Position the bed for transfer from stretcher or wheelchair.
    3. Hang signs above the bed related to care, such as NPO status.
    4. Ask the patient if he/she needs special equipment, such as walker.
    5. Store belongings, such as jewelry, watch, or wallet, in bedside table.
    6. Assist patient to arrange desired items, such as eyeglasses, within reach.

14. The patient tells the nurse that he would like to be transferred to hospital X, because his cardiologist doesn't come to hospital Y. What should the nurse do? *(322)*
    1. Obtain an against medical advice form and have the patient sign it.
    2. Call hospital X and advise that the patient desires transfer.
    3. Advise the patient that the cardiologists in hospital Y are good.
    4. Advise the patient that a transfer requires an order from the health care provider.

15. A patient with Alzheimer's disease is being transferred from a long-term care facility to an acute care hospital for possible sepsis and change in mental status. Which question is the most important to ask the nurse who is giving the report? *(322)*
    1. "Has the family been advised about the reason for the transfer?"
    2. "What is the patient's baseline mental status and behavior?"
    3. "When is the patient scheduled to be transferred?"
    4. "Will the patient be accompanied by a nurse or family member?"

16. Which patient is likely to have the most complex discharge plan? *(323-325)*
    1. A 73-year-old man with chronic disease who has no family in the area
    2. A 23-year-old mother who just delivered her first healthy baby
    3. A 17-year-old adolescent who broke his leg during a ski trip
    4. A 35-year-old woman who had an emergency appendectomy

17. The nurse is giving instructions to a family caregiver of an older patient who will need help after discharge from the hospital. The nurse senses tension, resentment, and unwillingness from the caregiver. What should the nurse do first? *(326)*
    1. Continue to give the instructions and ask for feedback from the caregiver.
    2. Notify the health care provider for an order for home health.
    3. Get a social services consult to resolve family tensions and problems.
    4. Assess the caregiver's attitude toward the patient and the circumstances.

CRITICAL THINKING ACTIVITIES

18. The patient is admitted through the emergency department for an exacerbation of a chronic respiratory disorder. When the patient arrives to the room, he appears very tired. He has oxygen per nasal cannula and demonstrates labored breathing. He is able to speak, but his sentences are short and he takes a breath after every few words. How would the nurse modify the nursing actions related to the admission in order to meet the needs of this particular patient? *(316-318)*

   a. Checking and verifying of ID band: _____

   _____

   b. Assessing immediate needs: _____

   _____

   c. Explaining hospital routines, such as visiting hours, mealtime, and morning wake-up: _____

   _____

   d. Orienting the patient to the room: _____

   _____

   _____

19. A 45-year-old woman was admitted to the hospital for chronic infection of a stasis ulcer on her leg. She will be discharged after completing antibiotic therapy and consultation with the wound care specialist.

   a. Identify examples of health care disciplines other than nursing that are involved in referrals, and explain their role in the discharge process. *(323-326)*

   _____

   _____

   b. Provide the rationale for each of the following nursing actions in the discharge of a patient. *(337)*

   i. Makes certain there is a written discharge order: _____

   _____

   ii. Arranges for patient and family to visit the business office and check to see that a release has been given:

   _____

   iii. Notifies the family or person who will be transporting the patient home: _____

   _____

   iv. Gathers equipment, supplies, and prescriptions that the patient is to take home: _____

   _____

   v. Assists the patient with dressing and packing items to go home: _____

   _____

Surgical Wound Care

Answer Key: Textbook page references are provided as a guide for answering these questions. A complete Answer Key is provided in your Additional Learning Resources on Evolve.

MATCHING

Directions: Match the terms related to wound complications on the left with the descriptions on the right. Indicate your answers in the spaces provided. (347)

Term		**Description**
_____ 1.	abscess	a. Infection of the skin characterized by heat, pain, erythema, and edema
_____ 2.	adhesion	b. Protrusion of an internal organ through a wound or surgical incision
_____ 3.	cellulitis	c. Band of scar tissue that binds together two anatomical surfaces that are normally separated
_____ 4.	dehiscence	d. Passage or escape into the tissues; usually of blood, serum, or lymph
_____ 5.	evisceration	e. Cavity containing pus and surrounded by inflamed tissue
_____ 6.	extravasation	f. Collection of extravasated blood trapped in the tissues, resulting from incomplete hemostasis after surgery or injury
_____ 7.	hematoma	g. Separation of a surgical incision or rupture of a wound closure

SHORT ANSWER

Directions: Using your own words, answer each question in the space provided.

8. What are the time frames and characteristics of the three phases of wound healing? *(334)*

    a. Inflammatory phase: _____

    b. Reconstruction phase: _____

    c. Maturation phase: _____

9. Describe the three types of wound healing. *(334, 335)*

    a. Primary:_____

    b. Secondary:_____

    c. Tertiary: _____

10. What is the purpose of each of the following types of dressings? *(338, 341)*

    a. Gauze: _____

    b. Semiocclusive: _____

    c. Occlusive: _____

    d. Dry dressing: _____

    e. Transparent: _____

11. Identify the type of bandage turns that should be used for the following body areas. *(358-360)*

    a. Finger or wrist: _____

    b. Calf or thigh: _____

    c. Joints: _____

    d. Scalp: _____

MULTIPLE CHOICE

Directions: Select the best answer(s) for each of the following questions.

12. Which lunch tray is best for providing protein, vitamins A and C, and zinc, the nutrients required for wound healing? *(335)*
    1. A peanut butter sandwich with a glass of milk
    2. A bowl of bean soup with crackers and iced tea
    3. Broiled seafood with spinach salad and tomato juice
    4. Stir-fried mixed vegetables with rice and hot tea

13. The patient has no contraindications for fluid intake; over a 24-hour period, he drank 16 ounces of decaffeinated coffee, 10 ounces of juice, 6 ounces of milk, and a half a liter of soda. What instructions does the nurse give the patient about fluid intake to promote wound healing? *(335)*
    1. Instructs the patient to continue drinking the same amount as he drank today
    2. Tells the patient that tomorrow he should try to drink twice as much as today
    3. Advises the patient that drinking excessive fluid is likely to decrease appetite for food
    4. Suggests that he drinks 2-3 additional 8-oz servings of his favorite fluid every day

14. The nurse is caring for a patient who has a large abdominal incision. The patient tells the nurse that she is afraid to sit up or even move because of the pain and the strain on the incision site. What instructions should the nurse give to the patient? *(335)*
    1. "Rest in bed until the incision site is less tender and healing has progressed."
    2. "Roll to one side, use your elbow as a lever, and push to a sitting position."
    3. "Hold a pillow next to your abdomen and roll forward into a sitting position."
    4. "Call for assistance whenever needed and someone will help you sit up."

15. A patient has just returned from surgery. What is/are the initial assessment(s) that the nurse would make related to the surgical site? (Select all that apply.) *(335, 351)*
    1. Inspect the protective dressing that was placed by the surgical team.
    2. Look at the area around the dressing and record observations.
    3. Check under the patient to make sure that exudate is not pooling.
    4. Carefully remove the dressing and inspect the suture line for intactness.
    5. Expect and note amount of serous drainage that is coming from the wound.

16. A patient had surgery 4 days ago and now re-ports an increase in pain and has a temperature of 101.6° (38.7° C). The incision site looks red compared to yesterday and a small amount of purulent drainage is seeping around the suture line. Which laboratory result will the nurse check before contacting the health care pro-vider? *(337)*
    1. Hemoglobin and hematocrit
    2. White blood cell count
    3. Platelet count
    4. Blood glucose level

17. Which patient is most likely to benefit from the application of a triangular binder? *(358)*
    1. Has a chronic pressure ulcer on the sacral area
    2. Has a possible fracture in the forearm
    3. Has venous stasis ulcer on left ankle
    4. Has a surgical wound on the lateral chest area

18. The nurse is preparing to remove the patient's staples, but after assessment, the nurse decides that the staples should not be removed. The decision was based on which finding? *(348)*
    1. The wound edges were partially separated.
    2. Dried serous drainage was noted around the staples.
    3. The patient was anxious about staple re-moval.
    4. Early keloid formation was observed.

19. The nurse is preparing to change the patient's dry sterile dressing. Upon attempting the re-moval of the old dressing, it adheres to the site. What should the nurse do? *(339)*
    1. Notify the health care provider.
    2. Leave the dressing in place.
    3. Pull the dressing off quickly.
    4. Moisten the dressing with saline.

20. The patient returned to the unit 3 hours ago after having surgery on the abdomen, and the dressing is now saturated with red, watery drainage. What should the nurse do first? *(347)*
    1. Notify the charge nurse and the health care provider.
    2. Take the patient's vital signs and assess for pain.
    3. Securely reinforce the dressing with layers of gauze.
    4. Remove the dressing and observe the wound site.

21. After a total abdominal hysterectomy, a post-operative patient develops a wound eviscera-tion. What should the nurse do first? *(347)*
    1. Check patency of the intravenous (IV) site for delivery of fluids.
    2. Place the patient in a supine position to re-duce strain on the wound.
    3. Prepare the patient for surgery and contact the health care provider.
    4. Cover the wound with a sterile dressing moistened with saline.

22. A postoperative patient who was happy and cheerful earlier now demonstrates restless-ness and anxiety. He reports feeling "a little lightheaded." He is mildly diaphoretic and his pulse feels thready. What assessments does the nurse perform to identify a suspected compli-cation? *(347)*
    1. Checks the pulse rate, blood pressure, and assesses for pain
    2. Assesses for localized warmth or redness with tenderness
    3. Observes the incision site for wound edge approximation
    4. Takes the temperature and checks for pu-rulent drainage

23. The patient has a T-tube in place following an abdominal cholecystectomy. What is the ex-pected output of bile in the first 24 hours? *(353)*
    1. 30 mL per hour
    2. 250-500 mL
    3. 10-50 mL
    4. 1-2 L

24. The nurse is observing a new staff member perform a sterile dry dressing change. The nurse would intervene if the staff member per-formed which action? *(340)*
    1. Loosens tape and gently pulls towards the incision
    2. Uses sterile gloves to remove the old dress-ing
    3. Cleanses wound by starting at incision moving outward
    4. Allows antiseptic cleansing solution to air-dry

25. A nurse is supervising a nursing student who is doing a wet-to-dry dressing change. What does the nurse do when the student applies a dry dressing over the wet gauze? *(342, 343)*
    1. Directs the student to moisten all of the layers.
    2. Hands the student an occlusive dressing.
    3. Tells the patient that the student is doing a great job.
    4. Suggests removal of all layers and starting over.

26. The nurse is assessing the amount of drainage that the patient has from a surgical wound and finds that 650 mL has drained from 9:00 AM until now, 11:40 PM. What should the nurse do first? *(351)*
    1. Record the amount and appearance of the drainage and continue to observe.
    2. Take the patient's vital signs, assess for other symptoms, and inform the provider.
    3. Make sure that the patient's linens are clean and dry and empty the drainage receptacle.
    4. Apply a pressure dressing and place the patient in a supine position.

27. The patient needs an abdominal binder. What is the most important consideration for the nurse when implementing this application? *(359)*
    1. Respiratory function must not be restricted.
    2. Vomiting and nausea are a contraindication.
    3. Binders cannot be used for patients who are obese.
    4. Older patients have difficulty tolerating the binder.

28. The nurse is applying a dressing over the insertion site of a peripheral intravenous catheter. Which dressing is the best choice? *(343)*
    1. Sterile tape with dry gauze
    2. Moistened gauze with paper tape
    3. Transparent dressing
    4. Sterile pad with chevron taping

CRITICAL THINKING ACTIVITIES

29. The nurse is caring for a 72-year-old patient who is being treated for a chronic ulcer on the right lower leg. The patient lives alone. He is diabetic and reports poor vision. The nurse notes that the patient has trouble with fine motor control. He reports that he does his own meal preparation, although he admits that he doesn't make the effort to prepare fresh produce. He is 15 pounds underweight and he has "cut down on his smoking."

    a. Identify factors that may impair wound healing for this patient. *(332, 335)* _____

    _____

    _____

    b. Discuss how the nurse applies knowledge about older adults to help this patient achieve wound healing. *(363)*

    _____

    _____

    _____

    _____

    _____

    _____

30. The student nurse is preparing to implement wound irrigation for a patient. The nursing instructor asks the student to answer the following questions before starting the procedure. *(343, 345, 346)*

a. What is the purpose of wound irrigation?_____

_____

b. What equipment is needed for irrigation at the patient's bedside? _____

_____

c. How is the syringe positioned for the irrigation?_____

_____

d. What is the direction of cleansing ? _____

_____

e. What findings should be immediately reported to the health care provider? _____

_____

Specimen Collection and Diagnostic Testing

Answer Key: Textbook page references are provided as a guide for answering these questions. A complete Answer Key is provided in your Additional Learning Resources on Evolve.

MATCHING

Directions: Match the suffix on the left to the correct definition on the right and give an example for each. (385)

Suffix	**Definition**
_____ 1. -oscopy	a. Procedure involving puncture of a body cavity
_____ 2. -ogram	Example _____
_____ 3. ography	b. Procedure in which an image is produced
_____ 4. -centesis	Example _____
	c. Actual image or results of a test
	Example _____
	d. Procedure in which body structures are visualized
	Example _____

FILL-IN-THE-BLANK SENTENCES

Directions: Complete each sentence by filling in the blank with the correct word or phrase.

5. Nursing responsibilities while assisting during a procedure/testing include anticipating the needs of the _____ performing the procedure, having the proper _____ ready, and assisting the _____ through the procedure. *(368)*

6. Written consent is not always necessary for individual tests if it is considered noninvasive; _____ is adequate in many cases. *(368)*

7. Wear gloves when collecting specimens of blood or other body fluids to prevent spread of _____, _____, and other pathogens. *(385)*

8. Even when using safety needles, the nurse should never _____ needles and always carefully discards them in _____. *(400)*

9. If the patient's language skills inhibit communication, assistance from _____, word signs, or charts may be necessary. *(384)*

10. It is essential to maintain _____ when disclosing results from testing and diagnostic procedures. *(368)*

11. It is the responsibility of the nurse to notify the prescribing health care provider when laboratory and diagnostic studies are _____ and intervention is necessary. *(383)*

12. A patient who is modest and self-conscious about the body will need _____ before some procedures and tests. *(384)*

FIGURE LABELING

13. Directions: Label the veins of the arms and hands on the figure. *(401)*

Basilic vein
Cephalic vein
Median cubital vein
Radial vein
Median vein of forearm
Superficial dorsal vein
Dorsal venous arch

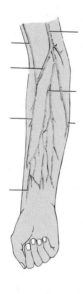
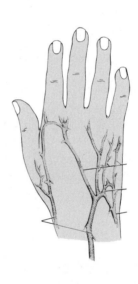

SHORT ANSWER

Directions: Using your own words, answer each question in the space provided.

14. Identify the general guidelines for specimen collection. *(385)* _____

_____

_____

15. Describe the general nursing responsibilities related to caring for a patient who needs diagnostic testing. *(367, 368)*

_____

_____

16. What general assessments need to be performed prior to diagnostic testing? *(368, 404)* _____

_____

_____

_____

17. Identify considerations for the older adult in regard to specimen collection and diagnostic testing. *(384)*

_____

_____

_____

18. Proper labeling of specimens requires: *(390)* _____

_____

_____

FIGURE LABELING

19. Directions: Label the placement of the chest (precordial) leads on the figure. *(409, 410)*

V_1—Fourth intercostal space (ICS) at right sternal border
V_2—Fourth ICS at left sternal border
V_3—Midway between V_2 and V_4
V_4—Fifth ICS at midclavicular line
V_5—Left anterior axillary line at level of V_4 horizontally
V_6—Left midaxillary line at level of V_4 horizontally

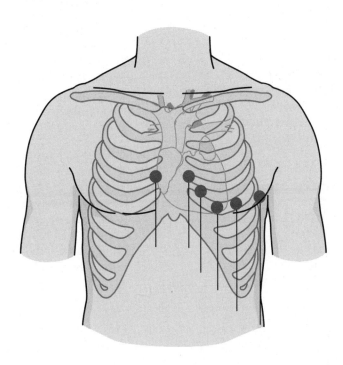

DELEGATION

20. Directions: Determine which specimen collections are usually possible to delegate to unlicensed assistive personnel (UAP), and indicate yes or no in the space provided. *(404)*

_____ a. Urine by midstream collection

_____ b. Gastric secretion from nasogastric tube

_____ c. Blood sample by venipuncture

_____ d. Sputum specimen by suctioning

_____ e. Blood sample for glucose

_____ f. Wound cultures

_____ g. Stool for ova and parasites

_____ h. Throat culture

_____ i. Sputum specimen by expectoration

_____ j. Nasal culture

_____ k. Emesis

_____ l. Nasopharyngeal culture

_____ m. Cerebrospinal fluid

_____ n. Stool for hemoccult

_____ o. Stool from colostomy

MULTIPLE CHOICE

Directions: Select the best answer(s) for each of the following questions.

21. The nurse is using a commercially prepared tube for the collection of an aerobic wound specimen for culture. After collecting the specimen with the swab, the nurse should: *(395)*
    1. place the swab into the collection tube, close it tightly, and keep the specimen warm.
    2. take the swab and mix it with the special color-changing reagent in the collection tube.
    3. place the swab into the collection tube and add the liquid culture medium.
    4. crush the ampule at the end of the tube and put the tip of the swab into the solution.

22. Following a lumbar puncture, what does the nurse do to prevent a postpuncture spinal headache? *(378)*
    1. Reduces the patient's fluid intake
    2. Places the patient in a high Fowler's position
    3. Informs the health care provider if headache develops
    4. Instructs the patient to lie in the supine position

23. The patient is to have a thoracentesis performed. The nurse assists the patient to which position for this test? *(382)*
    1. Dorsal recumbent
    2. Supine with the arms held above the head
    3. Sitting up and leaning over a table
    4. Side-lying with the knees drawn up

24. The health care provider has ordered a magnetic resonance imaging (MRI) study for the patient. The patient is concerned about the procedure and requests information from the nurse. The nurse informs the patient to expect: *(379)*
    1. to have nothing to eat or drink for 4 hours before the test.
    2. to hear humming and loud thumping sounds.
    3. minor discomfort to the area being tested.
    4. frequent position changes.

25. The nurse is teaching the patient how to collect a specimen for blood glucose monitoring. The patient demonstrates correct technique when: *(389)*
    1. allowing the blood specimen to drop onto the test strip.
    2. using the center of the finger for the puncture.
    3. holding the finger upright after puncture.
    4. vigorously squeezing the fingertip after puncture.

26. Instruction to the patient for collection of a midstream urine sample includes: *(386)*
    1. use of a clean specimen cup.
    2. collection of 200 mL of urine for testing.
    3. voiding some urine first and then collecting the sample.
    4. washing the perineal area with Betadine before collection.

27. When obtaining a urine specimen from a patient with an existing indwelling catheter, the nurse should: *(387)*
    1. apply sterile gloves for the procedure.
    2. clamp the drainage tubing for 30 minutes before specimen collection begins.
    3. disconnect the catheter from the drainage tubing and collect the urine in a specimen cup.
    4. insert a small-gauge needle directly into the catheter tubing to draw up the urine.

28. The patient will be catheterized for residual urine. What is the correct technique for this procedure? *(385)*
    1. Catheterize the patient when the bladder is full.
    2. Obtain an order for an indwelling catheter.
    3. Catheterize the patient within 10 minutes of voiding.
    4. Use clean technique to obtain the sample.

29. A patient requires venipuncture to obtain a blood sample for diagnostic testing. Which laboratory result is the greatest concern related to the venipuncture? *(398)*
    1. High blood glucose level
    2. Low platelet count
    3. Elevated blood urea nitrogen
    4. Low sodium level

30. A tourniquet is used when performing a venipuncture. The nurse is aware that the tourniquet should be: *(401)*
    1. tied into a knot.
    2. left in place for no more than 1-2 minutes.
    3. placed 6-8 inches above the selected site.
    4. tight enough to occlude the distal pulse.

31. The patient is suspected of having a urinary tract infection (UTI). The health care provider has ordered a urine specimen for culture and sensitivity testing. The patient asks, "Can't I just get a prescription for antibiotics?" What is the best response? *(390)*
    1. "This is just a routine test for any patient suspected of having a UTI."
    2. "Your health care provider feels this test is necessary in determining your diagnosis."
    3. "I can contact your health care provider if you would like to ask for a prescription."
    4. "Different bacteria can cause a UTI and the test results will indicate the best antibiotic."

32. When performing a Hemoccult slide test to determine the presence of occult blood in a stool specimen, the nurse would be correct in performing which action? *(392)*
    1. Use two separate areas of the stool when obtaining the specimen.
    2. Obtain the specimen from the toilet bowl.
    3. Perform the test control before obtaining the specimen.
    4. Take the specimen immediately to the laboratory to prevent hemolysis.

33. An older patient had a bronchoscopy several hours ago and now seems restless and confused compared to baseline behavior. Which assessment is the most important? *(384)*
    1. Orientation to person, place, and time
    2. Pulse oximeter reading and respiratory rate
    3. Use of antianxiety medications during procedure
    4. Time of last food and fluid ingestion

34. An elderly female patient is supposed to have diagnostic testing that requires NPO status for 12 hours prior to the test and a bowel preparation. The test has been cancelled two days in a row; once for a large amount of retained stool and once because of equipment problems. Which intervention is the priority? *(384)*
    1. Explain the cancellations to the patient using terms that she can easily understand.
    2. Call the diagnostic technician to ensure that the test gets done.
    3. Assess the patient for dehydration and fluid and electrolyte imbalances.
    4. Call the health care provider and ask if the test can be postponed for a few days.

35. The nurse has just informed the patient that he should collect a sputum specimen in the morning. Which additional instruction will the nurse give? *(384)*
    1. "Brush your teeth and use mouthwash just prior to collecting the specimen."
    2. "Drink extra water the day before collection to decrease the thickness of mucus."
    3. "Inhale and cough deeply and then spit the clear saliva into the sterile cup."
    4. "Do not eat any red meat or drink any caffeinated beverages."

36. The nurse has just received laboratory results for an unfamiliar test, so he is unsure if the results are within normal limits. What should the nurse do first? *(383, 385)*
    1. Call the health care provider and read the results exactly as they are shown.
    2. Ask the patient if he is having any unusual symptoms or complaints.
    3. Call the laboratory technician and ask for an explanation of the results.
    4. Check the facility's laboratory manual for information about the test.

37. The nurse has orders for voided midstream urine specimens for several patients. Which patient is most likely to require an order for a straight catheterized specimen rather than a voided midstream specimen? *(385)*
    1. A 25-year-old female who finished her menstrual period yesterday
    2. A 55-year-old female diabetic patient who is very overweight
    3. A 63-year-old male who has difficulty with urination due to prostate problems
    4. An 18-year-old male who is comatose because of a drug overdose

38. The nurse sees that several patients require stool specimens for diagnostic testing. Which patient's stool specimen must be taken immediately to the laboratory after it has been obtained? *(387, 389)*
    1. Patient traveled to a foreign country and reports abdominal cramping with diarrhea.
    2. Patient saw very dark black stool several days ago, but now stool seems normal.
    3. Patient (small child) is suspected of swallowing a plastic marble 3 days ago.
    4. Patient saw stool floating in toilet and there was an oily film in the water.

39. The nurse is suctioning the patient to obtain a sputum specimen. During the 10 seconds of suctioning, the cardiac monitor shows bradycardia and the patient becomes very diaphoretic. What is the best explanation for this occurrence? *(390)*
    1. Patient demonstrated anxiety due to the procedure.
    2. Nurse caused hypoxia by suctioning for a prolonged time.
    3. Cardiac changes are unrelated to the procedure.
    4. Catheter caused direct stimulation of vagal nerve fibers.

40. The nurse notes purulent drainage from a wound and decides to obtain an order for a wound culture. Prior to contacting the health care provider, what other data will the nurse obtain? (Select all that apply.) *(395)*
    1. Check oral temperature.
    2. Look at trends of white blood cell count.
    3. Ask about subjective symptoms, such as chills or fatigue.
    4. Assess for pain at the wound site.
    5. Review the previous documentation about the wound.

41. A patient is newly admitted for pneumonia with possible early sepsis. The nurse is reviewing the admission orders. Which order should be done first? *(400)*
    1. Intravenous antibiotics
    2. Blood cultures from two sites
    3. Chest x-ray
    4. Blood chemistries

42. The nurse is supervising a nursing student who will perform venipuncture to obtain a blood sample for blood chemistries. The nurse will intervene if the student performs which action? *(389, 399)*
    1. Applies a warm compress to the arm on the side of a mastectomy
    2. Obtains a Vacutainer and different colors of collection tubes
    3. Applies a tourniquet 3 inches above elbow and palpates the antecubital space
    4. Releases the tourniquet after 2 minutes of trying to locate a vein

43. A patient had a diagnostic study with a contrast medium 4 hours ago. Now he has swelling and itching around the eyes, a rapid pulse, and mild dyspnea. What should the nurse do first? *(368)*
    1. Administer a PRN dose of diphenhydramine (Benadryl) and call the health care provider.
    2. Call the Rapid Response Team and bring resuscitation equipment to the bedside.
    3. Contact the health care team member who administered the contrast medium.
    4. Apply a cool compress to reduce the swelling and instruct the patient to rest.

44. The UAP made two attempts to test a patient's blood glucose but was unable to get enough blood to adequately cover the test strip. What factor(s) will nurse assess that could interfere with getting an adequate drop of blood? (Select all that apply.) *(384)*
    1. Environmental temperature of the room
    2. Technique used to obtain the sample
    3. Position of the patient's arm
    4. Improper calibration of the glucometer
    5. Problems with peripheral circulation
    6. Condition of the skin on hands and fingers

45. The nurse is supervising a new nurse who must collect gastric secretions from a nasogastric (NG) tube. The nurse would intervene if the new employee: *(393)*
    1. uses an alcohol swab to scrub the NG tube prior to inserting a sterile needle.
    2. assists the patient to a high Fowler's position and places a towel underneath the NG tube.
    3. disconnects the NG tube from the suction or the gravity drainage.
    4. verifies NG tube placement to ensure aspiration of gastric contents.

46. The nurse is suctioning a patient to obtain a sputum specimen. Which occurrence is expected? *(394, 395)*
    1. As the suction catheter is inserted into the tracheostomy, there is resistance.
    2. As the suction catheter is inserted into the trachea, the patient begins to cough.
    3. As suction is applied, oxygen saturation drops below normal for several minutes.
    4. As the suction catheter is withdrawn, the patient begins to exhale very deeply.

47. The nurse has tried several times to obtain a throat culture on a patient, but the patient has gagged, moved, and contaminated the tip of the swab during each attempt. What should the nurse do first? *(398)*
    1. Have the patient look in the mirror, give him the swab, and coach him through the procedure.
    2. Inform the health care provider that several unsuccessful attempts have been made.
    3. Instruct the patient to open mouth and say a very long "ahhhhh" and avoid using a tongue blade.
    4. Obtain an order for a mild local anesthetic that will temporarily suppress the gag reflex.

48. The nurse needs to perform venipuncture to obtain a blood sample for blood chemistries. What factor(s) influence(s) the nurse's choice of sterile needles? (Select all that apply.) *(405)*
    1. Age of patient
    2. Condition of veins
    3. Nurse's familiarity with product
    4. Syringe method versus vacuum tube method
    5. Type of blood chemistry test ordered
    6. Color of the collection tube

49. Nurse A is aware that Nurse B, who is not very skilled at venipuncture, is sticking her patients more than the recommended two times as stated by hospital policy. What should Nurse A do first? *(406)*
    1. Report Nurse B to the nurse manager for violating hospital policy.
    2. Watch Nurse B and offer to perform venipunctures after two attempts.
    3. Assess Nurse B's understanding and skill in performing venipuncture.
    4. Ask the charge nurse to assess Nurse B's understanding of hospital policy.

50. As the nurse is performing an electrocardiogram (ECG), the patient reports very mild left anterior chest pain. What should the nurse do first? *(374)*
    1. Stop the procedure and obtain the crash cart and other emergency equipment.
    2. Continue the procedure, but ask the patient to report worsening.
    3. Stop the procedure and obtain an order for pain medication.
    4. Continue procedure and make notation of pain on the request slip or ECG strip.

CRITICAL THINKING ACTIVITIES

51. The nurse is caring for a patient who is scheduled to have a thoracentesis.

    a. What assessments should be performed prior to the procedure? *(382, 410)* _____

    _____

    _____

    _____

    _____

    b. Why would it be particularly important to assess this patient's lung sounds and presence of cough before the procedure? *(382)*

    _____

    _____

    _____

    _____

    c. Describe the nursing responsibilities related to the care of the patient before and during the thoracentesis. *(382)*

    _____

    _____

    _____

    _____

    d. Describe the assessments and care that the nurse should perform after the thoracentesis procedure. *(382, 403)*

    _____

    _____

    _____

52. The nurse is caring for a 68-year-old woman who is scheduled to have a urinalysis, blood chemistries, and an intravenous pyelogram. The patient is alert and cooperative. She is thin and reports a poor appetite and fluid intake. The patient demonstrates some trouble with fine motor movements of the hands and some mobility issues related to arthritis, but she is able to independently perform most ADLs. Identify considerations for this older patient with regards to the urinalysis, blood chemistries, and intravenous pyelogram (IVP). *(384)*

_____

_____

_____

_____

_____

_____

_____

_____

Care of Patients Experiencing Urgent Alterations in Health

chapter

16

Answer Key: Textbook page references are provided as a guide for answering these questions. A complete Answer Key is provided in your Additional Learning Resources on Evolve.

WORD SCRAMBLE

Directions: Unscramble the terms that describe different types of shock and then match each term with the correct associated characteristics. (423)

	Scrambled Word	Unscrambled Term that Describes a Type of Shock	Associated Characteristics
1.	lpnaaayctich		
2.	gdarioenicc		
3.	oypvolhmice		
4.	erognenciu		
5.	shgcenioycp		
6.	espict		

Associated characteristics of shock

a. Prolonged vomiting, diarrhea, or loss of fluid due to surgery, trauma, or burns
b. Sudden release of histamine, which creates capillary hyperpermeability
c. Nervous system's reaction to an emotional stimulus
d. Toxins from the microorganisms cause loss of fluid through the blood vessel walls
e. Heart unable to maintain sufficient blood pressure to all body parts
f. Common causes are spinal anesthesia, quadriplegia, or medications that cause vasodilation

SHORT ANSWER

Directions: Using your own words, answer each question in the space provided.

7. The nurse is at a community event and several people are injured when a large tent structure is blown over by the wind. What information is essential to convey when calling the emergency medical system for help? *(415)*

_____

_____

_____

8. The health care provider directs the nurse to call Poison Control to get advice for a patient who comes to the health care facility for "feeling sick after spraying the yard with insect spray." What information is necessary to report when calling Poison Control? *(430)*

_____

_____

_____

9. Identify areas that should be included in a teaching plan for safety and response to an emergency in the home environment. *(441)*

_____

_____

_____

10. Directions: Refer to the figure and use the Rule of Nines to determine how much of the body surface is burned for an adult patient who has severe burns to the anterior and posterior thorax and both upper extremities. _____% *(438)*

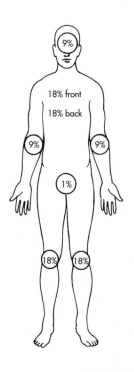

MULTIPLE CHOICE

Directions: Select the best answer(s) for each of the following questions.

11. The nurse arrives outside of the public library and finds a person lying on the ground. What is the first action to take? *(416)*
    1. Check if the victim is unconscious.
    2. Check the carotid or brachial pulse.
    3. Move the victim to a flat, hard surface.
    4. Direct someone to call 911.

12. A patient is unresponsive to normal verbal stimuli and not breathing. When assessing for a carotid pulse, the nurse should assess: *(417)*
    1. the location of the pulse for a maximum of five seconds.
    2. strength of the pulse for 5 seconds and then compare it to the opposite side.
    3. the pulse rate for 10 seconds and then check for 3-second capillary refill.
    4. the rate, rhythm, and strength of the pulse for a maximum of 10 seconds.

13. Which sign or symptom of a foreign body airway obstruction is of greatest concern? *(421)*
    1. Says, "I think I swallowed something."
    2. Is coughing so hard that he can't speak.
    3. Makes a wheezing sound between coughs.
    4. Demonstrates a high-pitched inspiratory noise.

14. The person gives the universal sign for choking. The nurse prepares to perform abdominal thrusts by placing the fist: *(421)*
    1. over the ribs.
    2. over the sternum.
    3. slightly above the navel.
    4. over the xiphoid process.

15. For an unconscious adult victim with a foreign body airway obstruction, the nurse should: *(422)*
    1. apply a series of three quick chest thrusts.
    2. repeat 10 abdominal thrusts and attempt to ventilate.
    3. perform finger sweeps between abdominal thrusts.
    4. visually look for object each time before providing a breath.

16. Which intervention(s) is/are appropriate for a victim who is in hypovolemic shock at the scene of an accident? (Select all that apply.) *(424)*
    1. Establish airway.
    2. Control bleeding.
    3. Keep the head elevated.
    4. Cover with a blanket or coat.
    5. Provide oral fluids, such as water.
    6. Administer over-the-counter analgesics.

17. During a camping trip, a person who is allergic to bee stings is stung by a bee. The nurse immediately scrapes the skin to remove the stinger. Which question should the nurse ask first? *(433)*
    1. "What happens when you get stung by a bee?"
    2. "Do you want to go to the hospital?"
    3. "Where is your epinephrine pen?"
    4. "Do you have any diphenhydramine (Benadryl)?"

18. The nurse finds a person lying at the bottom of a long staircase. The person is conscious, but appears dazed and confused. There are no obvious injuries or signs of bleeding. What should the nurse do first? *(415)*
    1. Assist the person to sit up and suggest that he rest on a step.
    2. Instruct the person to remain still and ask for permission to assist.
    3. Initiate spinal cord precautions and hold head and neck in alignment.
    4. Ask the person what happened and if he is having pain or distress.

19. Two nurses are shopping together in a mall and they witness a person collapse and become unresponsive. Based on assessment, they initiate two-rescuer CPR. Under which circumstance(s) can the two nurses discontinue the CPR? (Select all that apply.) *(417)*
    1. Relative of the unresponsive person tells them to stop.
    2. Mall personnel arrive with the automated external defibrillator (AED).
    3. Curious crowd pushes in and bystanders are loud and unruly.
    4. Trained medical personnel arrive and take over CPR.
    5. Person remains unconscious but spontaneous pulse and breathing occur.
    6. A layperson offers to take over the role of doing compressions.

20. The health care provider informs the wife that her husband has suffered brain death and is in an irreversible coma, even though his heart is still beating. Which comment indicates that the wife has understood what the provider said? *(417)*
    1. "His heart is still beating, so there is still has a chance he'll recover."
    2. "He is in a coma, but do you think that he can hear what I say?"
    3. "I must notify the family so that everyone can come and say goodbye."
    4. "How long do you think he will have to stay in the intensive care unit?"

21. Which assessment finding confirms cardiac arrest? *(417)*
    1. Absence of radial pulse
    2. Absence of carotid pulse
    3. Absence of spontaneous respirations
    4. Unresponsiveness to normal stimuli

22. The latest recommendation for CPR is to go "hard and fast" when performing chest compressions. What is the best rationale for maintaining the recommended 100 compressions/minute? *(418)*
    1. The rescuer will become fatigued if compressions exceed 100/minute.
    2. Lacerations of the liver or spleen are more likely to occur if speed is excessive.
    3. Releasing external chest compression allows time for blood to flow back into the heart.
    4. A smooth motion is required to prevent rocking and rolling that decrease the force.

23. The nurse is performing CPR on an infant. What is the most common event that could occur? *(420)*
    1. Fracture of the rib
    2. Gastric distention
    3. Aspiration of emesis
    4. Laceration of spleen

24. An infant is observed picking up something from the floor and putting it into his mouth before the mother can stop him. He demonstrates coughing, gagging, stridor, and respiratory distress. What should the nurse do first? *(422)*
    1. Instruct the mother to hold the child and look into the mouth with a flashlight.
    2. Place the infant in a supine position and deliver five chest thrusts.
    3. Place two fingers just above the navel and deliver five abdominal thrusts.
    4. Hold the infant with the head lower than trunk and deliver five back blows.

25. The nurse is assessing a trauma patient who was treated for shock in the emergency department. Oliguria is noted and immediately reported to the health care provider. Which complication is most related to this finding? *(423)*
    1. Right-sided heart failure
    2. Kidney failure
    3. Paralytic ileus
    4. Electrolyte imbalance

26. The nurse hears a scream; a patient has slipped in the bathroom. There is bright-red blood spurting from her forearm. What should the nurse do first? *(425)*
    1. Don sterile gloves and apply firm pressure using a sterile gauze pad.
    2. Use layers of sterile dressing material and wrap them snugly with an elastic bandage.
    3. Don clean gloves, and use a clean towel to apply direct pressure; elevate the arm.
    4. Locate the brachial artery and use the heel of the hand to compress the artery.

27. Under what circumstances would the nurse use a tourniquet? *(425, 426)*
    1. The nurse is acting in good faith and conforms to Good Samaritan principles.
    2. The health care provider gives a telephone order to apply a tourniquet.
    3. The victim tells the nurse to apply a tourniquet.
    4. Pressure and elevation have failed to control life-threatening bleeding.

28. An elderly patient comes to the clinic for epistaxis. It is readily controlled with steady pressure applied to the bridge of the nose. What additional assessment is most important for this patient? *(426)*
    1. Measuring the blood pressure
    2. Understanding of self-care measures
    3. First-aid attempts performed by patient
    4. Checking an oral temperature

29. Which patient has the greatest risk for internal bleeding? *(426)*
    1. A 20-month-old child who stumbled and struck his forehead on a coffee table
    2. A 70-year-old woman sustained a hip fracture and takes an anticoagulant
    3. A 25-year-old man who was punched and kicked in the stomach
    4. A 30-year-old woman who was admitted for postpartum hemorrhage

30. A young man who is injured is brought to the clinic by his friends. They are all very excited, but they are able to point out that he has a stick poking out of the anterior chest wall. Which symptom(s) indicate(s) that the patient has a pneumothorax? (Select all that apply.) *(429)*
    1. Pain worsens with inspiration and expiration efforts.
    2. Breathing is labored and difficult.
    3. A hissing sound is audible as air flows in and out of chest.
    4. Patient is unconscious and unresponsive to normal stimuli.
    5. Pulse is weak, rapid, and thready.
    6. Chest does not expand on side of injury during inspiration.

31. The home health nurse sees the patient lying on the floor. On entering the house, the nurse can smell a strong odor of gas and the house is extremely hot. What should the nurse do first? *(432)*
    1. Step out of the house and call 911.
    2. Call Poison Control and describe situation.
    3. Establish responsiveness and start cooling measures.
    4. Open the windows and move the patient out of the house.

32. The nurse comes home and finds that her teenage son and his friends have been challenging each other to chug large shots of whiskey. Which adolescent needs to be taken to the hospital for serious alcohol intoxication? *(433)*
    1. Face appears flushed and seems sleepy.
    2. Demonstrates slurred speech and continuously giggles.
    3. Is loudly singing and starting to remove clothes.
    4. Is incontinent of bowel and bladder and is hallucinating.

33. It's the Fourth of July and the nurse is working at a walk-in clinic. Several people who were viewing a parade come in and report abdominal cramps, headache, weakness, nausea, and diaphoresis. All are alert and oriented. Which intervention would the nurse use first? *(434)*
    1. Establish peripheral intravenous sites on everyone.
    2. Give everyone several cool compresses.
    3. Assist everyone to remove constrictive clothing.
    4. Move everyone into a cool environment.

34. A person sustains full-thickness burns to both forearms while lighting an outdoor grill. The nurse would intervene if a bystander attempts to perform which action? *(439)*
    1. Removes smoldering clothing
    2. Removes wedding ring
    3. Applies an antiseptic cream to the burns
    4. Elevates the forearms

CRITICAL THINKING ACTIVITIES

35. The nurse comes upon the scene of a motor vehicle accident. Several people are standing around a woman who is lying on the ground in a supine position. She is crying and trying to sit up. The right sleeve of her blouse is torn and blood is pooling on the asphalt underneath her arm.

   a. How does the Good Samaritan law affect the nurse in the situation? *(415)* _____

   _____

   _____

   b. What actions should the nurse take first in order to help this victim? *(415)* _____

   _____

   _____

   c. What assessments would lead the nurse to believe the victim is in shock? *(415)* _____

   _____

   _____

   d. What interventions are appropriate for a victim in shock at the scene of an accident? *(415, 416)*

   _____

   _____

36. The nurse is hiking with a group of friends on a cool, windy autumn day. They come across a man who is sitting in the middle of the trail. He is alert, but his speech is slurred. His clothes are wet and muddy and he is not wearing any shoes. Others in the group look around to see if they can find any additional clues about what happened to the man. The nurse starts to assess the man and notes that he is shivering and decides to assess him for additional signs of hypothermia.

   a. What factors in the scenario helped the nurse to identify that hypothermia might be occurring? *(435)* _____

   _____

   _____

   _____

   _____

   b. What are the signs and symptoms of hypothermia? *(435)* _____

   _____

   _____

   c. For the conscious victim with hypothermia, what interventions can be provided at the scene? *(436)*

   _____

   _____

   _____

37. Review Box 16-2 and think about the events that necessitate cardiopulmonary resuscitation. Select one (or two) of the events that you are most likely to encounter because of your work or family situation and mentally "rehearse" how you would respond. Based on your mental rehearsal of the event, identify information, equipment, skills, or safety precautions that you want to have available if the actual event happens. *(416)*

_____

_____

_____

_____

_____

_____

_____

_____

_____

Complementary and Alternative Therapies

Answer Key: Textbook page references are provided as a guide for answering these questions. A complete Answer Key is provided in your Additional Learning Resources on Evolve.

FILL-IN-THE-BLANK SENTENCES

Directions: Complete each sentence by filling in the blank with the correct word or phrase.

1. _____ are treatments used in addition to conventional health care regimens recommended by a person's health care provider. *(444)*

2. _____ often include the same interventions as complementary therapies, but frequently become the primary treatment modality that replaces conventional medicine. *(444)*

3. Holistic nursing addresses and treats the _____ of the patient. *(445)*

4. The strength of _____ is its effectiveness in treating certain physical ailments (e.g., bacterial infections, structural abnormalities, acute emergencies). *(445)*

5. _____ involves an interdisciplinary, multiple-professional treatment group that a patient consults as a cooperative entity. *(459)*

TRUE OR FALSE

Directions: Write T for true or F for false in the blanks provided.

_____ 6. A doctor of chiropractic medicine can prescribe medications that will provide relief for back pain and gently manipulate an area of disturbed structural integrity. *(450)*

_____ 7. Acupuncture and acupressure are therapies based on the belief that there is a form of energy or Qi that flows through the body along meridians. *(450)*

_____ 8. Reflexologists are qualified to diagnose certain medical conditions such as anxiety or depression. *(455)*

_____ 9. All systems of yoga recognize certain basic principles, including control of the body through correct posture and breathing, control of the emotions and the mind, and meditation and contemplation. *(457)*

_____ 10. A patient complains of right lower abdominal pain, nausea, and vomiting. The nurse, suspecting appendicitis, should recommend the benefits of relaxation and herbal therapy. *(459)*

MULTIPLE CHOICE

Directions: Select the best answer(s) for each of the following questions.

11. The nurse is collecting data for the health history of a new patient. What is the best rationale for directly asking the patient about the use of complementary and alternative medicine (CAM) therapies? *(445)*
    1. About 50% of patients use herbal supplements, but they rarely report usage.
    2. A complete health history is essential for every patient.
    3. CAM therapies must be listed to be eligible for insurance coverage.
    4. Nurses should be advocates for holistic care for patients.

12. The nurse is seeking evidence-based practice information related to CAM therapies for cancer patients. What would be the best source for this information? *(445)*
    1. Consult an updated comprehensive medical-surgical nursing textbook.
    2. Use the Internet to search for "cancer" and "CAM therapies."
    3. Access National Center for Complementary and Alternative Medicine website.
    4. Talk to the local chapter of the American Cancer Society.

13. What issue(s) of herbal products could potentially cause problems for consumers? (Select all that apply.) *(446)*
    1. Do not have the same rigorous study as pharmaceuticals
    2. Reduced level of accountability of their manufacturers
    3. Not required by law to demonstrate safety, efficacy, or quality of products
    4. Wide variations in potency, quality, and chemical content
    5. No standardized dosages have been established for most herbs
    6. More potent than pharmaceuticals because the whole plant is used

14. Which patient statement indicates a correct understanding of the patient teaching information about using herbal preparations? *(447)*
    1. "Herbal preparations are made from plants and are natural and safe."
    2. "These are over-the-counter products so they don't have dangerous side effects."
    3. "If I follow the package instructions on dosage, I'll be okay."
    4. "The herbs should be discontinued at least 2 weeks before any surgery."

15. The patient has a history of congestive heart failure and receives a prescription for digoxin. The nurse cautions the patient against the use of which herb? *(448, 449)*
    1. Evening primrose oil (*Oenothera biennis*)
    2. Goldenseal (*Hydrastis canadensis*)
    3. Ginkgo, maidenhair tree (*Ginkgo biloba*)
    4. Kava (*Kava-Kava*)

16. A 42-year-old female patient has a family history of osteoporosis and would like advice about the use of CAM for prevention of osteoporosis. Which therapy would the nurse provide information about? *(450)*
    1. Acupuncture
    2. Chiropractic therapy
    3. Reflexology
    4. T'ai chi

17. Which patient statement indicates understanding of a therapy that could help with smoking cessation? *(450, 451)*
    1. "I could consult an herbalist and smoke herbal leaf instead of tobacco."
    2. "Acupuncture stimulates acupoints and has been used to treat addictions."
    3. "Inhalation of lavender oil relieves stress and decreases craving for a cigarette."
    4. "Biofeedback would increase my awareness about my physiologic cravings."

18. Which patient would not be a candidate for therapeutic massage? *(453)*
    1. A pregnant woman who would like to have a foot massage
    2. A postsurgical patient who wants the legs massaged to relieve cramping
    3. An older patient who has an ache in the upper back after prolonged sitting
    4. A school-aged child who has been confined to bed for several days

19. The elderly patient disrobes to take a shower. The young nursing student who is assigned to assist with hygiene is shocked and repulsed by the appearance and condition of the patient's skin. What should the student do? *(453)*
    1. Quickly excuse herself and step out into the hall to recover composure.
    2. Smile and avoid looking at the patient directly, but continue to assist with care.
    3. Apologize to the patient and then seek out the instructor for advice.
    4. Make eye contact, smile, and assist the patient to maintain safety in the shower.

20. The nurse is working in a long-term care center and recognizes that elderly residents are at risk for "skin hunger." What would the nurse do to address this problem? *(453)*
    1. Ensure that herbal lotion enriched with vitamins and protein is applied after bathing.
    2. Identify residents who are comfortable with hugging and touching by staff members.
    3. Consult with a holistic nutritionist to design meals that supply nutrition for the skin.
    4. Apply herbal sunscreens to protect the skin and take residents into the sun.

21. Which patient should be cautioned that inhalation of essential oils could exacerbate symptoms? *(454)*
    1. Takes PRN medication for asthma
    2. Recently diagnosed with major depression
    3. Currently experiences excessive stress related to work
    4. Underwent chiropractic treatments for back pain

22. The patient has myasthenia gravis and tells the nurse that she has been using magnet therapy because her aunt recommended it would increase circulation. Which assessment is the most essential? *(455)*
    1. Blood pressure and pulse
    2. Memory and judgment
    3. Muscle strength and balance
    4. Oral temperature and infection signs

23. The nursing student has severe test anxiety. She is using guided imagery to help reduce anxiety just before the beginning of each test. What is the desired outcome of this type of therapy? *(455)*
    1. Controls response to stimuli by regulating expectations and perceptions
    2. Learns to deep-breathe and include all senses during times of stress
    3. Visualizes warmth entering the body on inspiration and tension leaving on expiration
    4. Creates an image of self successfully passing the exam

24. What is/are the advantage(s) of animal-assisted therapy? (Select all that apply.) *(457)*
    1. Research indicates that animals have a calming effect.
    2. Animals can stimulate mental activity through interaction.
    3. Most families have a pet that will be familiar to the patients.
    4. Everyone likes animals because they decrease loneliness.
    5. Patients who like animals are usually not allergic to them.
    6. Being around an animal can reduce blood pressure and anxiety.

25. The patient suffered a traumatic event as a child; however, the event is not something the patient ever thinks or talks about. Which therapy would be most likely to trigger a memory that would require psychological intervention? *(457, 458)*
    1. Biofeedback
    2. Reflexology
    3. Yoga
    4. Accupressure

CRITICAL THINKING ACTIVITIES

26. The nurse is caring for a patient who is from a different culture than the nurse. The patient requests some ginseng tea and there is a vial of tea tree oil on the bedside table.

   a. What should the nurse ask the patient about in regard to complementary and alternative therapies, and why is it important to ask? *(460)*

   _____

   _____

   b. Identify cultural considerations that arise in relation to complementary and alternative therapies. *(460)*

   _____

   _____

   c. What information should the nurse include in teaching this patient about complementary and/or alternative therapies in the treatment regimen? *(460)*

   _____

   _____

27. Consider the cognitive skills of focusing, passivity, and receptivity and discuss the use of relaxation therapy with the following patients. *(456)*

   a. A 77-year-old woman with advanced dementia is frequently restless. She will pace and demonstrate nonpurposeful movements. Her family has asked the nurse to help her to be calmer and relax.

   _____

   _____

   _____

   b. A 23-year-old college student is extremely anxious about doing well. At times, he has studied to the point of exhaustion. He reports taking "uppers" so that he can stay awake and study. Currently, it appears that he is under the influence of stimulants because he is talking very fast about a math problem that he is working on and he appears jittery and nervous.

   _____

   _____

   _____

   c. A 62-year-old retired military officer appears very tense, but he tells the nurse that he doesn't have any problems with anxiety, tension, or stress. Furthermore, he informs the nurse that if he did have any problems, he would control them on his own. His wife tries to tell the nurse that he does need some help to relax, but he cuts her off abruptly.

   _____

   _____

   _____

Pain Management, Comfort, Rest, and Sleep

Answer Key: Textbook page references are provided as a guide for answering these questions. A complete Answer Key is provided in your Additional Learning Resources on Evolve.

FILL-IN-THE-BLANK SENTENCES

Directions: Complete each sentence by filling in the blank with the correct word or phrase.

1. Pain is an unpleasant sensation caused by _____ stimulation of the sensory nerve endings. *(464)*

2. Patients with _____ pain often describe pain for which little or no tissue damage can be found. *(465)*

3. Acute pain is intense and of short duration, usually lasting less than _____ months. *(465)*

4. The combination of fatigue, sleep disturbance, and depression has the potential to markedly change a person's _____ of pain. *(465)*

5. Pain relief measures such as transcutaneous electric nerve stimulation (TENS), acupuncture, and placebos, are believed to cause the release of _____. *(466)*

TRUE OR FALSE

Directions: Write T for true or F for false in the blanks provided.

_____ 6. A predictable relationship exists between identifiable tissue injury and the sensation of pain. *(464)*

_____ 7. Approximately 10% of people who suffer moderate to severe pain will continue to suffer, primarily because nurses fail to assess pain. *(467)*

_____ 8. Morphine and other opioid analgesics are the most widely available and frequently used analgesic group. *(468)*

_____ 9. Bedrest does not necessarily mean a patient is resting. *(478)*

_____ 10. Older adults require less sleep than younger people, but they are more likely to take naps. *(478)*

MULTIPLE CHOICE

Directions: Select the best answer(s) for each of the following questions.

11. The patient had a surgical procedure this morning and is requesting pain medication. The nurse assesses the patient's vital signs and decides to withhold opioid medication based on the finding of: *(469)*
    1. pulse = 90/min.
    2. respirations = 10/min.
    3. blood pressure = 130/80 mm Hg.
    4. temperature = 99° F rectally.

12. The nurse is caring for a patient who has arthritis. Which medication does the nurse anticipate the health care provider will prescribe? *(469)*
    1. propoxyphene (Darvon)
    2. diphenhydramine (Benadryl)
    3. ibuprofen (Motrin)
    4. morphine (MS Contin)

13. The patient is receiving an epidural opioid. The nurse is alert for a complication of this treatment and observes the patient for: *(472)*
    1. diarrhea.
    2. hypertension.
    3. urinary retention.
    4. increased respiratory rate.

14. An older adult patient diagnosed with osteoarthritis suffers from chronic pain. Based on the patient's age and condition, which pain medication(s) will the health care provider most likely avoid? (Select all that apply.) *(469)*
    1. Meperidine
    2. Acetaminophen
    3. Morphine sulfate
    4. Nonsteroidal antiinflammatory drugs
    5. Combinations of opioid drugs

15. Which nursing intervention demonstrates the application of the gate control theory of pain? *(465)*
    1. Performs a back massage using warmed lotion
    2. Administers a placebo to release endorphins
    3. Obtains an order for opioid medication
    4. Advocates for patient-controlled analgesia pump

16. Which nursing action demonstrates that the nurse is complying with the Joint Commission (TJC) standards of pain management? *(466)*
    1. Documents that medication is given after the patient receives it.
    2. Incorporates knowledge of the patient's culture in pain management.
    3. Assesses the patient's pain and reassesses pain after interventions.
    4. Stays current with the latest information about pain therapies.

17. The nursing student reports to the nurse that a postoperative patient is asking for pain medication. What is the most important question that the nurse will ask the student to answer? *(467)*
    1. "Can you give the medication yourself?"
    2. "What did the patient tell you about his pain?"
    3. "Did you try any nonpharmacologic interventions?"
    4. "What do you know about the ordered medication?"

18. The patient agrees to try guided imagery as a noninvasive method of pain relief. Before they begin the therapy, which instruction is the nurse most likely to give? *(467)*
    1. "I'll use a combination of firm and light strokes during the therapy."
    2. "The skin will be stimulated with a mild electric current that reduces pain."
    3. "Tell me about a place and time where you felt relaxed and peaceful."
    4. "We have to use specialized equipment to identify your biologic responses."

19. What is the greatest advantage of using noninvasive pain management techniques as an adjunct to pain medication? *(467)*
    1. Inexpensive and easy to perform
    2. Based on the gate control theory
    3. Low risk and few side effects
    4. Gives patients some control over pain

20. The nurse is talking to a patient who wants to try transcutaneous electric nerve stimulation (TENS). The nurse would alert the health care provider if the patient reveals he has a: *(468)*
    1. cardiac pacemaker device.
    2. hearing aid.
    3. metallic hip joint.
    4. history of a broken back.

21. The health care provider orders 1000 mg acetaminophen every 4 hours as needed for pain. What should the nurse do? *(468)*
    1. Assess the patient every 4 hours and give the medication as needed.
    2. Give the medication as needed during the daytime hours only.
    3. Call the health care provider and ask for clarification of the order.
    4. Call the pharmacy and ask if the medication comes in 1000-mg tablets.

22. The nurse is caring for several patients who are receiving morphine. Which patient is most likely to have respiratory depression? *(469)*
    1. Patient with a history of chronic back pain who is receiving epidural morphine for an acute exacerbation
    2. Elderly patient who is postoperative for a fractured hip and is receiving patient-controlled analgesia
    3. Child who received an intramuscular injection prior to having fracture reduction of the forearm
    4. Elderly patient with end-stage uterine cancer who is receiving an oral form of morphine

23. What is the physiologic rationale for avoiding use of meperidine (Demerol) for patients with sickle cell disease? *(469)*
    1. There is a direct action that causes sickling of blood cells.
    2. Renal insufficiency will be present to some degree.
    3. Underlying respiratory distress results in respiratory depression.
    4. Patients with sickle cell disease are more prone to seizures.

24. The home health nurse sees an order for meperidine (Demerol) for a 63-year-old patient with cancer who requires long-term opioid treatment. What is the best rationale for the nurse to question this medication order? *(469)*
    1. Meperidine (Demerol) is an older drug that is now rarely prescribed for any condition.
    2. The patient cannot be continuously monitored for adverse effects in the home setting.
    3. The patient is not young nor healthy and is therefore more likely to suffer side effects.
    4. Repeated administration of meperidine (Demerol) increases the risk of accumulation.

25. The nurse hears in report that the patient with diabetes has reported a tingling, burning sensation in the lower extremities. Which drug is the nurse mostly likely to administer for this type of discomfort? *(470)*
    1. ketorolac tromethamine (Toradol)
    2. tramadol (Ultram)
    3. acetaminophen (Tylenol)
    4. duloxetine (Cymbalta)

26. The patient now reports that the prescribed opioid dose does not seem to provide the same relief for his acute pain that it did when he first started to take the medication 4 weeks ago. Based on the nurse's knowledge of pharmacology, the nurse recognizes that the patient has developed: *(469)*
    1. a physical tolerance.
    2. a psychological dependence.
    3. an addiction.
    4. chronic pain.

27. The nurse is talking to an older adult who reports feeling tired and not getting enough sleep. Which question related to the patient's medication is most relevant to designing interventions for the patient's problem? *(478)*
    1. "Which NSAID medication has the health care provider suggested?"
    2. "Has there been a recent increase in the dosage of your opioid medication?"
    3. "What time of the day do you usually take your diuretic medication?"
    4. "Are you taking your antiemetic medication before or after meals?"

28. The new nurse is looking at nursing jobs to consider after graduation. Which shift is most likely to cause the nurse to have sleep-wake cycle disruption? *(478)*
    1. Straight night shift
    2. Rotating day to night shift
    3. Weekends-only evening shift
    4. Monday to Friday day shift

29. The health care provider has ordered blood pressure, pulse, and respirations q2h x 12 hours. It is currently 8:00 PM and the nurse knows that the patient has been having a lot of problems sleeping in the hospital. What strategy should the nurse try first? *(481)*
    1. Clarify the necessity of the order with the health care provider.
    2. Explain to the patient that q2h vital signs will only be taken for 12 hours.
    3. Tell the UAP to be very quiet and quick while taking the vital signs q2h.
    4. Apply an automatic blood pressure cuff that can programmed for q2h.

30. The nurse enters the patient's room at 3:00 AM and finds that the patient is awake and sitting up in a chair. The patient tells the nurse that she is not able to sleep. The nurse should first: *(478)*
    1. obtain an order for a hypnotic.
    2. instruct the patient to return to bed.
    3. provide a glass of warm milk with honey.
    4. ask about methods that have helped her sleep.

CRITICAL THINKING ACTIVITIES

31. a. The patient has identified to the nurse that she is experiencing pain. What should the nurse do to fully assess the patient's pain? *(467)*

    _____

    _____

    b. What problem(s) can occur if the nurse does not respond to and treat the patient's pain? *(467)*

    _____

    _____

    c. Identify nursing interventions that may be implemented to reduce or eliminate the patient's pain. *(467)*

    _____

    _____

    _____

    _____

    _____

32. The patient is experiencing difficulty sleeping while in the hospital. She reports this is the first time she has been in the hospital and the sounds and smells seem very strange. In addition, she reports feeling mildly anxious because "so many people come in and out of the room at all hours of the day and night." She looks tired and seems mildly irritable.

    a. Identify and briefly describe the usual phases and stages of the sleep cycle and describe what is happening to patient when NREM and REM sleep are interrupted. *(478)*

       _____

       _____

    b. Write a patient outcome for the nursing diagnosis Disturbed sleep pattern related to unfamiliar hospital environment. *(482)*

       _____

       _____

    c. Identify nursing interventions that may be implemented to promote sleep. *(481)* _____

       _____

       _____

33. a. Think about the patients that you have cared for thus far during your clinical experiences and identify at least five possible causes for the discomfort that your patients were experiencing. *(463)*

       _____

       _____

       _____

       _____

       _____

    b. Describe what you did to relieve your patients' discomfort. *(472)* _____

       _____

       _____

       _____

       _____

       _____

Nutritional Concepts and Related Therapies

Answer Key: Textbook page references are provided as a guide for answering these questions. A complete Answer Key is provided in your Additional Learning Resources on Evolve.

MATCHING

Directions: Match the term on the left to the correct definition on the right.

Terms

_____ 1. amino acids *(492)*

_____ 2. anabolism *(493)*

_____ 3. basal metabolic rate (BMR) *(510)*

_____ 4. catabolism *(493)*

_____ 5. enteral nutrition *(522)*

_____ 6. essential nutrients *(487)*

_____ 7. glycogen *(489)*

_____ 8. nutrient-dense foods *(502)*

_____ 9. total parenteral nutrition (TPN) *(525)*

_____ 10. dietary reference intakes *(486)*

Definition

a. Energy required to maintain necessary, involuntary body functions, to digest nutrients, and for physical activity

b. Building blocks of protein

c. Nutrients that our bodies are not able to make in the amounts essential for good health

d. Building more tissue

e. Foods that contain large amounts of nutrients relative to kilocalories

f. Used when the body's blood sugar is low

g. Breaking down tissue

h. Set of nutrient-based values that serve for both assessing and planning diets

i. Administration of nutrients into the GI tract

j. Administration of a hypertonic solution into the superior vena cava by way of a catheter

SHORT ANSWER

Directions: Using your own words, answer each question in the space provided.

11. Identify the six classes of nutrients and their general function. *(487)*_____

_____

_____

12. What are the calories provided and the recommended percentage of intake for each of the following nutrients? *(487)*

    a.　Protein: _____

    b.　Carbohydrates: _____

    c.　Fats: _____

13. For each of the following vitamins, identify a food source, its function in the body, and signs and symptoms of a deficiency and toxicity (if applicable). *(495)*

    a.　Vitamin A: _____

    _____

    b.　Vitamin D: _____

    _____

    c.　Vitamin K: _____

    _____

14. For each of the following minerals, identify a food source, its function in the body, and signs and symptoms of a deficiency and toxicity (if applicable). *(498)*

    a.　Calcium: _____

    _____

    b.　Potassium: _____

    _____

    c.　Sodium: _____

    _____

TRUE OR FALSE

Directions: Write T for true or F for false in the blanks provided.

_____　15.　The sole purpose of fat in the body is for storage of excess nutrients. *(490)*

_____　16.　In the United States, high-sodium, high-protein, and low-potassium diets appear to contribute to osteoporosis by increasing the amount of calcium that is excreted in the urine. *(499)*

_____　17.　Increased fluid intake is a common dietary treatment for renal failure and urinary retention. *(520)*

_____　18.　For healthy Americans, a well-planned diet provides adequate nutrition without supplementation. *(532)*

_____　19.　Laxatives decrease absorption of calcium, potassium, and fat-soluble vitamins (especially vitamin D). *(509)*

_____　20.　Current American Heart Association recommendations for healthy individuals older than 2 years are to eliminate saturated fats and *trans*-fatty acids from the diet. *(519, 520)*

_____ 21. In the United States, nearly 60% of adults and over 30% of children and adolescents are obese. *(510)*

_____ 22. If unable to aspirate gastric contents from a nasogastric tube, the nurse first obtains an order to have the tube replaced. *(527)*

_____ 23. Complications such as aspiration pneumonia, pneumothorax, and peritonitis can be avoided by checking placement of a feeding tube prior to giving any medication or feeding. *(524)*

TABLE ACTIVITY

24. Directions: Complete the table below with the missing numerical value or the interpretation of the numerical value. The first block is done for you. *(492)*

Numerical Value	Interpretation of Numerical Value
LDL Cholesterol	
<100	Optimal
100-129	
	Borderline high
160-189	
	Very high
Total Cholesterol	
	Desirable
200-239	
≥240	
HDL Cholesterol	
<40 men; <50 women	

FIGURE LABELING

25. Directions: Label the figure below with the correct tube feeding sites. *(522)*

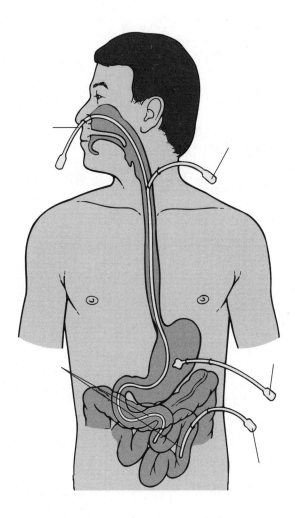

MULTIPLE CHOICE

Directions: Select the best answer(s) for each of the following questions.

26. The patient is going to be discharged with a prescription for an anticoagulant medication. Which question should the nurse ask? *(497)*
    1. "How many servings of leafy green vegetables would you normally consume during the week?"
    2. "Do you drink at least 8 glasses of fluid every day?"
    3. "What would you typically eat for breakfast every morning?"
    4. "Are you having any problems with constipation or adequate fiber intake?"

27. The patient reports noticing that his gums bleed very easily. If the bleeding is caused by a nutritional deficiency, which types of food will correct the problem? *(496)*
    1. Milk, egg yolks, and liver
    2. Broccoli, peppers, and tomatoes
    3. Cereals, legumes, and nuts
    4. Poultry, fish, and brown rice

28. Which patient is at risk for pernicious anemia and is most likely to be prescribed a vitamin B_{12} supplement? *(497)*
    1. Frequently tries different weight-loss plans
    2. Eats small amounts of a variety of foods
    3. Prefers meat and potatoes, with very few vegetables
    4. Adheres to a strict vegan diet

29. The nurse is working with a patient who requires an increase in complete proteins in the diet. The nurse will recommend the intake of: (Select all that apply.) *(520)*
    1. chicken.
    2. eggs.
    3. peanuts.
    4. beans.
    5. fish.

30. A patient reports routinely taking high doses of vitamin supplements. Which vitamin has the greatest potential for toxic effects related to high dosage? *(494)*
    1. A
    2. B_1 (thiamine)
    3. B_2 (riboflavin)
    4. C

31. The patient tells the nurse that the ads on television are talking about zinc and its importance. The patient says that he doesn't know anything about zinc and would like to find out what foods have it. The nurse tells the patient that a good source of zinc is: *(499)*
    1. fruit.
    2. liver.
    3. poultry.
    4. cheese.

32. A patient in the hospital who is placed on a clear liquid diet may have: *(508)*
    1. orange juice.
    2. gelatin.
    3. sherbet.
    4. creamed soup.

33. Which patient is most likely to be prescribed a carbohydrate-modified diet? *(515)*
    1. Has heart failure
    2. Has hypertension
    3. Has cirrhosis of the liver
    4. Has diabetes mellitus

34. An Asian-American patient reports experiencing nausea, a bloated feeling, and flatulence after eating. Which question is the most relevant? *(518)*
    1. "Do you have any food allergies?"
    2. "Are you following the MyPlate guidelines?"
    3. "What did you eat just before the onset of the symptoms?"
    4. "Is anyone who ate the same food having the same symptoms?"

35. Patients with nasogastric (NG) tubes may develop otitis media. To prevent this occurrence, the nurse will: *(525)*
    1. increase fluid intake.
    2. remove and reinsert the tube every 24 hours.
    3. suction the nose and mouth.
    4. turn the patient side to side every 2 hours.

36. The nurse is evaluating the performance of a UAP who is feeding a patient. Which action indicates a need for correction? *(530-532)*
    1. Offering the patient the bedpan before the meal.
    2. Placing the patient in a recumbent position.
    3. Providing opportunity for hand hygeine before the meal.
    4. Talking with the patient during the feeding.

37. Which admission assessment(s) should be performed for long-term care residents in relation to potential nutritional problems? (Select all that apply.) *(485, 486, 508)*
    1. Problems with fine motor movements
    2. Ability to chew and swallow different textures of foods
    3. Typical daily fluid intake
    4. Ability to obtain and prepare own food
    5. Dietary restrictions related to chronic health problems
    6. Food preferences or rituals related to cultural background

38. The nurse sees an order for "clear liquid diet, advance as tolerated to regular diet." What does the nurse do to get the best food selection for the patient? *(508)*
    1. Contact the health care provider for clarification of order.
    2. Ask the patient if he is hungry and what he prefers to eat.
    3. Assess the patient's overall response to the clear liquid diet.
    4. Call the nutritionist and ask for an individualized diet plan.

39. The mother asks the nurse about giving strained fruits to her infant. The nurse tells the mother that this food should be introduced at around: *(505)*
    1. 2 months.
    2. 5 months.
    3. 8 months.
    4. 12 months.

40. The patient is taking a diuretic medication every day. The nurse observes the patient for signs of a decrease in: *(509)*
    1. chloride.
    2. sodium.
    3. phosphorus.
    4. potassium.

41. What are nursing responsibilities in promoting nutrition for patients? (Select all that apply.) *(486)*
    1. Assisting patients to eat or drink
    2. Designing diet plans for patients with chronic health problems
    3. Recording the patient's fluid and food intake
    4. Observing the patient for signs of poor nutrition
    5. Communicating dietary concerns to other members of the health care team
    6. Monitoring laboratory values that are related to nutritional intake

42. The patient has just ordered lunch at a restaurant. According to the USDA MyPlate recommendations, which food item should the patient plan to divide and take a portion home in a carry-out box? *(486, 487)*
    1. 10 ounces grilled skinless chicken breast
    2. 1 cup of steamed vegetables
    3. ¾ cup of mixed fruit salad
    4. ¾ cup of brown rice pilaf

43. The older patient is trying to understand the difference between dietary reference intakes (DRIs) and recommended dietary allowances (RDAs). Which patient statement best indicates an understanding of DRIs? *(486)*
    1. "DRIs replace the RDAs, but are essentially the same thing."
    2. "Using DRIs could help me prevent disease and improve my health."
    3. "RDAs apply mostly to the average-sized adult American; DRIs apply to everyone."
    4. "DRIs incorporate adequate intake, excessive intake, and average intake."

44. The patient was directed by the health care provider to consume 1500 kcal/day to achieve weight-loss goals. If the patient consumes 60% carbohydrates, 20% protein, and 20% fats, calculate the total number of grams/day for carbohydrates _____ g; fats _____ g; and protein _____ g. *(487)* (Recall that carbohydrates and protein will provide 4 kcal/g. Fats provide 9 kcal/g.)

45. The patient has sustained severe injuries in an accident. Which food sources supply the nutrient that plays the biggest role in helping the patient to build and repair injured tissue? *(487)*
    1. Green vegetables and bright-colored fruits
    2. Pasta and breads made from whole grains
    3. Beans, legumes, and soy products
    4. Lean meats, poultry, and fish

46. The nurse routinely participates in long distance endurance sports, such as running, swimming, and cycling. Which foods should the nurse eat in order to have energy over a longer period of time? *(489)*
    1. Corn and potatoes
    2. Milk and citrus fruits
    3. Honey and table sugar
    4. Chocolate and electrolyte drinks

47. The nurse is talking to a patient who has high cholesterol and a family history of cardiovascular disease. Which foods are most likely to counteract the high cholesterol? *(489)*
    1. Wheat bran and celery
    2. Orange juice and white rice
    3. Lettuce and pears
    4. Oats and barley

48. The patient reports sensations of bloating, gas, and constipation after adding lots of fruits, vegetables, and whole grains to her diet. So she has decided to go back to her former dietary pattern and exclude these foods. What is the best advice that the nurse can give the patient? *(490)*
    1. "Resume former dietary patterns and contact the health care provider."
    2. "Slowly increase intake of fiber foods and drink at least 8 glasses of water each day."
    3. "Start with a fiber supplement instead of fruits, vegetables, and whole grains."
    4. "Excessive fiber intake can lead to osteoporosis and anemia in women."

49. The patient expresses a strong preference for beef that is marbled with fat at every meal, because of the flavor and the feeling of fullness and satisfaction. Nurse would advise that this eating habit is likely to increase risk for which health condition? *(491)*
    1. Osteoporosis
    2. Cirrhosis of the liver
    3. Diabetes mellitus
    4. Atherosclerosis

50. The patient tells the nurse that he has problems with his cholesterol, so a friend told him to eat avocadoes. What is the best response? *(491)*
    1. "Avocadoes are very high in fat so the total cholesterol will increase."
    2. "Avocadoes are a source of monounsaturated fats, which are thought to lower LDL cholesterol."
    3. "Avocadoes are yellow fruits, and fruits generally do not affect cholesterol levels."
    4. "Avocadoes are a source of trans-fatty acids, which will increase the HDL levels."

51. The patient was advised by the health care provider to "watch intake of cholesterol." Which question is the most useful in assessing the likelihood of the patient's adherence to the provider's advice? *(492)*
    1. "Do you understand what 'watch your intake of cholesterol' means?"
    2. "How do you plan to manage your intake of cholesterol?"
    3. "Would you like a list of foods that contain high amounts of cholesterol?"
    4. "What do you normally eat in a 24-hour period?"

52. Which laboratory value would the nurse check to evaluate the protein status of a patient who has been receiving medical nutrition therapy? *(492)*
    1. Hemoglobin
    2. Albumin
    3. White blood cell count
    4. Electrolyte values

53. According to the DRI, the protein requirement for healthy adults is 0.8 g/kg of body weight per day. How many grams of protein does a man require if he weighs 185 pounds? *(492)*
    _____ g

54. The nurse is talking to a 17-year-old female whose parents have reluctantly allowed her to start a vegan diet if she agrees to talk to a health care provider before beginning the diet. The provider is most likely to monitor her for which nutrition-related condition? *(491)*
    1. Anorexia nervosa
    2. Rickets
    3. Iron deficiency anemia
    4. Marasmus

55. Which patient is at the greatest risk for a negative nitrogen balance that will lead to atrophy of muscles? *(493)*
    1. Patient is NPO for several days due to intractable nausea and vomiting.
    2. Patient is in the first trimester of a normal pregnancy.
    3. Patient sustained severe burns to 50% of the body surface.
    4. Patient has been fasting for several days for a religious ritual.

56. During a trip to a developing country, the nurse observes that many of the toddlers appear very fat with enlarged abdomens and swollen extremities. Which nutritional deficiency is associated with these symptoms? *(493, 494)*
    1. Carbohydrates
    2. Fats
    3. Vitamins
    4. Protein

57. The patient reports a habit of smoking at least one pack of cigarettes every day. Which foods would the nurse encourage the patient to eat, because of the heavy smoking habit? *(494)*
    1. Fish and poultry
    2. Milk products
    3. Citrus fruits
    4. Whole grains

58. A 69-year-old patient reports frequently taking antacids. Why does this patient have an increased risk for developing pernicious anemia? *(497)*
    1. Low stomach acidity blocks the absorption of vitamin B_{12} from foods.
    2. Antacids interfere with the body's ability to use heme iron.
    3. Elderly people who take antacids are less likely to produce intrinsic factor.
    4. Antacids inhibit the digestion of foods that supply vitamin C.

59. The mother reports that her child took a few extra chewable vitamins, because he thought they were gummy candies. Which question is the most important to assess for potential toxicity? *(501)*
    1. "Does the product contain vitamin C?"
    2. "How much does the child weigh?"
    3. "Is iron listed as one of the ingredients?"
    4. "Did you induce vomiting?"

60. Which patient should not be offered low-fat milk? *(505)*
    1. 15-year-old female with type 1 diabetes
    2. 26-year-old female who is in the third trimester of pregnancy
    3. 68-year-old female who has hip fracture related to osteoporosis
    4. 18-month-old female who is transitioning to cow's milk

61. Which parental action encourages good dietary habits in the child? *(506)*
    1. Allow the child to eat whenever he is hungry and skip meals if he is not hungry.
    2. Give the child whatever the rest of the family is eating; do not cater to special requests.
    3. Encourage the child to help with food preparation and create a positive environment.
    4. Give everyone the same serving size and quietly remove leftover food.

62. The nurse is talking to an adolescent girl about nutrition, but the girl seems bored, uninterested, and unlikely to try any of the nurse's suggestions. What should the nurse do? *(506)*
    1. Delay the discussion until the girl initiates interest.
    2. Explain the science of physiology and nutrition.
    3. Assess the girl's interest in other health topics.
    4. Describe how nutrition improves skin and facial appearance.

63. The UAP brings holiday cupcakes to the long-term care center and passes them out to all of the residents before checking with the nurse. What should the nurse do first? *(507)*
    1. Ask the UAP to collect the cupcakes and then determine who is allowed to have one.
    2. Praise the UAP for bringing seasonally appropriate good cheer to the residents.
    3. Remind the UAP that not all residents should have too much sugar, so next time, ask first.
    4. Sit with the residents, enjoy the cupcakes, and make the food into a social occasion.

64. Calculate your own body mass index (BMI). _____ *(510, 511)*

65. The patient is trying to lose weight because he is obese and has been told that he has a high risk for diabetes, coronary heart disease, and stroke. What is the most important point that the nurse should emphasize? *(512)*
    1. Strictly adhere to 1500 kcal/day, but eat a variety of foods.
    2. Take a multivitamin and mineral supplement while dieting.
    3. Exercise 60-90 minutes most days of the week.
    4. A weight loss of 5% to 15% can reduce health-related risks.

66. Which patient is most likely to be a candidate for bariatric surgery? *(512)*
    1. Body mass index of 40 or higher
    2. Body mass index of 35 or higher
    3. Body mass index of 23 with severe cardiovascular disease
    4. Body mass index of 17 with diabetes

67. The nurse is assessing a patient and notices tooth erosion and calloused knuckles. Which behavior would the nurse watch for around mealtimes? *(514)*
    1. Hiding the food or throwing it away
    2. Pushing the food around the plate
    3. Eating an extraordinarily large amount
    4. Self-induced vomiting

68. The patient is newly diagnosed with type 2 diabetes. In talking to the patient about diet management, what would the nurse suggest? *(516)*
    1. Suggest the patient follow a standardized preprinted menu for each meal.
    2. Indicate that two or more servings of fried fish would be beneficial.
    3. Closely monitor and control intake of table sugar and desserts.
    4. Emphasize consistent mealtimes; approximately every 4-5 hours.

69. A patient who is a known diabetic presents with weakness, diaphoresis, and disorientation. What should the nurse do first? *(517)*
    1. Encourage the patient to drink a lot of water.
    2. Give the patient a glass of milk.
    3. Establish intravenous access and give glucose.
    4. Have the patient suck on a hard candy.

70. A patient has symptoms of steatorrhea and flatulence. Which diet is the health care provider most likely to recommend? *(520)*
    1. Carbohydrate-modified diet
    2. Protein-restricted diet
    3. Sodium-restricted diet
    4. Fat-controlled diet

71. A patient is on fluid restrictions because of renal failure. Which intervention(s) would the nurse use? (Select all that apply.) *(522)*
    1. Encourage the patient to drink most of the fluid allowance in the morning.
    2. Explain the various sources of fluid such as IV fluids, gelatin, and fluids taken with medications.
    3. Suggest chewing gum and sucking on breath mints.
    4. Explain the rationale for fluid restrictions.
    5. Show the volume of fluid that is allowed for the shift.
    6. Post a sign in the room so that visitors are aware of fluid restrictions.

CRITICAL THINKING ACTIVITIES

72. The nurse is working on a medical-surgical unit and has identified several patients who may need enteral feeding.

    a. What are the indications for the use of enteral feeding? *(522)* _____

    _____

    _____

    b. Identify the nursing assessments and interventions for enteral feeding in the following situations. *(526)*

       i. Patient assessment before feeding: _____

       _____

       ii. Assessment of gastric aspirate:_____

       _____

       iii. Gastric residual above 150 mL:_____

       _____

       iv. Formula is cold: _____

       _____

    v. Occlusion of the tubing is suspected: _____

_____

    vi. After feeding is given: _____

_____

    vii. Documentation: _____

_____

  c. What are the possible complications or problems associated with enteral feeding? *(525)*_____

_____

_____

_____

73. The nurse is talking to a 25-year-old woman who is approximately 10 pounds underweight for her age and height, but is otherwise in good health. She would like some information about healthy diet and lifestyle, because she and her husband are thinking about trying to have a baby.

  a. Explain to this young woman why there is an increased need for nutrients during pregnancy. *(502)*

_____

_____

  b. Which vitamins would be recommended for the pregnant patient and what is the function of these vitamin supplements? What are the food sources for each vitamin? *(503)*_____

_____

_____

  c. What can the nurse tell the patient about her current weight in relation to getting pregnant? *(502)*

_____

_____

_____

  d. What can the nurse tell the patient about foods and lifestyle activities that should be avoided? *(504)*

_____

_____

_____

Fluids and Electrolytes

Answer Key: Textbook page references are provided as a guide for answering these questions. A complete Answer Key is provided in your Additional Learning Resources on Evolve.

MATCHING

Directions: Match the terms on the left to the correct definition on the right.

Term

_____ 1. active transport *(541)*

_____ 2. adenosine triphosphate (ATP) *(539)*

_____ 3. blood buffers *(550)*

_____ 4. diffusion *(539)*

_____ 5. filtration *(541)*

_____ 6. homeostasis *(538)*

_____ 7. hydrostatic pressure *(541)*

_____ 8. milliequivalent *(541)*

_____ 9. osmosis *(540)*

_____ 10. passive transport *(539)*

Definition

a. Natural tendency of a substance to move from an area of higher concentration to one of lower concentration

b. Passage of substances across the cell membrane that requires energy expenditure

c. Force of fluid pressing outward on a vessel wall

d. Water moves across a membrane from low particle concentration to high particle concentration

e. Produced in the mitochondria of cells from nutrients

f. Circulate throughout the body in pairs, neutralizing excess acids or bases by contributing or accepting hydrogen ions

g. Measure of the chemical activity of an ion

h. Transfer of water and dissolved substances from an area of higher pressure to an area of lower pressure

i. Process of keeping body fluids in balance

j. Move substances through the cell membranes by diffusion, filtration, and osmosis

SHORT ANSWER

Directions: Using your own words, answer each question in the space provided.

11. What does the intracellular fluid compartment contain? *(537)* _____

_____

12. What does the extracellular fluid compartment contain? *(537)* _____

_____

_____

13. Where is the interstitial fluid? List several examples. *(537)* _____

_____

_____

_____

14. What does the intravascular fluid contain? *(537)* _____

_____

_____

_____

TABLE ACTIVITY

15. Directions: List the normal value range for the electrolytes.

Electrolyte	Normal Value Range
Sodium *(542)*	a.
Potassium *(543)*	b.
Chloride *(544)*	c.
Calcium *(545)*	d.
Phosphorus *(546)*	e.
Magnesium *(548)*	f.
Bicarbonate *(548)*	g.

MULTIPLE CHOICE

Directions: Select the best answer(s) for each of the following questions.

16. The patient is experiencing hyperkalemia. The nurse anticipates that the treatment will include: *(545)*
    1. intravenous (IV) calcium.
    2. fluid restrictions.
    3. foods high in potassium.
    4. administration of loop diuretics.

17. Following an auto accident and a significant hemorrhage, the patient was given a large infusion of citrated blood. The patient is assessed for the development of: *(546)*
    1. urinary retention.
    2. poor skin turgor.
    3. increased blood pressure.
    4. positive Chvostek's sign.

18. The best food source for calcium is: *(546)*
    1. milk.
    2. meat.
    3. whole grains.
    4. green leafy vegetables.

19. The patient has experienced a prolonged episode of diarrhea. Which clinical observation is consistent with the development of metabolic acidosis? *(550)*
    1. Increased perspiration
    2. Increased respiratory rate
    3. Increased urinary output
    4. Decreased heart rate

20. The patient has had emphysema for a number of years. Which set of arterial blood gas values indicates that the patient is in respiratory acidosis? *(550)*
    1. pH 7.35, $Paco_2$ 40, HCO_3^- 22
    2. pH 7.40, $Paco_2$ 45, HCO_3^- 30
    3. pH 7.30, $Paco_2$ 50, HCO_3^- 24
    4. pH 7.48, $Paco_2$ 55, HCO_3^- 18

21. While in the delivery room with his wife, the father-to-be begins to develop an anxiety reaction and lightheadedness. Which intervention does the nurse use to prevent respiratory alkalosis? *(551)*
    1. Lay him down.
    2. Provide nasal oxygen.
    3. Have him breathe into a paper bag.
    4. Have him cough and deep-breathe.

22. A child has gotten into the medicine cabinet in the home and ingested the remaining contents of an aspirin (acetylsalicylic acid) bottle. What is the life-threatening condition that can occur as a result of excessive aspirin ingestion? *(552)*
    1. Metabolic acidosis
    2. Metabolic alkalosis
    3. Respiratory acidosis
    4. Respiratory alkalosis

23. The patient has had continuous gastric suction. The nurse recognizes that acid-base imbalances can occur with this treatment. Which laboratory data confirms metabolic alkalosis? *(553)*
    1. pH elevated, $Paco_2$ normal, and HCO_3^- elevated
    2. pH elevated, $Paco_2$ elevated, and HCO_3^- decreased
    3. pH decreased, $Paco_2$ decreased, and HCO_3^- decreased
    4. pH decreased, $Paco_2$ normal, and HCO_3^- decreased

24. The best way for the nurse to determine the patient's fluid balance is to: *(539)*
    1. assess vital signs.
    2. weigh the patient daily.
    3. monitor IV fluid intake.
    4. check diagnostic test results.

25. The patient used excessive antacids, which resulted in a serum sodium level of 150 mEq/L. Why would the health care provider instruct the nurse to give an IV hypotonic solution? *(541)*
    1. To correct intracellular dehydration
    2. To correct intravascular volume
    3. To increase the sodium level
    4. To pull fluid from the cells

26. The nurse is caring for a postoperative patient. Which solution is the health care provider most likely to order to replace the fluid deficiency related to the NPO status in the pre- and postoperative period? *(540, 541)*
    1. Hypotonic solution
    2. Hypertonic solution
    3. Isotonic solution
    4. Parental nutrition

27. What purpose(s) do the electrolytes serve in the body? (Select all that apply.) *(541)*
    1. Maintenance of normal body metabolism
    2. Regulation of water balance in the body
    3. Regulation of water and electrolyte contents within cells
    4. Formation of hydrochloric acid in gastric juice
    5. Transportation of nutrients to cells and waste products from cells

28. The patient has been placed on a low-sodium diet to assist in the treatment of hypertension. Which patient statement indicates an understanding of the diet teaching? *(541)*
    1. "Cheese is a good between-meal snack for me."
    2. "It is okay for me to eat at my favorite seafood restaurant."
    3. "In order for me to eat enough vegetables, I can prepare canned peas and corn."
    4. "I use a a lot of fresh vegetables, although I should give up table salt."

29. Which patient has the greatest risk for developing hypokalemia? *(543)*
    1. Has a small bowel obstruction
    2. Has renal failure
    3. Consumes excessive alcohol
    4. Takes prescribed loop diuretic

30. Diet and fluid restriction and medications have been administered to the patient to decrease excess fluid volume. On the first day, the patient's weight was 150 pounds. After therapy, the patient's weight is 145.5 pounds. Assuming that the weight change represents fluid loss, how much fluid did the patient lose? _____ liters *(539)*

31. The nurse receives notification from the laboratory that a patient's potassium level is 6 mEq/L. The nurse has paged the health care provider and is awaiting a call back. What should the nurse do first? *(544)*
    1. Attach the patient to a cardiac monitor.
    2. Encourage foods and fluids that contain potassium.
    3. Ensure that intravenous calcium gluconate is available.
    4. Check medications for association with potassium level.

32. The nurse is checking the laboratory data of a woman who is at risk for osteoporosis. Which electrolyte value is most relevant to this condition? *(545)*
    1. Sodium level of 145 mEq/L
    2. Calcium level of 3.0 mEq/dL
    3. Potassium 3.5 mEq/dL
    4. Phosphorus of 3.4 mEq/dL

33. The nurse hears in report that the patient has been receiving Amphojel (aluminum hydroxide) to correct an electrolyte imbalance. Which electrolyte value indicates that the therapy is working? *(547)*
    1. Phosphorus level of 4.1 mEq/dL
    2. Magnesium level of 1.5 mEq/dL
    3. Bicarbonate level of 22 mEq/dL
    4. Calcium level of 4.5 mEq/dL

34. The nurse is caring for a patient who had surgery on the parathyroid glands. Which electrolyte level in the low-normal range is the greatest concern? *(547)*
    1. Calcium level of 4.6 mEq/dL
    2. Sodium level of 127 mEq/dL
    3. Potassium level of 3.7 mEq/dL
    4. Magnesium level of 1.7 mEq/dL

35. The patient has a medical diagnosis of diabetic ketoacidosis (DKA). Which clinical manifestation indicates that the blood buffer system is exhausted? *(550)*
    1. Urinary output is decreased.
    2. Respiratory rate is increased.
    3. Heart rate is decreased.
    4. pH is increased.

36. The patient is on mechanical ventilation. The arterial blood gas results indicate that the patient has respiratory alkalosis. What would the nurse do first? *(552)*
    1. Suction the airway for excessive secretions or a mucus plug.
    2. Notify the RN or the health care provider.
    3. Check the ventilator settings and compare to the orders.
    4. Deliver breaths using a bag-valve-mask with high-flow oxygen.

CRITICAL THINKING ACTIVITIES

37. The nurse is caring for an elderly patient who was brought to the hospital for confusion. Family reports that the patient lives alone and is usually alert and independent, but recently complained of stomach cramps, vomiting, and diarrhea. Nurse notes that home medications include a diuretic and blood pressure medication. Mucous membranes are dry. Laboratory results show potassium 3.4 mEq/L and serum sodium 127 mEq/L.

    a. Identify at least two considerations for the older adult patient regarding fluid, electrolyte, and acid-base balance. *(537)*

    _____

    _____

b. What is the clinical significance of a serum potassium of 3.4 mEq/L? *(543)* _____

_____

_____

c. For this patient, what factors are likely to be contributing to the current serum potassium value? *(543)*

_____

_____

d. What are the most common signs/symptoms associated with hypokalemia, and what are the nursing interventions for the imbalance? *(543)*

_____

_____

e. What is the clinical significance of a serum sodium of 127 mEq/L? *(542)* _____

_____

_____

f. Identify the most common signs and symptoms of hyponatremia, and nursing interventions for the imbalance. *(542)*

_____

_____

g. The nurse is monitoring the patient's intake and output (I&O). What should be counted as part of the output? *(538)*

_____

_____

38. The nurse is caring for a patient with pneumonia. The patient is having dyspnea. The following laboratory data are available for review.

pH	7.30
$Paco_2$	50 mm Hg
Pao_2	70 mm Hg
O_2 saturation	90%
HCO_3^-	22 mEq

a. What do these laboratory values suggest for this patient? *(551)* _____

_____

_____

b. What signs and symptoms are likely to be associated with the laboratory values? *(551)* _____

_____

_____

_____

c. What treatment does the nurse anticipate will be ordered for this patient? *(551)* _____

_____

_____

_____

Dosage Calculation and Medication Administration

Answer Key: Textbook page references are provided as a guide for answering these questions. A complete Answer Key is provided in your Additional Learning Resources on Evolve.

BASIC MATH REVIEW

Directions: Use basic math functions (e.g., addition, subtraction, conversion, rounding, etc.) to solve the review problems.

1. Change the improper fraction to a mixed number: $\frac{8}{5} =$ _____ *(561)*

2. Change the mixed number to an improper fraction: $7\frac{5}{8} =$ _____ *(561)*

3. Reduce the fraction to the lowest term: $\frac{25}{100} =$ _____ *(561)*

4. Add the fractions and reduce the sum to its lowest term: $2\frac{1}{3} + 5\frac{1}{4} =$ _____ *(562)*

5. Subtract the fractions and reduce the answer to its lowest term: $\frac{1}{2} - \frac{1}{3} =$ _____ *(563)*

6. Multiply the fractions and reduce the product to its lowest term: $\frac{1}{3} \times \frac{3}{12} =$ _____ *(563)*

7. Divide the fractions and reduce the answer to its lowest term: $\frac{3}{10} \div \frac{5}{25} =$ _____ *(563)*

8. Add the decimals: $57.629 + 14.22 =$ _____ *(564)*

9. Subtract the decimals: $0.089 - 0.0057 =$ _____ *(564)*

10. Round the decimal to hundredths and then to tenths: $5.753 =$ _____ _____ *(560)*

11. Multiply the decimals: $64.75 \times 22.9 =$ _____ *(564)*

12. Divide the decimals and round to the nearest hundredth: $2.9 \div 0.218 =$ _____ *(564)*

13. Convert the fraction into a decimal: $\frac{1}{2} =$ _____ *(565)*

14. Convert the fraction into percent: $\frac{75}{100} =$ _____ *(565)*

15. Solve for X: $20 : 40 = X : 5$ $X =$ _____ *(566)*

TABLE ACTIVITY

16. Directions: In the table below, fill in the metric measures that are equivalent to the amount given as apothecary measures, according to the conversion information in your textbook. *(560)*

Equivalents for Metric and Apothecary Measures

Metric	Apothecary
_____ milligrams	1 grain
_____ kilograms	1 pound
_____ kilograms	2.2 pounds
_____ milliliters	1 fluid ounce
_____ milliliters	1 pint
_____ milliliters	1 quart

17. Directions: Convert and calculate the following equivalents using the equivalent measure information from your textbook for conversion. *(559, 560)*

    a.   30 mL = _____ ounces

    b.   1000 mL = _____ liters

    c.   1 L = _____ quarts

    d.   500 mL = _____ pints

    e.   60 mg = _____ grains

    f.   1 kg = _____ pounds

    g.   400 mL = _____ liters

    h.   2 mcg = _____ milligrams

    i.   4 mg = _____ grams

    j.   44 pounds = _____ kilograms (round to whole number)

    k.   5 mg = _____ micrograms

    l.   1 inch = _____ centimeters

    m.   25 inches = _____ centimeters

    n.   225 pounds = _____ kilograms (round to whole number)

    o.   8 ounces = _____ milliliters

    p.   24 ounces = _____ milliliters

    q.   250 mcg = _____ milligrams

    r.   3 teaspoons = _____ milliliters

    s.   2 tablespoons = _____ milliliters

MATCHING

Directions: Match the abbreviations on the left to the correct meaning on the right. (576)

Abbreviation		Meaning
_____ 18.	bid	a. Three times a day
_____ 19.	tid	b. After meals
_____ 20.	qid	c. Four times a day
_____ 21.	ac	d. Two times a day
_____ 22.	pc	e. Before meals

CLINICAL APPLICATION OF MATH

Directions: Calculate the math problems using the equivalent measures from your text (i.e., 1 inch = 2.5 centimeters, 1 pound = 2.2 kilograms, 30 milliliters = 1 ounce, etc.).

23. The patient's height is 25 inches. What is the patient's height in centimeters? *(559)* _____ centimeters

24. The patient's height is 36 inches. What is the patient's height in centimeters? *(559)* _____ centimeters

25. The patient's abdominal girth is 38 inches. What is the patient's abdominal girth in centimeters? *(559)* _____ centimeters

26. The patient weighs 158 pounds. What is the patient's weight in kilograms? *(560)* _____ kilograms (round to whole number)

27. The patient weighs 57 pounds. What is the patient's weight in kilograms? *(560)* _____ kilograms (round to whole number)

28. The patient weighs 12.2 kilograms. What is the patient's weight in pounds? *(560)* _____ pounds (round to whole number)

29. Calculate the patient's total fluid intake for breakfast: 8 ounces of milk, 6 ounces of juice, and 10 ounces of coffee. *(560)* _____ mL

30. Calculate the patient's total fluid intake for 24 hours: 16 ounces of milk, 10 ounces of coffee, 6 ounces of juice, 2 liters of water, 500 mL of IV fluid. *(560)* _____ mL

31. Calculate the patient's total fluid intake and output for 24 hours: 6 ounces of milk, 16 ounces of coffee, 3 liters of water, 250 mL of IV fluid. *(560)* Intake _____ mL
Urine 2950 mL, wound drainage 200 mL. Output _____ mL

32. The prescription is for Tegretol 200 mg po tid. *(566)*
Available—Tegretol 100-mg tablets
How many tablets should be given per dose? _____

33. The prescription is for Aldomet 250 mg po bid. *(566)*
Available—Aldomet 125-mg tablets
How many tablets should be given per dose? _____

34. The prescription is for V-Cillin K suspension 500,000 units po. *(566)*
    Available—V-Cillin K suspension 200,000 units/5 mL
    How much should be prepared? _____

35. The prescription is for morphine 4 mg IM PRN for pain. *(566)*
    Available—morphine 10 mg/mL
    The nurse prepares _____ mL.

36. The prescription is for heparin 5000 units subQ. *(566)*
    Available—heparin 10,000 units/mL.
    How much should be given? _____

37. The prescription is for Solu-Medrol 50 mg IV. *(566)*
    Available—Solu-Medrol 125 mg/2 mL.
    How much is prepared? _____

38. Using Young's rule, identify the dose for a child who is 3 years old when the adult dose is 75 mg. *(568)*
    _____ mg

39. Using Clark's rule, identify the dose for a child who weighs 30 pounds when the adult dose is 50 mg.
    (568) _____ mg

40. Using Fried's rule, identify the dose for a child who is 10 months old when the adult dose is 100 mg.
    (568) _____ mg

41. Using the body surface area calculation, identify the dose for a child with a body surface area of 1.1 m^2
    when the adult dose is 10 mg. *(568)* _____

42. An IV is prescribed to infuse at 75 mL/hr. The drip factor is 10 gtt/mL. The rate of infusion should be
    _____ gtt/min. *(608)*

43. An IV is prescribed to infuse at 125 mL/hr. The drip factor is 10 gtt/mL. The rate of infusion should be
    _____ gtt/min. *(608)*

44. An IV is prescribed to infuse at 30 mL/hr with a microdrip set. The rate of infusion should be
    _____ gtt/min. *(608)*

45. An IV of 1000 mL is to infuse over 6 hours. The drip factor is 15 gtt/mL. The rate of infusion should be
    _____ gtt/min. *(608)*

46. An IV of 1000 mL is to infuse at 125 mL/hour and the nurse will use an infusion pump that can be set to
    deliver fluid in mL/hour. What is the pump setting in _____ mL/hour? *(608)*

47. An IV of 250 mL contains potassium to be infused over 2 hours. The nurse will use an infusion pump
    that can be set to deliver fluid in mL/hour. What is the pump setting in _____ mL/hour? *(608)*

48. An IV of 100 mL contains an antibiotic to be infused over 30 minutes. The nurse will use an infusion
    pump that can be set to deliver fluid in mL/hour. What is the pump setting in _____ mL/hour?
    (608)

49. An IV of 250 mL contains an antibiotic to be infused over 1 hour and 30 minutes. The nurse will use an
    infusion pump that can be set to deliver fluid in mL/hour. What is the pump setting in _____ mL/
    hour? *(608)*

50. The health care provider orders 8 units of regular insulin. Indicate on the insulin syringe how many units the nurse will draw for the correct dose. *(596)*

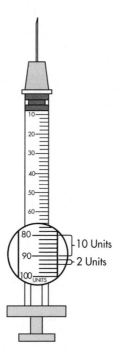

51. The health care provider orders 0.07 mg of epinephrine. Epinephrine Injection, USP 1:1000 (1 mg/mL) is supplied in a 1-mL ampoule single-dose container. Indicate on the tuberculin syringe how many milliliters the nurse will draw up. *(596)*

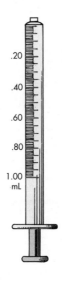

SHORT ANSWER

52. What are the Six Rights of medication administration? *(575)* _____

_____

_____

53. What are the Three Label Checks of medication administration? *(575)* _____

_____

_____

54. A medication order should include the following: *(573, 611)*_____

_____

_____

55. What factors can influence a patient's response to a medication? *(571)*_____

_____

_____

MULTIPLE CHOICE

56. Put the following terms in order of priority. *(569)*

_____ a.   PRN

_____ b.   now

_____ c.   stat

_____ d.   one time only

57. A prescription for codeine gr ½ is written for the patient. The medication is supplied in mg. The nurse should administer: *(560)*
   1. 3 g.
   2. 30 g.
   3. 3 mg.
   4. 30 mg.

58. An IV of 500 mL D$_5$W is to infuse over 4 hours. The administration set is 15 gtt/mL. How many gtt/min should the infusion run? *(608)*
   1. 19 gtt/min
   2. 24 gtt/min
   3. 31 gtt/min
   4. 42 gtt/min

59. The nurse determines the location for an injection by identifying the greater trochanter of the femur, the anterosuperior iliac spine, and the iliac crest. The injection site being used by the nurse is the: *(599)*
   1. rectus femoris.
   2. ventrogluteal.
   3. dorsogluteal.
   4. vastus lateralis.

60. Upon getting the assignment for the evening, the nurse notices that two patients on the unit have the same last name. The best way to prevent medication errors for these two patients is to: *(576)*
   1. ask the patients their names.
   2. check the patients' ID bands.
   3. ask another nurse about their identities.
   4. verify their names with the family members.

61. The nurse is working in the newborn nursery and will be giving vitamin K injections to the babies. The site preferred for these injections is the: *(599)*
   1. deltoid.
   2. dorsogluteal.
   3. ventrogluteal.
   4. vastus lateralis.

62. When preparing an opioid medication, the nurse drops the pill on the floor. The nurse should: *(574)*
    1. discard the medication in the biohazard container.
    2. notify the pharmacy for a replacement dose.
    3. wipe off the medication and administer it.
    4. have another nurse witness the disposal of the pill.

63. The Z-track technique is used by the nurse when the patient is: *(602)*
    1. extremely obese.
    2. younger than 5 years old.
    3. receiving an irritating medication.
    4. having a large dose of medication given.

64. A tuberculin test will be given to the patient. In selecting the site for this intradermal injection, the nurse assesses the: *(603)*
    1. upper outer aspect of the arm.
    2. anterior aspect of the forearm.
    3. middle third of the anterior thigh.
    4. 2-inch diameter around the umbilicus.

65. How does the nurse determine what the drip factor is for an IV set? *(608)*
    1. Ask the charge nurse.
    2. Calculate the IV rate.
    3. Look in a reference book.
    4. Check the IV tubing box.

66. The nurse is observing the patient self-administer medication with a metered-dose inhaler (MDI). What action by the patient requires correction and further instruction? *(591)*
    1. Inhaling slowly
    2. Inhaling one puff with each inspiration
    3. Spraying the back of the throat
    4. Using an aerochamber spacer for a better fit

67. The nurse is aware that certain types of medications cannot be crushed for ease in administration. These medications include: (Select all that apply.) *(581)*
    1. extended-release capsules.
    2. tablets.
    3. sublingual tablets.
    4. enteric-coated tablets.
    5. sustained-release capsules.

68. The nurse identifies that a patient is having an idiosyncratic reaction to a medication. Which patient's report is consistent with the nurse's analysis? *(570)*
    1. Hypnotic medication causes him to be awake most of the night.
    2. Antianxiety medication seems to make the pain medication more effective.
    3. Previous dosage of pain medication does not seem to be working like it used to.
    4. Antibiotic medication seems to cause an uncomfortable, itchy rash.

69. Which route of drug administration will achieve the fastest onset of action? *(592)*
    1. Intradermal
    2. Buccal
    3. Subcutaneous
    4. Enteral

70. The nurse has five stable patients and each needs many medications. All of the medications are scheduled to be administered at 9:00 AM. What should the nurse do first? *(575)*
    1. Inform the RN that some of the medications were given late, despite best efforts.
    2. Start at 08:30 AM and give medications to the most cooperative patients first.
    3. Administer as many medications at 9:00 AM as possible and then write an incident report.
    4. Ask the RN to change patient assignments so that medications are given on time.

71. An IV of 1000 mL 5% dextrose and 45% saline is to infuse over 8 hours. The IV fluid is started at 0800 hours. At 1400 hours, how much IV fluid has the patient received if the nurse correctly set the flow rate? *(608)*
    1. 1000 mL
    2. 750 mL
    3. 625 mL
    4. 500 mL

72. The nurse hears in report that 1000 mL of normal saline was started at 3:00 AM to infuse at 125 mL per hour. At 7:30 AM, the nurse evaluates the patient and the IV infusion, which is running by gravity; the IV fluid bag shows that approximately 200 mL has been infused. What should the nurse do first? *(608)*
    1. Calculate the amount of fluid that should have infused and then give it.
    2. Report the error to the charge nurse and write an incident report.
    3. Document the amount of fluid infused and the appearance of the site.
    4. Recalculate the drops/minute and reset the rate of flow to 125 mL/hour.

73. The health care provider orders two medications and suggests to the nurse that they could be mixed together in the same syringe to prevent the patient from having to get two separate injections. The nurse mixes the drugs, but a precipitate forms in the syringe. What should the nurse do? *(570)*
    1. Ask the health care provider to verify the request to mix the drugs.
    2. Gently rotate the syringe between the palms of the hands to mix the solution.
    3. Discard the syringe and call the pharmacy for information about compatibilities.
    4. Administer the medications as ordered and document the injection site.

74. The nurse is giving a patient the morning medications. The patient says, "I don't recognize this pill." What should the nurse say? *(579)*
    1. "The medications that you will get in the hospital may be different than the ones you take at home."
    2. "The medications are made by different manufacturers. They can be chemically identical, but have a different appearance."
    3. "Let me review the list of your home medications and I'll find out if anything new was ordered for you."
    4. " I carefully checked all of your medications against the health care provider's orders and these are correct."

75. The patient reports having an anaphylactic reaction to an IV medication, but cannot remember the name. The nurse informs the health care provider and the provider tells the nurse to go ahead and administer the ordered medication. What should the nurse do? *(609)*
    1. Refuse to administer the medication, because the allergy history is not clarified.
    2. Take baseline vital signs and recheck the patient frequently during the infusion.
    3. Inform the charge nurse or RN about the potential for an adverse reaction.
    4. Call the pharmacy and see if they have any records of the patient's allergies.

76. The nurse has performed a medication calculation and has determined that to give the ordered dose, 15 tablets would have to be administered to the patient. The nurse has asked two other nurses to recheck the calculations and the answer is always 15. What should the nurse do first? *(569)*
    1. Give the 15 tablets because the calculations have been checked and rechecked.
    2. Call the pharmacy and ask if the medication comes in a different strength.
    3. Call the health care provider and ask for verification of the order.
    4. Consult a reliable drug reference to see if the ordered dose is within safe range.

77. Two nurses are standing in the medication area. Nurse A is preparing medication, but hears an alarm indicating that an unstable patient needs help right away. She hands the prepared medication to Nurse B and asks her to give it to the correct patient. What should Nurse B do? *(575)*
    1. Go ahead and give it because she witnessed all the preparations that Nurse A made.
    2. Inform the charge nurse that Nurse A needs assistance because of a critical patient.
    3. Give the medication, but later indicate to Nurse A that she should do the documentation.
    4. Discard the prepared medication and prepare another dose and give it to the patient.

78. The nurse is supervising a nursing student who must give several medications. The nurse would intervene if the student performed which action? *(581)*
    1. Puts a suppository in a uniform pocket
    2. Used aseptic technique to handle pills
    3. Looked at the meniscus when pouring a liquid
    4. Read the label of the bottle as she took it off the shelf

79. The patient has an order for a medication that is to be delivered via a metered-dose inhaler. Which chronic health condition is the patient most likely to have? *(589)*
    1. Hypertension
    2. Chronic bronchitis
    3. Diabetes mellitus
    4. Arteriosclerotic heart disease

80. Which factor would be the most important in the nurse's decision to choose a Luer-Lok tip over a plain slip tip syringe? *(596)*
    1. Viscosity of solution
    2. Age of patient
    3. Length of needle
    4. Weight of patient

81. The nurse is assessing an existing IV that seems to have stopped infusing. What should the nurse do first? *(608, 609)*
    1. Recalculate the drip rate and then count the number of drops per minute.
    2. Discontinue the IV and inform the RN or health care provider.
    3. Check for infiltration and ask the patient about pain or discomfort.
    4. Try repositioning the patient's extremity or adjusting the height of the IV bag.

82. The nurse is performing an intradermal injection for an allergy test. She does not aspirate for this type of injection. What is the best rationale for the nurse's technique? *(602)*
    1. This is standard procedure and she is following the procedure manual.
    2. Aspirating can cause bruising and the patient will receive many allergy tests.
    3. There are no major veins or arteries in the intradermal tissues.
    4. The needle is so fine and short that it is unlikely to cause tissue damage.

83. The nurse is assessing a patient who is receiving IV fluid and medication. Which finding is the most serious? *(609)*
    1. Patient complains of pain at the insertion site.
    2. Patient is dyspneic and has a weak, thready pulse.
    3. Patient's arm is swollen and the skin is cool to the touch.
    4. Patient is very scared and upset because the IV bag is empty.

84. The older patient is receiving a medication that is potentially nephrotoxic. Which assessment is the most relevant to prevent potential nephrotoxicity? *(572)*
    1. Change of mental status
    2. Reduced urinary output
    3. Nausea and vomiting
    4. Increased blood pressure

CRITICAL THINKING ACTIVITIES

85. Identify home health safety information that should be included in a teaching plan for medication administration. *(579)*

_____

_____

_____

86. Discuss ways to prevent medication errors and maximize safety in medication administration. *(579)*

_____

_____

_____

87. Look at the medication order below for patient John Smith and identify what parts of the order are missing. *(571)*

John Smith: BD 6/9/51

Pfizerpen 1.2 million units

Dr. James Jones

_____

_____

88. The patient needs a medication; however, to deliver the correct dose the nurse has to perform some calculations because the amount of medication in the vial exceeds the ordered dose. It's a very busy day. The nurse is trying to train a new nurse, there is a call light on, a health care provider wants to ask about a patient, the nurse left her calculator at home, and suddenly a patient falls on the floor. The nurse instructs the new nurse to perform the calculation and after a while they go to give the medication. The patient sustains no harm, but later the nurse thinks about her day and realizes that this situation could have harmed the patient. Analyze factors that could contribute to potential error and discuss what the nurse should have done in this situation. *(579)*

_____

_____

_____

_____

_____

_____

_____

_____

_____

_____

_____

_____

_____

_____

Care of Patients with Alterations in Health

Answer Key: Textbook page references are provided as a guide for answering these questions. A complete Answer Key is provided in your Additional Learning Resources on Evolve.

WORD SCRAMBLE

Directions: Unscramble the words that are related to performing various nursing skills and then match the word to the correct clue below.

Scrambled Term	Unscrambled Term	Correct Clue
1. zationcatheri *(662)*		
2. ymotso *(685)*		
3. secef *(685)*		
4. lencetualf *(685)*		
5. tionimpac *(685)*		
6. continencein *(673)*		
7. ationinfiltr *(636)*		
8. venintraous *(628)*		
9. vagela *(676)*		
10. ssionpredecom *(676)*		

Clues for words used in performing various nursing skills

a. To remove the air and fluids that build up when gastrointestinal (GI) motility is slowed
b. Introducing a rubber or plastic tube into the body
c. Seepage of a nonirritating solution or medication into tissue surrounding the vessel
d. Presence of air or gas in the intestinal tract
e. Inability to control bowel or bladder
f. Waste product expelled through the rectum
g. Instilling solutions into the stomach then suctioning it back out
h. An artificial opening
i. Can occur in the ear canal or in the rectum
j. Through the veins

FILL-IN-THE-BLANK SENTENCES

Directions: Complete each sentence by filling in the blank with the correct word or phrase.

11. The two most common complications of central venous catheters (CVCs) are _____ and _____ of the catheter cannula. *(634)*

12. Even when an ostomy pouch is adhering well, it is best to change it at least every _____ days to allow for observation of the stoma and the skin around the stoma. *(694)*

13. The maximum amount of fluid that should be administered to an adult during a tap-water enema is _____. *(687)*

14. For infants, the pressure of the wall suction should be set at _____ during suctioning of the airways. *(659)*

15. When inserting a urinary catheter into a female patient, the nurse knows that it should be inserted _____ inches. *(667)*

TRUE OR FALSE

Directions: Write T for true or F for false in the blanks provided.

_____ 16. Suctioning to keep the airway patent eliminates the need for the patient to perform coughing and deep-breathing. *(657)*

_____ 17. Intermittent urinary catheterization has a lower risk of infection than an indwelling urinary catheter due to the relatively shorter time the catheter remains in the bladder. *(693)*

_____ 18. The nurse should delegate to the UAP to routinely assist the home health patient with vaginal douching for hygiene. *(694)*

_____ 19. PICC lines pose less risk of pneumothorax, hemothorax, and air embolism than CVCs, are less expensive to maintain than CVCs, and pose less risk of phlebitis and infiltration than peripheral lines. *(635)*

_____ 20. Once nasogastric tube placement has been verified by x-ray, the nurse can safely use it for routine feedings. *(694)*

_____ 21. Patients with colostomies are at high risk for skin impairment at the site due to nearly continuous urine drainage. *(694)*

_____ 22. Oxygen will explode if someone lights a match while standing close to a patient who is using oxygen. *(646)*

SHORT ANSWER

Directions: Using your own words, answer each question in the space provided.

23. What are the five rights of delegation? *(614)*

    a. _____

    b. _____

    c. _____

    d. _____

    e. _____

24. Identify five purposes of intravenous (IV) therapy. *(627)*

    a. _____

    b. _____

    c. _____

    d. _____

    e. _____

25. Identify five potential complications of IV therapy. *(636, 637)*

    a. _____

    b. _____

    c. _____

    d. _____

    e. _____

CLINICAL APPLICATION OF MATH AND CONVERSION

Directions: Calculate or make the necessary conversions for math problems encountered in performing skills for patients.

26. At the beginning of the shift, the nurse inserts a urinary catheter and notes 300 mL of urine output into the drainage bag. One hour later, there is an order to send a urine sample, so the nurse uses the appropriate sterile technique and draws 20 mL from the port. At that time, the nurse notes 350 mL of urine in the bag, empties the bag, and records the urine output. At the end of the shift, the drainage bag contains 500 mL. How many mL of urine are recorded as the total output for the shift? *(663)* _____ mL

27. The patient vomits 200 mL of green bile drainage. Twenty minutes later, he vomits 100 mL. The health care provider orders the insertion of a nasogastric tube to decompress the stomach. During the procedure the patient vomits 50 mL. At the end of the shift there is 150 mL in the drainage container. What does the nurse record as the output of emesis for the shift? *(684)* _____ mL

28. The health care provider orders an enteral feeding to infuse at 30 mL/hour for 3 hours and then to check the residual and notify with the results. How many mL will the patient receive in 3 hours? *(676)* _____ mL

29. The health care provider orders an IV infusion of dextrose 5% and normal saline to infuse at 125 mL/hour for 8 hours. The nurse uses an electronic infusion pump to alarm every 2 hours. How many mL should the patient receive in each 2-hour period? *(636)* _____ mL

30. The patient is receiving continuous bladder irrigation through a three-way indwelling urinary catheter. Prescribed: 350 mL of normal saline irrigating solution infused. There are 475 mL in the urinary drainage bag. What is the patient's urinary output? *(671)* _____ mL

MULTIPLE CHOICE

Directions: Select the best answer(s) for each of the following questions.

31. The nursing student has the opportunity to perform urinary catheterization for a patient. What should the student do first? *(614)*
    1. Perform hand hygiene and don gloves.
    2. Explain the procedure to the patient.
    3. Obtain the necessary equipment.
    4. Check the health care provider's order.

32. In performing nursing skills and procedures for patients, which nursing action demonstrates the nurse's understanding and use of Standard Precautions? *(614)*
    1. Always checks the patient's armband and asks patient to state name
    2. Assesses the patient's understanding and teaches accordingly
    3. Performs hand hygiene before and after every patient encounter
    4. Evaluates the patient's response to and tolerance of the procedure

33. The nurse must perform catheter care. Prior to starting the procedure, the nurse raises the bed and lowers one side rail. What is the best rationale for this action? *(614)*
    1. Ensures patient safety and comfort
    2. Promotes good body mechanics
    3. Facilitates visualization of body
    4. Adheres to standard procedure

34. The nurse is at home and her husband accidental gets a caustic chemical splash in his eyes. What should the nurse do first? *(615)*
    1. Drive him to the hospital and flush his eyes with sterile normal saline.
    2. Call Poison Control and ask for advice about the specific chemical.
    3. Gently flush his eyes with tap water for at least 15 minutes.
    4. Assess him for burning, changes in visual acuity, or pain.

35. Which patient is the most likely candidate for the use of a Morgan lens to flush the eye? *(617)*
    1. Patient has allergic conjunctivitis in both eyes.
    2. Patient was sprayed in the eyes with pepper spray.
    3. Patient needs frequent eye irrigations at home.
    4. Patient has pain after prolonged use of contact lenses.

36. Which patient is an appropriate candidate for an ear irrigation? *(617)*
    1. A child who inserted a dried pinto bean into the ear canal
    2. A toddler who has a severe ear infection with exudate
    3. A teenager who has bleeding from the ear after a fight
    4. An elderly patient who reports a crackling noise in ear

37. The patient was diagnosed with a sprained ankle and the health care provider recommended a cold application for 20 minutes. Which condition would cause the nurse to question the order? *(621)*
    1. The patient's ankle is already slightly swollen.
    2. The pain medication has not had time to work.
    3. Patient has a history of peripheral vascular disease.
    4. The patient tells the nurse that 20 minutes is too long.

38. A cold application is ordered for the patient. The nurse is aware that a positive effect of this treatment is: *(620)*
    1. vasodilation.
    2. local anesthesia.
    3. reduced blood viscosity.
    4. increased metabolism.

39. There are principles to consider when using heat and cold therapy for patients. The nurse recognizes that the: *(627)*
    1. application usually lasts only 10-20 minutes.
    2. patient should adjust the temperature settings for comfort.
    3. patient should move the application around for relief.
    4. application is positioned for convenient observation.

40. The nurse applies heat to a fairly large area on the patient's trunk. The patient reports feeling slightly dizzy and his pulse is rapid. What is the best physiologic explanation for this systemic reaction? *(620)*
    1. The heat application has triggered a fever.
    2. The trunk contains some large blood vessels.
    3. The application is causing vasodilation.
    4. Antibodies and leukocytes are activated.

41. The nurse is giving instructions to the UAP about applying a warm, moist compress to a small abscess in the patient's axilla. What instruction(s) should the nurse give? (Select all that apply.) *(624)*
    1. Compress should be 105° to 110° F.
    2. Apply for 10-20 minutes.
    3. Report pain, exudate, or redness.
    4. Notify about completion of therapy.
    5. Evaluate the response to therapy.

42. The home health nurse is observing a family member assist the patient with a heat pad. The nurse would intervene if the family member performs which action? *(624)*
    1. Assists the patient to lie on the heating pad
    2. Adjusts the pad to the lowest temperature setting
    3. Places a cloth between the skin and the heating device
    4. Checks electrical cord for fraying or kinks

43. Just before IV line insertion, the nurse should: *(629)*
    1. shave the hair from the selected site.
    2. select a proximal site on the upper extremity.
    3. apply a tourniquet to impede venous flow.
    4. vigorously massage the extremity to be used.

44. Upon assessment of the IV insertion site, the nurse suspects that the patient has phlebitis. This is based upon the observation of: *(636)*
    1. edema at the site.
    2. erythema along the vein.
    3. cool skin around site.
    4. sluggish flow of IV fluid.

45. A blood transfusion is prepared for the patient. In setting up the IV, which solution does the nurse use to flush the tubing? *(644)*
    1. Normal saline
    2. 5% dextrose in water
    3. 10% dextrose in water
    4. Ringer's solution

46. The patient has had prolonged nausea and vomiting and requires IV hydration. On assessment, the skin turgor is poor and veins are flat and not easily palpated. Which IV catheter is the nurse most likely to use? *(632)*
    1. 16-gauge
    2. 18-gauge
    3. 20-gauge
    4. 22-gauge

47. The nurse is preparing the IV setup so that the IV solution will be immediately ready when the IV catheter is inserted. Place the steps of IV tubing preparation in the correct order. *(632)*
    _____ a. Select tubing based on patient condition and type of infusion.
    _____ b. Make sure the roller or slide clamp is functional.
    _____ c. Close the clamp.
    _____ d. Uncoil tubing and inspect it for kinks.
    _____ e. Remove the tubing from the sterile packaging.

48. Place the steps in the correct order for connecting the IV tubing to the ordered IV solution bag. *(632)*
    _____ a. Remove the solution from the package and check for expiration date, leaks, or contamination.
    _____ b. Hold the fluid bag upright and squeeze drip chamber to fill one-third to one-half.
    _____ c. Slowly open the clamp and prime the tubing.
    _____ d. Invert the bag to allow easy access to the tubing insertion port.
    _____ e. Remove the insertion port cover and remove the cover from the tubing spike.
    _____ f. Close the clamp when the tube is fully primed.
    _____ g. Insert the spike into the port until the plastic diaphragm covering the port is pierced.
    _____ h. As the fluid fills the tubing, invert injection ports to fill them.
    _____ i. Remove the tubing from the sterile packaging, inspect it for kinks and close the roller or slide clamp.

49. The nurse is monitoring an older patient who is receiving a fluid bolus for dehydration. The nurse notices that the patient suddenly has a slight cough and seems a little short of breath. The patient reports, "I'm okay." What should the nurse do first? *(636)*
    1. Notify the RN and the health care provider.
    2. Auscultate the lungs and compare to baseline.
    3. Stop the bolus infusion and establish a saline lock.
    4. Weigh the patient and compare to baseline.

50. The patient has an existing peripheral IV and develops chills, lethargy, headache, and nausea. What data does the nurse collect to help the health care provider differentiate sepsis caused by IV therapy versus other causes? (Select all that apply.) *(637, 638, 661, 675)*
    1. Review the white blood cell count results.
    2. Inspect the IV insertion site for infection signs.
    3. Compare the temperature to baseline values.
    4. Discontinue the IV and retain catheter and tubing for culture.
    5. Auscultate the lungs and assess respiratory effort.
    6. Ask the patient about urinary frequency, dysuria, or odor.

51. The patient requires suctioning of pulmonary secretions. An appropriate nursing diagnosis for this patient is: *(657)*
    1. Fluid volume excess.
    2. Ineffective breathing pattern.
    3. Ineffective tissue perfusion.
    4. Ineffective airway clearance.

52. Preparation for tracheostomy care in the acute care environment includes: *(653)*
    1. using clean technique and supplies for cleaning.
    2. preparing cotton balls to clean inside the ostomy.
    3. removing and cleaning the outer cannula.
    4. placing the patient in a semi-Fowler's position.

53. The nurse has inserted the urinary catheter into the patient and while the balloon is being inflated, the patient expresses discomfort. The nurse should: *(668)*
    1. remove the catheter and begin the procedure again.
    2. pull back on the catheter to determine tension.
    3. draw fluid out of the balloon and move the catheter forward.
    4. continue to inflate the balloon since discomfort is expected.

54. The nurse is providing instruction to the UAP on catheter care for the patient. An appropriate instruction is to: *(673)*
    1. maintain continuous tension on the external catheter tubing.
    2. empty the drainage bag every 24 hours.
    3. keep the drainage bag on the bed or attached to the side rails.
    4. clean the urinary meatus and 2 inches down the catheter.

55. The charge nurse delegates the removal of an indwelling urinary catheter to a new staff member. Which action requires correction? *(672)*
    1. Explaining the burning sensation with the first voiding
    2. Obtaining a final urine specimen from the drainage bag
    3. Deflating the balloon and pinching the catheter
    4. Using clean gloves and performing perineal care

56. Before the digital removal of a fecal impaction, the nurse checks the medical record. Which part of the patient's history alerts the nurse to be especially observant during the procedure? *(684)*
    1. Cardiac disease
    2. Hysterectomy
    3. Urinary infection
    4. Diabetes mellitus

57. The health care provider has ordered the application of a warm compress to a patient's leg wound. What does the nurse tell the patient about the compress? *(624)*
    1. "We soak your leg in a warm solution that has antibiotic medication for at least 30 minutes a day."
    2. "We wrap your leg with a towel and then apply a dry heating device that is similar to a heating pad."
    3. "We apply a hot water bottle to your leg and then wrap a towel around it to retain the warmth."
    4. "We apply a sterile, moist gauze dressing to the wound, then wrap it with a warm waterproof heating pad."

58. Upon assessment of a patient's IV site, the nurse determines that the site has become infiltrated. What are the sign(s) and symptom(s) that the nurse has most likely observed? (Select all that apply.) *(635)*
    1. Warmth at the insertion site
    2. Swelling at and above the insertion site
    3. Redness at the insertion site
    4. Coolness at and above the insertion site
    5. Sluggish flow of the IV fluid

59. The nurse is going to change the dressing of the peripheral IV line. Which action(s) is/are part of the correct technique for this procedure? (Select all that apply.) *(638)*
    1. Palpate the catheter site after the old dressing is removed.
    2. Leave catheter stabilization device (or tape) in place.
    3. Discontinue the infusion if there is erythema or edema at the site.
    4. Cover the insertion site with tape.
    5. Place tape over the transparent dressing.
    6. Label the dressing with the date, time, and nurse's initials.

60. There is less than 100 mL left in the IV bag and the nurse's shift will end in 30 minutes. The infusion pump is set to deliver 125 mL/hour. What should the nurse do? *(632)*
    1. Alert the oncoming nurse about the amount left in bag.
    2. Slow the infusion down so the fluid will last at least an hour.
    3. Hang a new bag and record IV fluid intake of 900 mL.
    4. Convert the IV to a saline lock to prevent an air emboli.

CRITICAL THINKING ACTIVITIES

61. Identify how the nurse achieves the following before, during, and after the performance of a procedure. *(614, 615)*

    a. Identify the patient: _____

    _____

    b. Reduce the spread of microorganisms: _____

    _____

    c. Provide privacy: _____

    _____

    d. Ensure the patient's safety: _____

    _____

62. The nurse has just finished inserting an IV catheter. The intravenous fluid is being regulated by an infusion pump. What would the nurse include in the patient teaching so that the patient knows what he/she should do during the IV therapy? *(633)*

_____

_____

_____

_____

_____

_____

_____

_____

63. Discuss special considerations for older adults who need intravenous therapy. *(634)*

_____

_____

_____

_____

_____

_____

_____

_____

_____

_____

Lifespan Development

Answer Key: Textbook page references are provided as a guide for answering these questions. A complete Answer Key is provided in your Additional Learning Resources on Evolve.

MATCHING

Directions: Match the terms on the left to the correct definition or characteristics on the right.

Terms

_____ 1. adoptive family *(701)*

_____ 2. nuclear family *(700)*

_____ 3. extended family *(701)*

_____ 4. single-parent family *(701)*

_____ 5. blended family *(701)*

_____ 6. cohabitation *(701)*

_____ 7. homosexual family *(701)*

_____ 8. grandfamilies *(701)*

_____ 9. foster family *(701)*

_____ 10. patriarchal family pattern *(702)*

Definition or Characteristics

a. Grandparents, grandchildren, aunts, and uncles living in the same household

b. Family with adopted children

c. Children may have loyalties to one parent

d. Same-sex couple

e. Parents and their biologic offspring

f. Unmarried couple living together and sharing responsibilities

g. Result of death, divorce, separation, or abandonment

h. Children may "age out" of system

i. Adult male makes most of the decisions

j. Related to increase of substance abuse, mental illness, military deployment, incarceration, and parental death

TRUE OR FALSE

Directions: Write T for true or F for false in the blanks provided.

_____ 11. It is estimated that a possible 5% to 25% of unfavorable outcomes in all pregnancies are attributable to smoking. *(699)*

_____ 12. Infants will speak spontaneously. *(705)*

_____ 13. The adolescent often requires fewer hours of sleep because of hormonal surge. *(721)*

_____ 14. According to the "Activity Theory" of aging, older adults choose to be less active and redirect energy toward internal needs. *(728)*

_____ 15. The fastest-growing segment of the U.S. population is the group aged 85 years and older. *(727)*

SHORT ANSWER

Directions: Using your own words, answer each question in the space provided.

16. Identify factors that have contributed to the changes that families of today have undergone and are still undergoing. *(700)*

_____

_____

17. Discuss the qualities of functional families. *(702)* _____

_____

_____

18. Three common causes of family stress are: *(703, 704)* _____

_____

19. Give an example of what happens during each of the six stages of family development. *(702, 703)*

   a. Engagement stage:_____

   b. Establishment stage: _____

   c. Expectant stage: _____

   d. Parenthood stage: _____

   e. Disengagement stage: _____

   f. Senescence stage: _____

TABLE ACTIVITY

20. Directions: Insert the expected values of vital signs for different age groups. *(707, 710, 716, 719)*

Age Group	Temperature	Pulse	Respirations (at Rest)	Blood Pressure
Infants at 12 months				
Toddler 1-3 years				
School age 6-12 years				
Adolescent 12-19 years				

MULTIPLE CHOICE

Directions: Select the best answer(s) for each of the following questions.

21. Which nursing action(s) contribute(s) to accomplishing the *Healthy People 2020* Health Indicators? (Select all that apply.) *(698)*
    1. Administers medication on time using the 6 rights
    2. Reinforces the need for preventive dental care
    3. Encourages patients to routinely exercise
    4. Assists patients to locate smoking cessation literature
    5. Shows respect and courtesy to elderly patients
    6. Teaches patients how to limit fats and sugar in the diet

22. The nurse is interviewing a woman who is from a different culture than the nurse's. The nurse directs the questions to the woman, but the woman consistently looks toward her husband and he gives all of the answers. What should the nurse do first? *(700)*
    1. Ask the husband to leave the room and continue the interview with the wife.
    2. Continue the interview and observe for additional nonverbal behaviors.
    3. Direct the questions to the husband, because the wife is deferring to him.
    4. Discontinue the interview and seek advice about how to interact with this couple.

23. The nurse determines that the family is primarily autocratic, based upon the observation of the: *(701, 702)*
    1. mother assuming dominance in decision-making.
    2. parents implementing strict rules and expectations.
    3. uncle controlling the finances.
    4. children participating in negotiations.

24. The nurse is assessing a 6-month-old infant, who was 21 inches at birth. Based on expected growth patterns, what height would the nurse expect on measuring this healthy baby? *(707)*
    1. 22 inches
    2. 27 inches
    3. 30 inches
    4. 31 inches

25. The nurse is assessing a 1-year-old child who weighed 9 pounds at birth. Based on expected growth patterns, how much should this healthy child weigh? *(707)* _____ pounds

26. Most of the weight gain in the first months of life is in the form of fat. What is the best physiologic explanation for this gain of fat? *(707)*
    1. Fat provides insulation and a source of nourishment if teething or other problems decrease food intake for a few days.
    2. In cephalocaudal growth, fat must be deposited in areas of the trunk and abdomen before growth in extremities can occur.
    3. Breast milk or prepared formulas are high in nutrients that are more readily converted to fat than to muscle or bone tissue.
    4. Muscle and bone require more protein and calcium, so development of these tissues is concurrent with intake of solid foods.

27. The mother of a 5-month-old infant reports the child is irritable; gums are red and edematous, and he demonstrates excessive drooling. What would the nurse recommend? *(707)*
    1. Advise the mother to contact the health care provider for treatment of infection.
    2. Suggest the mother wipe and massage the gums and offer sips of clear water.
    3. Teach the mother to brush the gums with a soft brush and fluoride toothpaste.
    4. Advise the mother to give an infant dose of acetaminophen for discomfort.

28. The nurse would advise the parents to contact the health care provider if their 1-year-old infant: *(709)*
    1. seems restless and makes little noises during short naplike periods.
    2. cries persistently during usual sleep periods and is inconsolable.
    3. sleeps 12 hours a night and takes one nap during the day.
    4. frequently kicks and stretches when in the supine position.

29. Which infant behavior is consistent with Piaget's theory that infants are in the sensorimotor stage of cognitive development? *(705)*
    1. Clings to the parent and protests any separation
    2. Reaches for objects and puts them into mouth
    3. Demonstrates shoulder control prior to hand control
    4. Frequently says, "me" and "no"

30. The working mother has an 8-month-old child who has to go to daycare while she works. How can the nurse best help the mother prepare for the first day of daycare? *(708)*
    1. Explain the likelihood of separation anxiety as a normal behavior.
    2. Emphasize that the child is likely to sleep most of the day, so he won't miss her.
    3. Describe the benefits of parallel play for cognitive development.
    4. Validate the mother's feelings of guilt and reassure that daycare is beneficial.

31. The nurse is teaching the parents of an infant the principles of introducing new foods. Which information should be provided? (Select all that apply.) *(709)*
    1. Citrus fruits may be given before the infant is 6 months of age.
    2. Foods should be mixed together to improve intake of nutrients.
    3. Cereals should be started before vegetables and meats.
    4. New foods should be introduced one at a time.
    5. Several days should pass between introducing new foods.

32. The nurse is watching a group of mothers interact with their young children. Which behavior by a mother would most suggest that additional assessment for potential child abuse might be required? *(711)*
    1. Retrieves toddler whenever he tries to run or jump or perform active movements
    2. Allows toddler to climb on a table space that is meant for snacks and drinks
    3. Berates and shames her toddler for refusing to share toys with other children
    4. Talks to other mothers and allows the toddler to fuss without comforting him

33. The nurse is interviewing the parents of a toddler who must be admitted for 23-hour observation for a febrile illness. What would be the most important question to ask about the child's bedtime? *(711)*
    1. "Would you prefer that he gets milk or juice in a night bottle?"
    2. "What do you usually do when you put him to bed?"
    3. "How many hours does he usually sleep?"
    4. "What would you like me to tell him about sleeping away from home?"

34. The mother is ordering lunch for her toddler. The nurse would intervene if the mother selected which food for the toddler? *(712)*
    1. Milk
    2. Peanut butter sandwich
    3. Carrot sticks
    4. Small banana

35. The parents report that their 3-year-old child has not started talking, but he seems happy and active and very interactive with the world in nonverbal ways. What should the nurse advise the parents to do? *(715)*
    1. Advise the parents to read to the child and ask him to name familiar objects.
    2. Suggest expanding opportunities for parallel play, such as at daycare or play groups.
    3. Reassure parents that children grow and develop at their own individual pace.
    4. Suggest consultation with the health care provider for possible hearing or speech problems.

36. The health care provider tells the nurse that he has to privately talk to the mother and asks if the nurse would please watch the 4-year-old child. What would be the best way for the nurse to interact with the child? *(715)*
    1. Take the child to the cafeteria and buy him a snack.
    2. Give him some crayons and paper and ask him to draw a picture.
    3. Ask him to "help" by sorting a bag of rubber bands by size and color.
    4. Explain why he has to wait and give him a book to read.

37. A mother reports that her child occasionally complains of pain in the legs particularly at night. Which question would the nurse ask to determine if this is an expected symptom? *(716)*
    1. "Has the child been running?"
    2. "How old is your child?"
    3. "Has your child appeared anxious?"
    4. "How much does your child weigh?"

38. The nurse must give the school-age child an immunization. Based on the nurse's awareness that the child is in the concrete operational stage, what would the nurse do prior to giving the child the injection? *(717)*
    1. Ask a helper to hold the child to prevent movement.
    2. Suggest that the child pretend that she is getting a fairy's kiss.
    3. Tell the child that it hurts a bit, but prevents sickness.
    4. Make extra efforts to protect modesty and privacy.

39. Which routine check-up(s) or screening (s) is/ are recommended for school-age children? (Select all that apply.) *(716)*
    1. Vision testing
    2. Dental every 6 months
    3. Hearing testing
    4. Scoliosis screening
    5. Cancer screening
    6. HIV testing

40. The nurse must perform a dressing change on a 7-year-old. The nurse explains that the procedure will not be painful, but the child appears apprehensive. What is the best approach for the nurse to use? *(717)*
    1. Demonstrate the procedure on a doll and answer questions.
    2. Ask the child to hold the tape strips and praise her.
    3. Premedicate with a mild anxiolytic medication and explain.
    4. Coach the parent through the procedure and stand back.

41. The school nurse is talking to a child who sustained an abrasion and bruise during recess. When the nurse asks the child what happened, he begins to cry, shakes his head, and refuses to answer. What should the nurse do first? *(717)*
    1. Tell him that all information is confidential, so he doesn't have to feel embarrassed or afraid.
    2. Call the parents and inform them that the child is emotionally overwhelmed and can't talk.
    3. Consult the school principal to see if something unusual happened on the playground.
    4. Talk to him while treating the wounds and give encouragement to establish rapport.

42. A parent expresses concern because her 11-year-old healthy, active son seems very short. She reports that all men on both sides of the family are tall. What is the best information that the nurse can give to the mother about growth and development? (Select all that apply.) *(717)*
    1. During the school-age period, the growth pattern is usually gradual and subtle.
    2. A second period of rapid growth is expected during adolescence.
    3. From ages 6-12, height increases by about 2 inches.
    4. He is probably lacking essential nutrients that contribute to height and weight.
    5. Distant genetic factors are likely to predispose him to a shorter height.

43. The parent reports that her 15-year-old daughter seems more moody than usual and she is concerned because there was a teenager in the neighborhood who recently committed suicide. What is the most important question that the nurse should ask to determine if the daughter has a high risk for suicide? *(422)*
    1. "Has she had a change in appetite?"
    2. "Does she seem to have an inability to concentrate?"
    3. "Is she preoccupied with thoughts of death?"
    4. "Has she talked about ways to commit suicide?"

44. The nurse is working with a group of parents of high school students. During the discussion, the following statements are made by the parents. Based on an understanding of the needs of adolescents, which statement requires follow-up by the nurse? *(721)*
    1. "We try to set reasonable limits on dating and are encouraging group activities."
    2. "The car has to be back home by 9:00 PM on school nights."
    3. "We are generally not in favor of allowing sex education to be taught at school."
    4. "The number of after-school activities are tremendous, so we suggest finding a focus."

45. Developmental tasks of early adulthood include: (Select all that apply.) *(722)*
    1. achieving financial and social independence.
    2. accepting self and others.
    3. maximizing personal worth and identity.
    4. making decisions regarding careers, marriage, and children.
    5. developing own value system.

46. Which behavior demonstrates that a 55-year-old adult is meeting his developmental task of generativity? *(724)*
    1. Ruminates over fears and lifetime failures
    2. Reorganizes personal belongings and assets
    3. Gives advice to nephew about succeeding in life
    4. Reviews will for distribution of worldly goods

47. The nurse is assessing the vision of an older adult patient. Which finding is not associated with the aging process? *(724)*
    1. Presbyopia
    2. Visualization of half the field
    3. Decreased depth perception
    4. Slowed accommodation

48. The nurse is working in a long-term care facility. Which activity will help the residents to meet the developmental task of ego integrity as described by Erikson? *(729)*
    1. Taking the residents out to lunch at a restaurant
    2. Reminiscing about past important events
    3. Assisting residents to maintain personal hygiene
    4. Leading the residents in an arts and crafts project

49. The home health nurse is interviewing an elderly patient who lives alone. The patient is underweight and the kitchen is so cluttered that it appears impossible to do any cooking or cleaning. What should the nurse do first? *(732)*
    1. Contact a local organization that will deliver meals to the house.
    2. Start an investigation to determine if elder abuse is an issue.
    3. Assess for additional factors that are contributing to the malnutrition.
    4. Weigh the patient and calculate the body mass index.

50. Based on knowledge of normal changes of the cardiovascular system, which recommendation would the nurse make to an older adult? *(730)*
    1. Maintain a low-fat, low-sodium diet.
    2. Obtain streptococcal pneumonia vaccine.
    3. Encourage coughing and deep-breathing.
    4. Change position frequently.

CRITICAL THINKING ACTIVITIES

51. Visit the home of friend, family member, or classmate who has an infant or very young child. Or visit a daycare center that cares for infants or very young children. Observe the setting, the way that the child interacts with the environment and other family members/people, and then review the safety rules for infants and children. Identify which rules that the family/daycare center already has in place and identify areas where safety could be improved. *(711)*

_____

_____

_____

_____

52. A young mother expresses frustration because she is having trouble toilet training her 18-month-old child. She reports that the child shows no interest in learning to use the "potty chair." She tells you that she has tried to sit the child on the potty chair and instructed the child to "urinate." She says that child frequently has temper tantrums when she places him on the chair.

   a. What can you tell the mother about physiologic development related to toilet training? *(711)*

_____

_____

_____

_____

   b. Use Erikson's stages of psychosocial development to explain how the mother can respond to the child during toilet training. *(711)*

_____

_____

_____

   c. What can you tell the mother about the child's temper tantrums? *(711)*

_____

_____

_____

_____

53. The nurse is working in an assisted-living facility. The majority of the residents are elderly and have some chronic health problems; however, many of the residents are active and only manifest changes associated with aging. Describe the physical changes that the nurse might observe in each of the following systems as a result of the aging process. *(729, 730)*

   a. Sensory: _____

_____

b.   Integumentary:_____

_____

c.   Cardiovascular: _____

_____

d.   Respiratory: _____

_____

e.   Gastrointestinal:_____

_____

f.   Genitourinary: _____

_____

g.   Musculoskeletal: _____

_____

h.   Neurologic: _____

_____

54. What influence does the aging process have on the following? *(729, 731)*

a.   Ability to cope:_____

_____

b.   Intelligence and learning: _____

_____

c.   Memory: _____

_____

55. Recall a recent interaction with an elderly person (patient, family member, neighbor, friend) and select one of the theories of aging that helps you understand an aspect of aging for that person. Describe what you saw and then explain how the selected theory supports your understanding. *(727, 728)*

_____

_____

_____

_____

_____

_____

_____

_____

Loss, Grief, Dying, and Death

chapter

24

Answer Key: Textbook page references are provided as a guide for answering these questions. A complete Answer Key is provided in your Additional Learning Resources on Evolve.

FILL-IN-THE-BLANK SENTENCES

Directions: Complete each sentence by filling in the blank with the correct word or phrase.

1. When any aspect of self becomes no longer available to a person, that person suffers a(n) _____. *(735)*

2. The process of adapting to and mourning a loss is called _____. *(735)*

3. _____ is a mental health treatment aimed at helping a patient deal with the pain of loss. *(737)*

4. _____ is defined as a common depressed reaction to the death of a loved one. *(737)*

5. _____ patterns include funerals, wakes, memorials, black dress, and defined time of social withdrawal. *(737)*

6. Hope is characterized as _____, even though the hopeful individual does not necessarily expect to achieve a specific goal. *(744)*

7. The most frequent symptoms experienced by the dying older adult are _____, _____, and _____. *(747)*

8. _____ is a deliberate action taken with the purpose of shortening life to end suffering or to carry out the wishes of a terminally ill patient. *(750)*

9. _____ are required in circumstances of unusual death (e.g., violent trauma or unexpected death in the home). *(756)*

10. Many believe that about a _____ must pass before the bereaved can begin to think of the deceased without feeling intense emotional pain. *(759)*

MULTIPLE CHOICE

Directions: Select the best answer(s) for each of the following questions.

11. Which person is mostly likely to suffer from a maturational loss? *(736)*
    1. A woman married to a police officer is informed that he has been shot and killed.
    2. A college student who has never been away from home goes to Europe to study.
    3. A school-aged child witnesses the family pet being killed by a speeding car.
    4. A middle-aged woman who was married for 30 years is divorced by her husband.

12. A student who normally gets "As" receives a "C" on her project and experiences a loss of confidence. Which behavior best indicates that the student is achieving growth because of this situational loss? *(736, 737)*
    1. Does the project over and over again until the teacher gives her an "A."
    2. Tells her parents to go to see the teacher and advocate for a grade change.
    3. Asks another teacher to look at the project and give an opinion about the grade.
    4. Requests a review of the project's strengths and weaknesses against the criteria.

13. Following the death of her husband, a wife feels that he is still with her. She also reports having dreams and vivid memories of him. Which question should the nurse ask to assess the sense of presence that the wife has described? *(738)*
    1. "Do you think he is trying to tell you something?"
    2. "What are your religious beliefs about life after death?"
    3. "How do you feel about these dreams and experiences?"
    4. "Would you like to see a doctor about these symptoms?"

14. On seeing the body of his little brother who just died from cancer, a 10-year-old sibling screams, "I won't go to the funeral! I won't go!" The mother is sobbing and the father begins to yell. What should the nurse do first? *(738)*
    1. Take the child aside and quietly talk to him about his feelings about death.
    2. Encourage the father to stop yelling because it is not helpful.
    3. Ask the mother to hold her child so that he can be supported and comforted.
    4. Calmly close the door and stay with the family while they express themselves.

15. A nurse is talking to a 63-year-old woman who underwent grief therapy for unresolved grief related to the death of her husband. Which behavior best indicates that the therapy is helping? *(741)*
    1. She frequently visits his grave site.
    2. She invites his old friends to dinner.
    3. She talks about things they used to enjoy.
    4. She cooks and serves his favorite foods.

16. As the nurse is performing medication teaching, the elderly woman begins to cry. "My grandson got into my pills and overdosed. He didn't die, but my daughter won't even speak to me." What is the most therapeutic response? *(738)*
    1. "Well, thank goodness he is okay; she should be happy about that."
    2. "I'm sure everything will work out; she'll get over it, give her time."
    3. "You feel like you were to blame for this, but accidents do happen."
    4. "Every time you look at your medicine, you think about your family."

17. The hospice nurse is visiting a family of a deceased patient. During the visit, the son displays symptoms of a grief attack. Which intervention would the nurse use? *(738)*
    1. Ensure that other members of the household do not get attacked.
    2. Reassure the son that he is safe and that no one will attack him.
    3. Help the son recognize that the attack is a type of grief response.
    4. Report the symptoms of the attack to the health care provider.

18. The UAP tells the nurse that the dying patient's family keeps calling for assistance with minor tasks that they could easily do for the patient. What should the nurse do? *(744)*
    1. Tell the UAP to do whatever the family or patient wants him/her to do.
    2. Encourage the family to participate in care to increase feelings of control.
    3. Ask the UAP to clarify what he/she means by "assistance with minor tasks."
    4. Assess the family's desire and ability to participate in the care of the patient.

19. Which statement by the family member of a dying patient best indicates a healthy retention of hope? *(744, 745)*
    1. "We are planning to take our father on one last trip to Europe next year."
    2. "My sister is coming from California next week; I know he wants to see her."
    3. "He really loves to golf and is looking forward to playing again this summer."
    4. "We know a man from our church who beat his cancer; Dad can do the same."

20. The patient is sobbing. When the nurse tries to find out what is wrong, the patient angrily says, "I'm dying! I have pain! My children are losing their mother! We are in debt up to our eyeballs! And God seems to be on a coffee break!" What does the nurse do first in order to use this data to identify and prioritize nursing diagnoses? *(745)*
    1. Use Maslow's Hierarchy and first address the physical issue of pain.
    2. Ask the RN to assume care because of multiple complex diagnoses.
    3. Collect additional data about each concern and consult with RN.
    4. Review the plan of care and determine if these are old or new issues.

21. Signs and symptoms that the nurse would expect to assess in the patient nearing death include: (Select all that apply.) *(754, 755)*
    1. lowered blood pressure.
    2. rapid, bounding pulse.
    3. irregular respiratory pattern.
    4. mouth-breathing with dry mucous membranes.
    5. rapid, anxious eye movements.

22. The terminally ill patient has been experiencing severe pain and has requested that the health care provider assist her to end her suffering. What should the nurse do if the provider orders a morphine dosage that could cause respiratory depression and respiratory arrest? *(759)*
    1. Administer the medication as ordered.
    2. Refuse to give the ordered dose.
    3. Tell the provider to administer the dose.
    4. Consult the nursing supervisor for advice.

23. On assessing the patient, the nurse notes that the pulse rate is 30/min, the respiratory rate is 8/min, and the systolic blood pressure is palpated at 60. The patient has a DNR order. What should the nurse do first? *(750, 751)*
    1. Call the family to the bedside.
    2. Make the patient comfortable.
    3. Initiate CPR and call for help.
    4. Start an IV and give a fluid bolus.

24. Which nursing action demonstrates that the nurse is performing his/her responsibilities according to the National Organ Transplantation Act (Public Law 98-507, 10-14, 1984) and the Uniform Anatomical Gift Act? *(751)*
    1. Assists the health care provider who certified death to remove suitable organs.
    2. Ensures that the clinical signs of death are present before death is certified.
    3. Explains the process of organ donation and transplant to the family.
    4. Contacts a qualified health care professional to ask family about organ donation.

25. Which action(s) indicate(s) the health care team is fulfilling the Dying Person's Bill of Rights? (Select all that apply.) *(751)*
    1. Nurse assesses pain and administers pain medication accordingly.
    2. Patient's choice of spiritual leader is contacted and rituals are allowed.
    3. Family is allowed to decide how much information is given to patient.
    4. Health care team creates a living will and advance directives for the patient.
    5. Nurse gives comfort measures and talks to a patient who is in a coma.
    6. Patient is allowed to make decisions, even though she seems indecisive.

26. Which nursing action is most likely to be affected by the patient's advance directives? *(751)*
    1. Instructing the UAP about how to perform select tasks of postmortem care
    2. Advising the health care provider that the pain medication is not working
    3. Assisting the health care provider to intubate for respiratory arrest
    4. Contacting the family if the patient dies unexpectedly during the night

27. The nurse is working in a pediatric outpatient clinic. There is an 8-year-old child whose grandfather has just died. The nurse anticipates, based on the developmental level, that the child will respond by saying the following: *(740)*
    1. "Grandpa will come back soon. He just went to see Grandma."
    2. "Grandpa was old and supposed to die. My cat was old; he died too. "
    3. "I was bad at school and talked back to Mom. That's why Grandpa died."
    4. "It was better that Grandpa died quickly and didn't have to suffer a long time."

28. The patient tells the nurse that he has a durable power of attorney for health care and medical treatment. What is the most important information to obtain from the patient? *(751)*
    1. The name and phone number of the person who will make health care decisions
    2. The name and phone numbers of the family member who is next of kin
    3. The patient's written permission to disclose information to the attorney
    4. The patient's wishes about his or her care when death is near

29. Number the following nursing actions in the order that they should be done for postmortem care, from first to last. *(755)*

    _____ a. Remove or secure all tubings according to policy.

    _____ b. Wash hands and don gloves.

    _____ c. Place patient in supine position.

    _____ d. Bathe patient as necessary.

    _____ e. Close patient's eyes and mouth if needed.

    _____ f. Allow family to view body and remain in the room.

CRITICAL THINKING ACTIVITIES

30. The patient lost her husband in an automobile accident a year ago. She is still experiencing insomnia and feelings of worthlessness and anger, and she continues to avoid family and social functions. A nursing diagnosis is identified: Grieving, dysfunctional related to death of husband manifested by insomnia, feelings of unworthiness, and avoidance of interpersonal interaction.

    a. Write a patient outcome and nursing interventions for this diagnosis. *(742)*_____

    _____

    _____

    _____

    b. Briefly use the concepts of loss and grief to explain the patient's behavior. *(740)*_____

    _____

    _____

    c. Identify at least seven factors that influence the experience of loss. *(737)* _____

    _____

    _____

d. Discuss how physical and social aspects of human functioning influence the grieving process. *(741, 743)*

_____

_____

e. What physical assessments will the nurse perform on this patient? *(741)* _____

_____

_____

_____

_____

31. Nurse A is a new nurse who recently started working on the unit. Nurse A likes and respects Nurse B, an experienced nurse who has been caring for terminal patients for a long time. Nurse A notices that Nurse B is efficiently caring for patients, but seems progressively cold, uncaring, and indifferent about everyone's feelings. Nurse B is particularly critical of one family because of how they act toward the staff and the dying family member.

a. Discuss what could be happening to Nurse B. *(738, 739)* _____

_____

_____

_____

_____

_____

b. What can Nurse A do to help Nurse B? *(739)* _____

_____

_____

_____

_____

_____

Health Promotion and Pregnancy

chapter

25

Answer Key: Textbook page references are provided as a guide for answering these questions. A complete Answer Key is provided in your Additional Learning Resources on Evolve.

MATCHING

Directions: Match the terms on the left to the correct definition on the right. (763)

		Term		**Definition**
_____	1.	conception	a.	Short vascular processes or protrusions growing on certain membranous surfaces
_____	2.	flagellation	b.	Cell formed by the union of two reproductive cells
_____	3.	zygote	c.	The embryonic form; a spherical mass of cells having a central fluid-filled cavity surrounded by two layers of cells
_____	4.	morula	d.	Developmental stage of the fertilized ovum in which there is a solid mass of cells resembling a mulberry
_____	5.	blastocyst	e.	Embedding of the fertilized ovum in the uterine mucosa
_____	6.	implantation	f.	Implantation of the fertilized egg outside of the uterine cavity
_____	7.	implantation bleeding	g.	Whiplike movements of sperm traveling through the mucus of the cervical canal
_____	8.	villi	h.	Medical term used to refer to the loss of a pregnancy prior to 20 weeks gestation
_____	9.	abortion	i.	Takes place when the sperm joins or fuses with the ovum
_____	10.	ectopic pregnancy	j.	Enzymes allow the blastocyst to enter the endometrium and implant; may cause slight bleeding in some individuals

FILL-IN-THE-BLANK SENTENCES

Directions: Complete each sentence by filling in the blank with the correct word or phrase.

11. The amniotic fluid acts as a cushion against _____, helps regulate fetal _____, allows the developing embryo or fetus room for growth promoting _____ development, and provides for fetal lung development. *(772)*

12. The very first fetal movements, characterized as "bubbling through a straw" in the stomach, may be experienced at _____ weeks. *(767)*

13. Chadwick's sign is a(n) _____. *(779)*

14. An early amniocentesis is performed to determine presence of _____. *(776)*

15. The embryonic stage lasts for _____ weeks. After this initial stage, the embryo is called the _____. *(764)*

TABLE ACTIVITY

16. Directions: For the parameters on the left, enter the expected change on the right. *(768)*

Cardiovascular Changes in Pregnancy

Parameter	Change
Heart rate	
Blood pressure	
Blood volume	
Red blood cell mass	
Hemoglobin	
Hematocrit	
White blood cell count	
Cardiac output	

MULTIPLE CHOICE

Directions: Select the best answer(s) for each of the following questions.

17. The pregnant woman reports blurring or diplopia. Which assessment should the nurse immediately perform? *(789)*
    1. Check the patient's blood pressure.
    2. Assess the patient's visual acuity.
    3. Auscultate the lungs and count respirations.
    4. Assess balance and coordination.

18. The woman has entered her 16th week of pregnancy and asks the nurse, "How is the baby growing?" The nurse provides accurate information by informing the mother that the baby will have: *(766)*
    1. development of head hair.
    2. attained a weight of about 27 ounces.
    3. settled into a favorite position.
    4. formed all organs and structures.

19. The nurse notices that the patient has facial swelling. What is the nurse's best response? *(783)*
    1. "This is a temporary condition caused by increased blood flow resulting from high estrogen levels."
    2. "An increased blood volume results in increased water retention, but the swelling should go away."
    3. "Facial swelling is something that has to be reported to your health care provider for follow-up care and evaluation."
    4. "This should be reported to your health care provider because swelling signals an increased amount of melanocyte-stimulating hormone."

20. The nurse notes in the health care provider's documentation that the patient is experiencing ptyalism. What should the nurse instruct the patient to do? *(783)*
    1. Eat small, frequent meals.
    2. Suck on hard candy.
    3. Sit up after eating.
    4. Avoid eating spicy foods.

21. The patient in the first trimester is advised to avoid exercising for more than 35 minutes in hot, humid weather. What is the best rationale for this advice? *(788)*
    1. An altered calcium and phosphorus balance could cause leg cramps.
    2. Maintaining balance and posture is more difficult during this time period.
    3. Prolonged or repeated fetal temperature elevation may result in birth defects.
    4. Stretching of the ligaments causes pain or tenderness in the lower abdomen.

22. The pregnant patient has been instructed to count fetal movements (kick count). Which statement demonstrates that the patient understands the procedure? *(782)*
    1. "I should count all movements during a 24-hour period."
    2. "I should choose a time of day after I have done my own exercises."
    3. "My baby should move at least 10 times in a 1- to 2-hour period."
    4. "I should feel the baby move at least 4 times after I have eaten a meal."

23. Which patient response indicates that she understands how to perform Kegel exercises? *(787)*
    1. "The exercises are most beneficial if they are done 10 times in a row, at least 3 times a day."
    2. "If I could perform the exercises 100 times in a row, I will only have to do them once a day."
    3. "I will perform the exercises whenever I have time to sit and concentrate for at least 20 minutes."
    4. "The exercises are most beneficial if I start performing them right after I deliver my baby."

24. After delivery, the nurse is examining the placenta. What is the most important observation that the nurse should note and document? *(764)*
    1. Weight of the placenta
    2. Presence of the placental barrier
    3. Appearance of the "Shiny Schultz"
    4. Intactness of the placenta

25. The nurse is examining the umbilical cord immediately after delivery. Which finding should be reported to the health care provider for further investigation of fetal anomalies? *(772)*
    1. The cord has two vessels, one artery and one vein.
    2. The cord contains a significant amount of Wharton's jelly.
    3. The cord is 50 cm long and 2.5 cm in diameter.
    4. The cord has a pale white, ropelike appearance.

26. The nurse is assessing fetal heart tones on a woman who is 12 weeks pregnant. What is the correct method for this procedure? *(772)*
    1. Use an amplified stethoscope and listen at the midline of the abdomen.
    2. Place the Doppler just above the symphysis pubis and apply firm pressure.
    3. Instruct the patient to drink a quart of water prior to abdominal ultrasound.
    4. Insert the transvaginal ultrasound probe into the vagina.

27. The nursing student is preparing to measure fundal height. At which step would the nurse intervene? *(772, 773)*
    1. Reviews the established protocol to measure this specific patient
    2. Verifies the patient's identity by asking name and birthdate
    3. Obtains a disposable paper tape measuring device
    4. Instructs the patient to lie supine on the examination table

28. The nurse is comparing today's fundal height measurement with the previous recording taken 5 weeks ago. What is the significance of a stable or decreased measurement? *(773)*
    1. Possible intrauterine growth restriction
    2. Possible multifetal gestation
    3. Possible excessive amniotic fluid
    4. Expected normal finding

29. The patient is at risk for a miscarriage. Which diagnostic test result is consistent with a miscarriage? *(774)*
    1. Elevated levels of maternal serum alpha-fetoprotein
    2. Declining levels of quantitative human chorionic gonadotropin
    3. Increasing levels of amniotic fluid
    4. Positive findings for chorionic villus sampling

30. The nurse is helping the woman prepare for an abdominal ultrasound. Which information is correct? *(774)*
    1. "You will have to drink several cups of water after the procedure to flush the bladder."
    2. "We will help you assume the lithotomy position for the examination."
    3. "The procedure is a little uncomfortable; just signal if you need to take a break."
    4. "You and your partner can watch the images on the screen if you would like to."

31. The mother has diabetes and is at risk for placental insufficiency. The results of the nonstress test shows 3 fetal movements accompanied by 2 increases of 15 bpm in a 20-minute period. The mother is so relieved that she starts crying. What should the nurse be prepared to do for the patient? *(726)*
    1. Encourage the mother to express feelings of anxiety or uncertainty.
    2. Prepare the mother for additional testing, such as the contraction stress test.
    3. Reassure the mother that crying with relief and joy is an understandable response.
    4. Support the mother through a repeat of the nonstress test for validation.

32. The mother is in her second trimester and reports "premilk" is leaking from her breasts. What should the nurse tell the mother? *(777)*
    1. "Any discharge from the nipples should be considered abnormal and evaluated by the health care provider."
    2. "Premilk or colostrum is not supposed to start until immediately after delivery."
    3. "Premilk will be pumped and discarded in order to stimulate the true breast milk."
    4. "If excessive leakage is a problem, breast pads can be useful."

33. The nurse is interviewing a woman who has just found out that she is pregnant. From a nursing standpoint, what is the best rationale for asking about insurance coverage for maternity and newborn care? *(778)*
    1. Information is used to determine the frequency of the prenatal visits.
    2. Admission to the hospital is based on the type of insurance coverage.
    3. Family will have additional stress related to finances if there is no insurance coverage.
    4. Number and frequency of diagnostic tests can be altered if there is no coverage.

34. The nurse is taking a health history and the information is likely to be used later during genetic counseling. Which question is the most appropriate in the initial data collection? *(764)*
    1. "How do you feel about undergoing genetic testing?"
    2. "What would you do if an abnormality is detected?"
    3. "Have you ever had rubella or have you had the vaccination?"
    4. "Would you like information about genetic defects?"

35. The patient had her last menstrual period (LMP) on August 18, 2014. Using Nägele's rule, when is the estimated date of birth (EDB)? _____ *(780)*

36. Define the parity of the pregnant woman using the GTPAL system: She has been pregnant four times, delivered three full-term infants, had no abortions or preterm deliveries, and has three living children. _____ *(781)*

37. The pregnant woman reports frequently feeling ill in the morning with bouts of nausea throughout the day. Which question is most important to differentiate between morning sickness and the more serious condition of hyperemesis gravidarum? *(783)*
    1. "How much and how frequently are you eating meals?"
    2. "Do you notice that you are salivating more than usual?"
    3. "Have you been vomiting? If yes, how frequently?"
    4. "Are you experiencing heartburn? If yes, when does it occur?"

38. The pregnant woman is a heavy smoker and she feels that it is unlikely that she will be able to quit. Because of the oxygen deprivation in utero, which outcome should the health care team be prepared to deal with? *(782)*
    1. Fetal respiratory distress requiring resuscitation
    2. Preterm delivery with low birth weight
    3. Intrauterine infection and fetal distress
    4. No change in fetal heart rate during contraction

39. The pregnant patient phones the clinic and reports having some symptoms that are causing discomfort and worry. Which symptom is the most serious and warrants immediate evaluation by the health care provider? *(783)*
    1. Shortness of breath when climbing the stairs
    2. Perineal discomfort and pressure with standing
    3. Muscle aches and difficulty walking
    4. Pain and burning sensation with urination

40. Which laboratory result should be reported to the health care provider because pregnancy increases the risk for blood clots? *(784)*
    1. Increase in the platelet count
    2. Decrease in the hematocrit
    3. Presence of protein and glucose in the urine
    4. Increased cholesterol level

41. The woman with a low-risk pregnancy tells the nurse that she frequently has to travel for her job. Which question(s) is/are most relevant? (Select all that apply.) *(793, 794)*
    1. "Will you have to travel to areas where the water is untreated?"
    2. "Will you be terminated if you refuse to travel?"
    3. "Have you checked the policies of the airline that you usually fly?"
    4. "Are you aware that magnetometers at airports are harmful to the fetus?"
    5. "Are you planning to travel to a foreign country?"
    6. "When you drive, do you use the lap belt and shoulder harness?"

CRITICAL THINKING ACTIVITIES

42. The nurse is working at an OB-GYN clinic and is aware that pregnancy is usually a time when women want to improve health habits and that expectant mothers are likely to want and welcome information about how to have a healthy baby.

    a. What counseling should the nurse give patients about self-care according to the trimester checklist? *(781)*

    _____

    _____

    _____

    _____

    b. Identify five drugs that the mother should avoid during pregnancy. *(765, 767)* _____

    _____

    _____

c.   In addition to selected medications, what are other activities or substances that the nurse will instruct the woman to avoid during pregnancy? *(782, 785, 788)*

_____

_____

_____

_____

_____

43. a.   Compare and contrast presumptive, probable, and positive signs of pregnancy. *(779, 780)*

_____

_____

_____

b.   Identify if the following are presumptive, probable, or positive signs of pregnancy. *(779, 780)*

Uterine enlargement:_____

Quickening: _____

Positive pregnancy test: _____

Amenorrhea:_____

Nausea and vomiting:_____

Goodell's sign: _____

Visualization: _____

Breast changes:_____

Hegar's sign:_____

44. The nurse is talking with a woman who is in the first trimester of pregnancy. The patient reports feeling "fat, sluggish, and bloated." She begins to cry and expresses feelings of guilt because she resents the pregnancy for making her feel this way and dreads what is coming, because "I'm just going to get bigger; then I'll start waddling like a duck and my skin will get all stretched out." The nurse recognizes that the patient has Situational low self-esteem related to perceived loss of control over lifestyle and Disturbed body image related to physiologic changes of pregnancy. What can the nurse do to assist the patient? *(788, 789)*

_____

_____

_____

_____

_____

Labor and Delivery

chapter
26

Answer Key: Textbook page references are provided as a guide for answering these questions. A complete Answer Key is provided in your Additional Learning Resources on Evolve.

MATCHING

Directions: Match the term/phrase on the left to the correct definition on the right.

Term	Definition
_____ 1. bloody show *(799)*	a. Begins with complete dilation at 10 cm and ends with the birth of the baby
_____ 2. effacement *(799)*	b. Involuntary uterine contractions that signal the beginning of labor
_____ 3. primary powers *(805)*	c. Turns and adjustments that occur as the fetus moves through the maternal pelvis
_____ 4. cardinal movements of labor *(808)*	d. Vaginal drainage and blood-tinged mucus typically increase as term approaches
_____ 5. second stage of labor *(809)*	e. Thinning and shortening or obliteration of the cervix that occurs during late pregnancy, labor, or both

FILL-IN-THE-BLANK SENTENCES

Directions: Complete each sentence by filling in the blank with the correct word or phrase.

6. Teaching about birth planning beginning in the _____ allows the family time to ask questions and retain information provided. *(797)*

7. The three primary options to consider for birth setting include _____, _____, or _____. *(797)*

8. The greatest advantage of birthing in the hospital is the _____ in the event that complications occur. *(797)*

9. The majority of home births are attended by _____. *(798)*

10. In most pregnancies, the uterus begins the process of labor once the fetus is _____. *(798)*

11. Several hormonal theories for the onset of labor are based on either an increase or a decrease in hormones. Some of the more common (but still unproven) theories relating to hormones are
(1) _____, (2) _____, (3) _____, and
(4) _____. *(798)*

12. True labor is marked by the onset of regular, rhythmic contractions that cause _____
_____. *(799)*

13. The five Ps of the complex process of labor and delivery include: (1) _____,
(2) _____, (3) _____, (4) _____, and
(5) _____. *(800)*

14. This reshaping of the skull bones in response to pressure against the maternal pelvis is called
_____. *(801)*

TRUE OR FALSE

Directions: Write T for true or F for false in the blanks provided.

_____ 15. Complications of a home birth are less than those statistically noted with hospital births. *(798)*

_____ 16. The mechanical theory of the cause of labor is a strong theory because there is a wide variation of uterine size between different pregnancies in the same woman. *(798)*

_____ 17. One of the signs of placental separation is a sudden gush of dark blood from the introitus. *(804)*

_____ 18. Fewer women suffered postdelivery emotional upset when their partners received support and assistance from parent education classes, health care providers, midwives, and nurses throughout the childbearing cycle. *(823)*

_____ 19. The woman should push to complete cervical dilation. *(806)*

FIGURE LABELING

20. Directions: Label the figure to indicate the fetal position in relation to the quadrant of the maternal pelvis. *(803)*

Right occipitoposterior ROP
Right occipitotransverse ROT
Right occipitoanterior ROA
Left occipitoposterior LOP
Left occipitotransverse LOT
Left occipitoanterior LOA

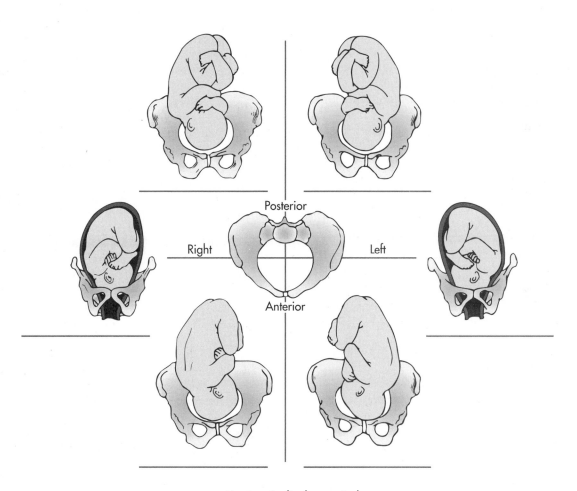

Posterior
Right
Left
Anterior

Lie: Longitudinal or vertical
Presentation: Vertex
Reference point: Occiput
Attitude: General flexion

MULTIPLE CHOICE

Directions: Select the best answer(s) for each of the following questions.

21. About 2 weeks before the due date, a nullipara patient reports that the "lightening" that was described in the prenatal classes has occurred. Which physical change is likely to occur because of the lightening? *(798)*
    1. Urinary frequency
    2. Decreased fetal movement
    3. Shortness of breath
    4. Leakage of amniotic fluid

22. The nurse informs the mother that the results of the nitrazine test are blue-green, pH 6.5. What additional information should the nurse give to the mother? *(799)*
    1. Advise her that precipitous labor is likely.
    2. Instruct her to go home and resume usual activity.
    3. Inform her that delivery should occur within 24 hours.
    4. Tell her that the test is nonreactive and that urine leakage is normal.

23. The patient in the first trimester reports an irregular tightening of the uterus and the health care provider informs her that these are Braxton Hicks contractions. What additional information should the nurse give the patient? *(799)*
    1. Call the health care provider whenever these occur.
    2. Expect Braxton Hicks to increase in frequency as pregnancy progresses.
    3. Anticipate that a headache and backache will accompany these contractions.
    4. Monitor these contractions for a few hours and then call the health care provider.

24. Which behaviors/symptoms would be considered normal and expected a few days before onset of true labor? *(799)*
    1. Depression and fatigue
    2. Vomiting and loss of appetite
    3. A loss of 5-10 pounds
    4. Renewed energy for cooking and cleaning

25. The nurse is assisting the health care provider to measure the pelvis of several patients. Which patient is most likely to undergo pelvimetry? *(800)*
    1. Patient is relatively thin and is in the early part of the first trimester.
    2. Patient is not currently pregnant, but has a history of pelvic fracture.
    3. Patient is in the second trimester and multiple fetuses are suspected.
    4. Patient is in the third trimester and placental location is questionable.

26. The patient gives a history of multiple pregnancies. What is the potential clinical significance for the fetus' attitude and lie within the womb? *(802)*
    1. A weakened abdominal wall increases the risk for a transverse lie.
    2. The fetus is more likely to be small and change positions frequently.
    3. The spine of the fetus will be parallel to the spine of the mother.
    4. The presentation is likely to be a complete breech.

27. The health care provider informs the nurse that there is a prolapsed umbilical cord. What should the nurse do first? *(803)*
    1. Assist the mother into a high Fowler's position.
    2. Apply a fetal monitoring device and count heart rate.
    3. Prepare the mother for a cesarean birth.
    4. Ensure that the health care provider has sterile gloves.

28. The nurse is caring for a patient who has completed the third stage of labor. What is the purpose and goal of massaging the fundus? *(805)*
    1. To achieve uterine atony
    2. To facilitate separation of the placenta
    3. To regain uterine muscle tone
    4. To determine the number and size of clots

29. The nurse is encouraging the mother to make frequent position changes during the first stage of labor. Which position promotes maternal cardiac output and placental perfusion? *(806)*
    1. Lateral side-lying
    2. Squatting
    3. Knee-chest
    4. Lithotomy

30. Put the following steps in the mechanism of labor in the order in which they occur for vertex positions. *(808)*

    _____ a. Extension

    _____ b. Flexion

    _____ c. Descent

    _____ d. Internal rotation

    _____ e. Expulsion

    _____ f. Engagement

    _____ g. External rotation and restitution

31. On examination, the patient is found to be 8 cm dilated with contractions every 3 minutes that last for 70 seconds. Which behavior is likely to occur in this transitional phase? *(809)*
    1. Alert and talkative
    2. Confused and disoriented
    3. Less talkative and focused on breathing
    4. Irritable and deeply focused

32. A woman who is in the mid- to active phase of labor will be expected to have: *(809)*
    1. 2-cm cervical dilation.
    2. contractions every 4 minutes.
    3. a desire to ambulate.
    4. very mild, easily controlled pain.

33. When coaching the patient through the early or latent phase of labor, the nurse uses the breathing technique of: *(829)*
    1. shallow panting.
    2. slow, deep chest or abdominal breathing.
    3. acceleration through contractions.
    4. holding the breath for 5 seconds and exhaling.

34. The baby is assessed after birth and the following are noted: heart rate 124/minute; respiratory effort good, crying; some flexion of the extremities; grimacing; body pink, extremities bluish. Based on this information, what is the Apgar score?_____ *(819)*

35. The nurse recognizes that which of the following is an acceptable practice in labor and delivery? *(821)*
    1. Maintenance of a full bladder
    2. Maintenance of supine position
    3. Ambulation before membrane rupture
    4. Administration of enemas in the presence of vaginal bleeding

36. The patient is receiving intravenous (IV) Pitocin for the stimulation of labor. The nurse notes that the fetal heart rate (FHR) is dropping below 100/min. The nurse should: *(830)*
    1. stop the infusion.
    2. slow down the infusion.
    3. monitor the FHR for 5-10 full cycles of contractions.
    4. do nothing, as this is an expected response.

37. Assessment of the amniotic fluid reveals yellow staining. The nurse is aware that this is associated with: *(819)*
    1. hydramnios.
    2. fetal hemolytic disease.
    3. abruptio placentae.
    4. meconium passage with a breech birth.

38. A birth plan includes the discussion of possible options related to: (Select all that apply.) *(797)*
    1. when to get pregnant.
    2. labor.
    3. delivery.
    4. the postpartum period.
    5. fetal development.
    6. genetic counseling.

39. The woman received general anesthesia by inhalation. Because the mother is at this increased risk for uterine relaxation, which action will the nurse perform? *(826)*
    1. Administer glycopyrrolate (Robinul) as ordered.
    2. Monitor for increased abdominal pain.
    3. Monitor for postpartum hemorrhage.
    4. Administer citric acid (Bictra).

40. Which patient(s) may be candidates for induction of labor? (Select all that apply.) *(829)*
    1. Patient had rupture of membranes 2 hours ago and labor has not started.
    2. Patient has high blood pressure with symptoms of headache and dizziness.
    3. Patient has a history of one stillbirth and one fetal demise.
    4. Patient has a history of diabetes mellitus.
    5. Patient has documented placenta previa.
    6. Patient has active herpes simplex infection.

41. Which patient(s) may be candidates for cesarean delivery? (Select all that apply.) *(831)*
    1. Cephalopelvic disproportion is present.
    2. Mother is a nullipara.
    3. Mother has a cardiac condition.
    4. Prolapse of cord is present.
    5. Presentation is breech.
    6. Fetus has a heart rate of 140 bpm.

CRITICAL THINKING ACTIVITIES

42. a. The admission assessment to the labor area includes: *(827)* _____

    _____

    _____

    b. Nursing assessment of a patient's status throughout labor includes: *(827)* _____

    _____

    _____

    c. For the fourth stage of labor, what are the nursing assessments and how often are they done? *(812)*

    _____

    _____

43. Discuss how the fetus is monitored and circumstances that would warrant notification of the health care provider. *(814, 817, 819)*

    _____

    _____

44. Discuss the use of Standard Precautions during childbirth. *(799, 800)* _____

    _____

    _____

45. The nurse is caring for a pregnant woman who is in the latent phase of labor. The woman becomes very agitated and panicky during the initial vaginal examination. She begins to cry and apologize after the health care provider leaves the room and confides in the nurse that she is a survivor of sexual abuse. She says, "I don't know how I am going to get through this. I feel so vulnerable and exposed."

    a. Discuss how history of sexual abuse may affect patients. *(823)* _____

    _____

    _____

    b. What can the nurse do to help this patient? *(823)* _____

    _____

    _____

Care of the Mother and Newborn

Answer Key: Textbook page references are provided as a guide for answering these questions. A complete Answer Key is provided in your Additional Learning Resources on Evolve.

FILL-IN-THE-BLANK SENTENCES

Directions: Complete each sentence by filling in the blank with the correct word or phrase.

1. The _____ lasts about 3-6 weeks, from the time the woman delivers the placenta until the reproductive organs return to the nonpregnant size and position. *(834)*

2. The decrease in size of the uterus is called _____. *(835)*

3. The tissue of light-skinned women, especially those with reddish hair, is not as readily _____ as that of darker-skinned women, and healing may be less efficient. *(836)*

4. In some cultures, including Chinese, Mexican, Korean, and Southeast Asian, there are certain postpartum rituals for mother and baby. These may include _____, _____, and _____ restrictions designed to restore the hot-cold (yin-yang) balance. *(858)*

5. Haitian women may request to take the _____ home to bury or burn. *(858)*

6. Newborns' and Mothers' Health Protection Act of 1996 requires all health plans to allow the new mother and the newborn to remain in the hospital for a minimum of _____ hours after a normal vaginal birth and _____ hours after a cesarean birth. *(859)*

7. Postpartum fatigue and _____ are common as a result of hormonal and physiologic changes. *(872)*

8. Parent-child _____ is the process by which parent and child come to love and accept each other. *(872)*

9. Motherhood is a(n) _____ skill. *(872)*

TABLE ACTIVITY

10. Directions: Complete the table below with the expected values for the newborn. *(859)*

Assessment of Newborn	Normal Value
Head circumference	
Relationship of head to chest circumference	
Temperature	
Pulse	
Respirations	
Blood pressure	

MULTIPLE CHOICE

Directions: Select the best answer(s) for each of the following questions.

11. The mother has lost a large volume of blood and appears to be in hypovolemic shock following the delivery. The nurse implements an appropriate action by: *(836)*
    1. raising the head of the bed to 80 degrees.
    2. discontinuing the oxytocic agent in the intravenous (IV) infusion.
    3. massaging the fundus firmly and continuously.
    4. providing oxygen by facemask at 8-10 L/min.

12. The nurse identifies that the mother requires additional teaching on the care of the infant's umbilicus if she: *(843)*
    1. gives a tub bath in the first 3 days after delivery.
    2. uses alcohol on the stump daily.
    3. folds the diaper down from the umbilicus.
    4. reports a foul odor or redness from the stump.

13. Care of the circumcision includes: *(868)*
    1. removing the yellow crusting right away.
    2. applying the diaper loosely.
    3. assessing for bleeding every hour for 4 hours.
    4. using petroleum gauze under the Plastibell.

14. An appropriate technique to teach the new mother about the baby's bath is: *(867)*
    1. vigorous removal of the vernix caseosa.
    2. use of plain water on the perineal area.
    3. washing the baby twice daily.
    4. having the bathwater at 100° F (37.7° C).

15. The nurse is discussing sexuality with the new mother. What information should the nurse provide? *(841)*
    1. Menses usually return in 3-5 months.
    2. Breastfeeding acts as an effective contraceptive.
    3. Discomfort and bleeding are expected with sexual activity.
    4. Avoid sexual activity until after the first postpartum office visit.

16. In teaching the new mother about breastfeeding, the nurse informs her to: *(843)*
    1. use one breast for two consecutive feedings.
    2. have the baby nurse for 5 minutes at each breast.
    3. put as much of the areolar tissue into the baby's mouth as possible.
    4. pull the breast straight away from the baby's mouth to break the suction seal.

17. The nurse is teaching the patient about the signs and symptoms that should be reported to the health care provider. The patient is instructed to notify the health care provider if, after 5 days from the delivery date, the patient experiences: *(842)*
    1. a temperature of 99° F.
    2. lochia that is light pink-brown in color.
    3. breast tenderness and redness.
    4. a fundus that feels like a softball.

18. The patient has opted to bottle-feed her newborn. The nurse is confident that the patient has understood discharge teaching related to breast engorgement when the patient states: *(842)*
    1. "I will most likely not experience breast engorgement if I manually express the milk."
    2. "If I experience engorgement, I should use ice to try to get some relief."
    3. "Engorgement will most likely occur about 10 days from my delivery date."
    4. "Breast engorgement is unlikely since I am not breastfeeding my baby."

19. The nurse is assessing a newborn infant who was just born at 30 weeks gestation. Which findings would be considered normal? (Select all that apply.) *(860)*
    1. Vernix caseosa
    2. Lanugo
    3. Desquamation
    4. Good skin turgor
    5. Good tissue elasticity

20. The mother reports that the new infant is making a weak, high-pitched crying sound. She has tried feeding, changing, rocking, and ignoring the baby, but the crying continues. What should the nurse do first? *(870)*
    1. Assess the mother-child interaction to see if there are problems with bonding.
    2. Try swaddling or bundling the baby to make him feel secure.
    3. Ask the mother to hold the baby while vital signs are obtained.
    4. Contact the health care provider, because the crying is excessive.

21. Normal variation(s) in the physical characteristics of a newborn that the parents should not be alarmed in seeing is/are: (Select all that apply.) *(859)*
    1. acrocyanosis in an infant that is 5 days old.
    2. the harlequin sign in a 2-day-old infant.
    3. jaundice during the first 24 hours after delivery.
    4. Epstein's pearls on the hard palate of a 2-week-old infant.
    5. lacy mottling on pale skin immediately at birth.

22. The home health nurse is assessing the mother's peripads 6 days after delivery. What is the expected finding? *(835)*
    1. Bright-red blood with tissue
    2. Thin pinkish-brown drainage
    3. Slightly yellow to white drainage
    4. Small clots with a fleshy odor

23. After delivery, which patient has the greatest risk for life-threatening postpartum hemorrhage? *(836)*
    1. Has a vaginal hematoma secondary to forceps-assisted delivery
    2. Has a vulvar hematoma associated with vulvar varicosity
    3. Has a vaginal hematoma related to primigravidity
    4. Has a retroperitoneal hematoma due to rupture of cesarean scar

24. Which treatment related to bowel function would the nurse question for a woman with a fourth-degree laceration of the perineum? *(836)*
    1. Administer stool softener for constipation as needed.
    2. Assist with ambulation in hall 3 or 4 times/day.
    3. Administer enema for constipation as needed.
    4. Encourage fluid intake of at least 3 liters/day.

25. The nurse is explaining to a mother who had an episiotomy how to use a Peri bottle to clean herself after urination or a bowel movement. Which information is correct? *(845)*
    1. "First, clean perineal area front to back with toilet tissue."
    2. "Use the whole Peri bottle of water to cleanse perineum."
    3. "Fill Peri bottle with sterile water warmed to approximately 98° F (37.7° C)."
    4. "Flush the perineal area twice a day for 20 minutes."

26. The nurse sees that the postpartum patient has an elevation in platelet count. Based on this observation, which action will the nurse perform? *(837, 847)*
    1. Observe the patient for fatigue, particularly after exertion.
    2. Monitor temperature and watch for signs of infection.
    3. Encourage the patient to get out of bed and walk around.
    4. Watch for signs and symptoms of hemorrhage.

27. In the postpartum period, the patient has no urge to void, but the nurse notes that the patient's bladder is distended. What complications are most associated with bladder distention in postpartum patients? *(837)*
    1. Uterine hemorrhage and urinary tract infections
    2. Rectocele and uterine prolapse
    3. Kidney dysfunction and painful sexual intercourse
    4. Urinary incontinence and perineal lacerations

28. The postpartum patient complains of a persistent headache. Which action would the nurse perform first? *(847)*
    1. Obtain an order for a mild analgesic, such as acetaminophen.
    2. Reassure that pregnancy-induced headaches will abate.
    3. Check the blood pressure and compare it to baseline measurements.
    4. Check the record for history of epidural or spinal anesthesia.

29. The nurse notes that the patient is profusely diaphoretic during the first night after delivery. Based on the nurse's knowledge of what is expected for the healthy mother in the immediate postpartum period, which action is the nurse mostly likely to take? *(839)*
    1. Assist the patient to change clothes and explain that diaphoresis is normal.
    2. Monitor the patient's temperature, because diaphoresis suggests a fever.
    3. Check the patient's blood sugar to validate that the patient is not hypoglycemic.
    4. Assist the patient to sit upright, to facilitate respiratory effort and oxygenation.

30. The nurse is trying to teach a 15-year-old mother how to swaddle the baby, but the young mother seems more interested in how her hair and makeup look. She states, "My boyfriend is coming in a little while." How should the nurse respond? *(840)*
    1. "Let's focus on the swaddling, then you can show him when he gets here."
    2. "You look very pretty. He will be delighted to see you and the baby."
    3. "Don't you want to spend some time holding and snuggling your baby?"
    4. "Well, you finish with your makeup and I'll take the baby back to the nursery."

31. The nurse hears in report that a patient who had a cesarean section should receive liquids for the first day with a gradual reintroduction to a regular diet. How does the nurse know when to offer solid foods? *(844)*
    1. Follow the protocol or clinical pathway for cesarean section patients.
    2. Give solid food when the dietary kitchen includes it on the meal tray.
    3. Call the health care provider and clarify specific parameters.
    4. Assess the abdomen and auscultate for bowel sounds.

32. The woman is interested in returning to her prepregnant weight as soon as possible. She has decided to breastfeed because "it's better for the baby and it will also help me lose weight." What information should the nurse give to the mother about nutrition and diet? *(844)*
    1. During breastfeeding, continue the diet recommended during pregnancy.
    2. For gradual weight loss, follow MyPlate suggestions and drink 3 L of fluid each day.
    3. Eliminate approximately 300-500 kcal/day for 6-8 weeks for weight loss.
    4. Breastfeeding does require extra calories, so weight loss is expected.

33. What is the most important nursing action to perform before assisting the woman to stand up and ambulate for the first time after the delivery of the baby? *(847)*
    1. Obtain a wheelchair and place it close to the bedside.
    2. Assist the patient to slowly sit and dangle legs while seated.
    3. Compare the blood pressure in the supine and upright positions.
    4. Assist the patient to apply a pair of slippers with a nonslip sole.

34. The patient received an epidural block. In the early recovery stage, what would be considered a normal finding? *(847)*
    1. Decreased sensation in both legs
    2. Altered level of consciousness
    3. Elevated blood pressure compared to baseline
    4. Low-grade fever

35. The woman's temperature is slightly elevated 12 hours after delivery of the baby. What additional assessment would the nurse perform first? *(847)*
    1. Check the appearance and odor of the lochia.
    2. Assess skin turgor and condition of mucous membranes.
    3. Palpate the fundus for height and firmness.
    4. Check a urine specimen for foul odor and cloudiness.

36. The unlicensed assistive personnel (UAP) tells the nurse that there was a gush of brownish vaginal drainage when the patient got out of bed and stood up. What should the nurse do first? *(847)*
    1. Inform the UAP that secretions pool in the supine position and flow is expected.
    2. Ask the UAP to describe the amount and color of the drainage and the patient's response.
    3. Check on the patient and assess for pain, dizziness, or continued vaginal flow.
    4. Tell the patient that there is nothing to worry about and help her clean up.

37. The mother reports to the nurse that the baby doesn't seem to be getting enough breast milk. What should the nurse do first? *(852)*
    1. Suggest that the mother supplement with formula feedings.
    2. Teach the mother how to manually pump the breasts.
    3. Assess the axillary region for engorgement of milk supply.
    4. Assess how the mother places the areola in the baby's mouth.

38. The nurse notices that the grandmother seems to be dominating the care of her own daughter and the new infant to the point of excluding the new father. What should the nurse do? *(854)*
    1. Gently suggest that the grandmother leave so that the new family can bond.
    2. Refer the family to counseling so that parental roles can be clarified.
    3. Assess the father's feelings about his role and his knowledge of child care.
    4. Wait until the grandmother leaves and then teach the father how to hold the baby.

39. The mother reports a mild cramping during the postpartum period. The nurse anticipates that the health care provider will write a PRN order for which medication? *(854)*
    1. Morphine
    2. Acetaminophen
    3. Aspirin
    4. Codeine

40. When is infant abduction most likely to occur? *(857)*
    1. During visiting hours
    2. In the middle of the night
    3. During the discharge process
    4. Upon admission to the nursery

41. Which assessment finding in a new infant should be reported to the health care provider for additional investigation? *(861)*
    1. Molding
    2. Strabismus
    3. Low-set ears
    4. Nystagmus

42. The nurse notes on assessing the newborn that there is a small tuft of hair at the base of the spine. What is the clinical significance of this finding? *(862)*
    1. This is the lanugo that frequently covers the newborn's body.
    2. This is part of the vernix caseosa that is usually left in place for 48 hours.
    3. Different skin colorations and hair patterns are related to genetic factors.
    4. Hair tufts indicate possible abnormalities of spinal column development.

43. Newborns are not able to synthesize vitamin K in the colon until they have adequate intestinal flora. Which action would the nurse take? *(866)*
    1. Monitor prothrombin levels and observe for bleeding signs.
    2. Administer an injection of vitamin K (AquaMEPHYTON) as ordered.
    3. Administer an injection of $Rh_o(D)$ immune globulin (RhoGAM) as ordered.
    4. Monitor the color, frequency, and consistency of bowel movements.

44. The newborn infant weighs 6.6 pounds. How much fluid does this healthy baby need every day? _____ mL *(866)*

45. The newborn infant has a blood glucose level of 40 mg/dL. The nurse prepares for which intervention? *(867)*
    1. Oral feeding of sterile glucose water
    2. Helping the mother to start breastfeeding
    3. Oral feeding of 15-30 mL of sterile water
    4. Administration of intravenous dextrose

46. Which nursing observation of the newborn's bowel function should be reported to the health care provider? *(869)*
    1. Initial stool is black-green with a sticky consistency
    2. Stool contains strands of lanugo, mucus, and vernix
    3. No stool is passed 24 hours after birth
    4. Newborn appears to be straining when passing stool

CRITICAL THINKING ACTIVITIES

47. What information would the postpartum nurse expect to get in a transfer report on a new patient who has delivered her baby and is being moved from the recovery area to the postpartum unit? *(839)*

_____

_____

_____

48. Identify the changes that occur in the mother's body systems after delivery. *(837-839)*

    a. Cardiovascular: _____

    _____

    b. Urinary: _____

    _____

c. Gastrointestinal:_____

_____

d. Endocrine:_____

_____

e. Integumentary:_____

_____

Care of the High-Risk Mother, Newborn, and Family with Special Needs

Answer Key: Textbook page references are provided as a guide for answering these questions. A complete Answer Key is provided in your Additional Learning Resources on Evolve.

CROSSWORD PUZZLE

1. Directions: Use the clues on the next page to complete the crossword puzzle.

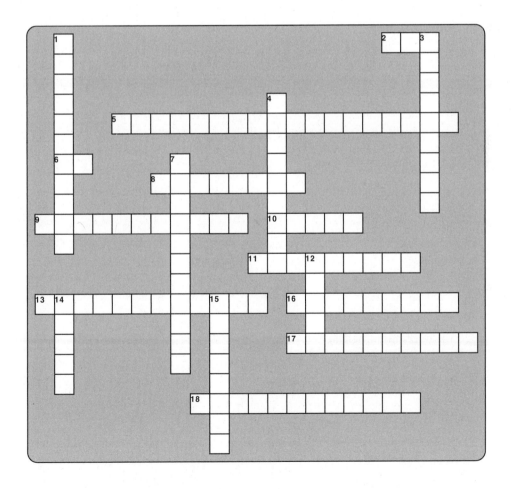

Across

2. Abbreviation for gestational diabetes mellitus *(898)*
5. Excess of bilirubin in the blood of the newborn *(912)*
6. Abbreviation for gestational hypertension *(889)*
8. Uses suture material to constrict the internal os of the cervix *(883)*
9. Phototherapy at home *(913)*
10. Organisms capable of crossing the placenta: toxoplasmosis, other infections, rubella virus, cytomegalovirus, and herpes simplex viruses *(894)*
11. Increased blood pressure after 20 weeks gestation with seizure activity *(889)*
13. Exposing the skin to fluorescent lights *(913)*
16. Number of deaths in a given population *(877)*
17. Excessive amount of amniotic fluid *(877)*
18. Increase in blood pressure *(889)*

Down

1. Twins begin with one fertilized ovum *(879)*
3. State of having disease *(877)*
4. Fertilization of two separate ova *(879)*
7. Abnormal toxic accumulation of bilirubin in central nervous system tissues *(912)*
12. Lack of normal tone or strength *(887)*
14. H, hemolysis; EL, elevated liver enzymes; LP, low platelet count *(893)*
15. Massive, generalized edema *(890)*

FILL-IN-THE-BLANK SENTENCES

Directions: Complete each sentence by filling in the blank with the correct word or phrase.

2. Factors primarily associated with mortality rates among neonates are _____ and _____. *(875)*

3. About 20% of cases of complete hydatidiform mole progress toward _____. *(880)*

4. About 95% of all ectopic pregnancies occur in the _____. *(881)*

5. Multiple pregnancy is suspected when _____ enlargement exceeds the norm. *(880)*

6. The preterm infant's greatest potential problem is _____. *(910)*

TRUE OR FALSE

Directions: Write T for true or F for false in the blanks provided.

_____ 7. It is still an immunologic mystery that a fetus is not rejected during pregnancy. *(893)*

_____ 8. Routine screening for gestational diabetes mellitus (GDM) is performed for most women during the second trimester. *(917)*

_____ 9. Prescribing oral contraceptives to postpartum adolescents is common because they are not likely to anticipate intercourse. *(902)*

_____ 10. A prominent feature of postpartum depression is rejection of the husband, often caused by abnormal jealousy. *(916)*

_____ 11. The woman who has gestational diabetes may have infections that compound the risk to the infant, including hepatitis; septicemia; and sexually transmitted infections (STIs), including AIDS. *(917)*

SHORT ANSWER

Directions: Using your own words, answer each question in the space provided.

12. Identify examples of high-risk factors in pregnancy for the following areas. *(876)*

    a. Biophysical:_____

    _____

    b. Psychosocial:_____

    _____

    c. Sociodemographic: _____

    _____

    d. Environmental:_____

    _____

13. Identify factors that place the postpartum mother and infant at risk. *(877)* _____

    _____

    _____

14. What are the characteristic physical manifestations of a preterm infant? *(909)* _____

    _____

    _____

MULTIPLE CHOICE

Directions: Select the best answer(s) for each of the following questions.

15. The patient is diagnosed with a missed abortion. Which signs and symptoms does the nurse expect to find during assessment of the patient? *(882)*
    1. Malodorous bleeding, increased temperature, and cramping.
    2. Some, but not all, products of conception are expelled.
    3. Amenorrhea continues, but no uterine growth is measurable.
    4. Bleeding increases and membranes rupture.

16. The nurse notes that the most appropriate outcome for a woman experiencing hyperemesis gravidarum is: *(917)*
    1. relief of painful uterine contractions.
    2. absence of fetal withdrawal symptoms.
    3. normalization of partial thromboplastin time.
    4. adequate caloric intake for maternal and fetal health.

17. In the care of a patient who has just been admitted for hyperemesis gravidarum, which task(s) can be delegated to the UAP? (Select all that apply.) *(878)*
    1. Assist with breakfast tray and encourage liquids.
    2. Measure and report frequency and amount of emesis.
    3. Assess for and report signs of dehydration.
    4. Assist with oral hygiene after episodes of vomiting.
    5. Assist the patient to maintain bedrest.
    6. Weigh the patient every day.

18. A patient is diagnosed with placenta previa. The health care provider indicates to the patient that she is stable enough to manage the condition at home. What instructions will the nurse give? *(885)*
    1. Take small amounts of clear fluid until vomiting subsides.
    2. Maintain bedrest, but getting up to the bathroom is allowed.
    3. Painless, bright-red bleeding is expected to continue.
    4. The prescribed tocolytic drug is used to relax the uterus.

19. The nurse's assignment on the postpartum unit includes patients with the following assessment data. Which patient should the nurse see first? *(890)*
    1. The patient has saturated one peripad within the last 2 hours.
    2. The patient has a blood glucose of 160 mg/dL.
    3. The patient had a spontaneous abortion and is experiencing moderate dark bleeding.
    4. The patient has had a continuous headache, upset stomach, and blurred vision.

20. The patient has a fasting blood glucose of 130 mg/dL. What sign/symptom would the nurse expect to finding in conjunction with laboratory result? *(898)*
    1. Cool, pale skin
    2. Increased appetite
    3. Frequent urination
    4. Irritability and tremors

21. The nurse is assisting an inexperienced health care provider who is in training to examine a patient with abruptio placentae. The nurse would intervene if the provider started to: *(886)*
    1. measure the fetal heart rate with a fetoscope.
    2. set up for a vaginal examination.
    3. place the patient in a side-lying position.
    4. order an ultrasound scan.

22. The nurse is getting change-of-shift report on several patients. Which patient is most likely to need vital signs every 15 minutes until stable and then every hour as indicated? *(886)*
    1. Has probable hydatidiform mole
    2. Had placement of prophylactic cerclage
    3. Has low-implantation placenta previa
    4. Has abruptio placentae requiring cesarean section

23. The nurse recognizes that the chance of hemolytic disease in the newborn is very low if which of the following findings are present? *(912)*
    1. Mother blood type O, infant blood type A
    2. Mother Rh negative, father Rh negative
    3. Mother Rh negative, infant Rh positive
    4. Mother blood type B, infant blood type A

24. The nurse is alert to a significant sign of gestational hypertension, which is: *(890)*
    1. edema.
    2. bradycardia.
    3. weight loss.
    4. hypoglycemia.

25. The nurse anticipates that the medication to be given to the patient who is experiencing severe gestational hypertension will be: *(891)*
    1. meperidine (Demerol).
    2. heparin (Lovenox).
    3. oxytocin (Pitocin).
    4. magnesium sulfate.

26. The nurse is working with an adolescent mother with her first child. A likely nursing diagnosis that is formulated for this patient is: *(903)*
    1. Knowledge deficit.
    2. Fluid volume deficit.
    3. Ineffective parenting.
    4. Cardiac output, decreased.

27. The nurse is teaching the pregnant woman about prevention of infection. In discussing toxoplasmosis with the patient, the nurse specifically highlights: *(895)*
    1. hand hygiene after using the bathroom.
    2. vaccination with an attenuated virus.
    3. reduction of sexual relations.
    4. avoidance of cat litter.

28. The nurse suspects that a postpartum patient being seen for her 6-week postdelivery checkup is experiencing postpartum depression (PPD). What patient behavior is evidence of PPD? *(916)*
    1. Demonstrates little interest in her baby
    2. Talks extensively about her labor experience
    3. Discusses her level of fatigue due to getting limited sleep
    4. Admits to having some problems with breastfeeding

29. A woman who had an incomplete abortion several days ago reports sudden onset of chest pain and dyspnea. The nurse notes bleeding gums, petechiae, and ecchymoses. To support suspicion of disseminated intravascular coagulation, which laboratory results will be immediately reported to the health care provider? *(887)*
    1. Cardiac enzymes
    2. Electrolyte levels
    3. Clotting factor studies
    4. Type, screen, and crossmatch

30. In the early postpartum period, the nurse notes a boggy uterus and the flow of lochia is heavy. What should the nurse do first? *(888)*
    1. Report suspected hemorrhage.
    2. Start intravenous oxytocin (Pitocin).
    3. Perform fundal massage.
    4. Continue routine assessments.

31. In the early postpartum period, the mother complains of severe, deep rectal pain. She has an increased pulse and respiratory rate and her skin is pale and cool. There are no obvious signs of hemorrhage that the nurse can see. What assessment should the nurse make to detect a possible hematoma? *(888)*
    1. Take the patient's blood pressure and compare it to baseline.
    2. Examine the vulva for a bulging mass or skin discoloration.
    3. Palpate the suprapubic area and listen for bowel sounds.
    4. Save all pads, linen savers, and linen to estimate blood loss.

32. The patient is diagnosed with gestational hypertension and is prescribed an antihypertensive medication. The AM blood pressure (BP) is 140/90 mm Hg. What should the nurse do first? *(891)*
    1. Administer the medication as ordered.
    2. Call the provider and clarify parameters for holding the medication.
    3. Compare BP to baseline; then administer medication.
    4. Call the pharmacy and ask for contraindications.

33. The pregnant patient with HELLP syndrome reports right upper quadrant and lower right chest pain, with nausea and vomiting. Which assessment technique should not be performed on this patient? *(893)*
    1. Auscultation of lung sounds
    2. Abdominal palpation
    3. Inspecting for hemorrhage
    4. Monitoring fetal status

34. To prevent mastitis, which teaching point would the nurse emphasize? *(894)*
    1. Take prophylactic antibiotics, as ordered.
    2. Increase fluid intake to flush organisms from breasts.
    3. Empty both breasts regularly by feeding or pumping.
    4. Apply cold packs between feedings to reduce edema.

35. In caring for an infant whose mother has tuberculosis, which condition will apply? *(897)*
    1. Neonates cannot metabolize tuberculosis medications because the renal and hepatic organs are too immature.
    2. Federal guidelines recommend that an infant not be exposed to the mother until cleared by health department.
    3. Tuberculin skin testing of the neonate is likely to yield false positives due to antibody exposure while in utero.
    4. Perinatal infection occurs frequently through exposure to amniotic fluids or by transmission through the umbilical vein.

36. The nurse is caring for a postpartum mother who was diagnosed and managed for peripartum cardiomyopathy. During labor, the mother required oxygen and demonstrated some transient arrhythmias, but otherwise had a normal delivery. What will the nurse plan to do in the care of this patient? *(902)*
    1. Routine care and assessment, because labor was the critical time for cardiac problems to surface.
    2. Obtain an order for oxygen as needed and continuous telemetry monitoring.
    3. Increase frequency of assessment for cardiac decompensation during the 48 hours after birth.
    4. Consult the health care provider to see if transfer to the cardiac care unit (CCU) is warranted.

37. In caring for the postpartum patient during the hospital stay, which intervention would the nurse use to prevent thrombolic disease? *(907)*
    1. Assist to elevate both legs.
    2. Gently massage the legs.
    3. Administer oral anticoagulant.
    4. Encourage early ambulation.

38. The nurse is reviewing the laboratory results for a woman who comes to the clinic for routine prenatal visits. The nurse sees that the mother is Rh negative. Which question is the most important to ask the mother? *(912)*
    1. "Is this your first time being pregnant?"
    2. "Do you know the blood type of the father?"
    3. "Have you ever received RhoGAM?"
    4. "Do you plan on having an amniocentesis?"

39. For a pregnant patient who is having a convulsion, place the nurse's responsibilities in the correct order. *(891, 892)*

    _____ Provide oxygen by mask at 8-10 L/min.

    _____ Notify the health care provider that a convulsion has occurred.

    _____ Note the time and sequence of the convulsion.

    _____ Insert an airway after the convulsion, and suction mouth and nose.

    _____ Remain with the woman and press the emergency bell for assistance.

    _____ Observe fetal monitor patterns for bradycardia, tachycardia, or decreased variability.

    _____ If she is not on her side already, turn the woman onto her side when the tonic phase begins.

CRITICAL THINKING ACTIVITIES

40. During a routine prenatal appointment, the patient's blood pressure is 140/90 mm Hg. The nurse sees that this is an elevated reading compared to the past several appointments. The patient is currently 22 weeks gestation.

    a. Describe the additional assessments that the nurse will make that will assist the health care provider in determining if the patient is developing gestational hypertension. *(890)*

    _____

    _____

    _____

    _____

    _____

    _____

    _____

    b. What is the treatment for mild preeclampsia? *(890)* _____

    _____

    _____

    _____

41. The nurse is interviewing a woman at the clinic who reports feeling more thirsty than before with frequent urination and excessive hunger. When the nurse performs urine testing, the results indicate the presence of glucose. The health care provider recommends testing for gestational diabetes.

a. Which diagnostic tests may be performed for gestational diabetes? *(898)* _____

_____

_____

b. What complications for mother and infant are related to gestational diabetes? *(901, 902)* _____

_____

_____

_____

_____

_____

Health Promotion for the Infant, Child, and Adolescent

Answer Key: Textbook page references are provided as a guide for answering these questions. A complete Answer Key is provided in your Additional Learning Resources on Evolve.

SHORT ANSWER

Directions: Using your own words, answer each question in the space provided.

1. Identify strategies to promote dental health for the following age groups. *(925, 926)*

    a. Infant: _____

    _____

    b. Preschooler: _____

    _____

    c. Adolescent: _____

    _____

2. Identify at least one nutritional consideration for the following age groups. *(920, 921)*

    a. Infant: _____

    b. Preschooler: _____

    c. Adolescent: _____

3. Identify three barriers to immunization for children. *(925)*

    a. _____

    b. _____

    c. _____

TRUE OR FALSE

Directions: Write T for true or F for false in the blanks provided.

_____ 4. Parents should be advised to monitor television shows that their children are viewing, because 61% of television shows depict violence. *(920)*

_____ 5. There is an increased risk of sudden infant death syndrome (SIDS) in infants placed in side-lying or prone positions. *(927)*

_____ 6. Fluoride supplementation for newborns should be initiated if the water in the residential area is not fluoridated. *(926)*

MULTIPLE CHOICE

Directions: Select the best answer(s) for each of the following questions.

7. The nurse is talking to an adolescent about responsible sexual behavior. Which question best demonstrates use of the principle of anticipatory guidance? *(919)*
   1. "What kind of precautions do you plan to use for protection during sexual intercourse?"
   2. "Are you sexually active now or thinking about having sex in the near future?"
   3. "Would you like to have information about HIV or other sexually transmitted infections?"
   4. "Abstinence is 100% effective; is this consistent with your beliefs and behavior?"

8. What would be the best way for the nurse to contribute to the overall achievement of the *Healthy People 2020* goals? *(919)*
   1. Administer immunizations to infants during routine well-baby visits.
   2. Teach health promotion classes for parents/children at a community center.
   3. Pass out healthy snack samples in the waiting room at a local children's hospital.
   4. Give burn prevention brochures to parents when children are treated for minor burns.

9. A young couple is seeking advice about how to help their toddler develop good lifelong health habits. What would the nurse recommend as the best method? *(920)*
   1. Schedule the child for regular medical and dental check-ups.
   2. Encourage the parents to obtain the recommended immunizations.
   3. Enroll the child in a daycare program that includes exercise.
   4. Role-model a lifestyle that includes exercise and healthy foods.

10. Which male child has the greatest risk for developing obesity? *(920)*
    1. A 3-year-old whose mother must work full-time
    2. A 9-year-old who eats at a fast-food restaurant every day
    3. A 13-year-old who spends 2-4 hours/day at the computer
    4. A 17-year-old who eats 5 meals a day with large portions

11. When an infant begins to transition from breastfeeding or formula to solid foods, which is recommended as the introductory food? *(921)*
    1. Strained applesauce
    2. Farina with whole milk
    3. Thinned rice cereal
    4. Strained bananas

12. The nurse is assisting a toddler to eat a healthy diet tray. Based on the child's developmental age, what would the nurse say? *(921)*
    1. "Drink your milk, then you can continue to play."
    2. "Let's have a race to see who can eat the most."
    3. "Would you like cheese or peanut butter on your bread?"
    4. "If you eat your vegetables, you will be strong like Daddy."

13. The nurse has a 14-year-old daughter who is refusing to wear sunscreen because "I want a tan just like my best friend has." What should the nurse say? *(921)*
    1. Tell the daughter that she can't go out unless she wears sunscreen.
    2. Review the dangers of skin cancer that are linked to sun exposure.
    3. Suggest that the best friend has heredity for naturally darker skin.
    4. Point out that red, peeling skin takes away from summer fashions.

14. Which age group is most at risk for foreign-body aspiration? *(928)*
    1. 1-5 months
    2. 6-12 months
    3. 1-2 years
    4. 2-4 years

15. The nurse is developing a nutrition plan with the parents of an overweight 12-year-old child. The parents demonstrate an understanding of the plan by stating: (Select all that apply.) *(920)*
    1. "Our child's calories from saturated fats should be no more than 7% daily."
    2. "We should not allow our child to drink milk that is less than 2% milk fat."
    3. "Our child should participate in physical activity for at least 60 minutes a day."
    4. "We should give our child foods from all the food groups except for grains."
    5. "Children outgrow obesity and complications when they reach adolescence."

16. Which statement by the child indicates an understanding of safety principles to reduce injury caused by motor vehicle accidents? *(923, 924)*
    1. "I won't play outside anymore unless somebody goes with me."
    2. "I will wear my helmet if I am going a long ways on my bike."
    3. "I will 'stop, look, and listen' if I have to run to get my ball."
    4. "I won't play behind parked cars or at the curbside of the street."

17. Which child has the highest risk for accidental ingestion of a poisonous substance? *(926)*
    1. Infant who is just learning to crawl
    2. A toddler who is visiting grandma
    3. A school-aged child who is cleaning paint brushes
    4. An adolescent who is studying chemistry

CRITICAL THINKING ACTIVITIES

18. Discuss benefits of physical activity and suggest ways that the nurse can promote physical activity for children. *(920, 921)*

_____

_____

_____

_____

_____

_____

_____

19. The nurse is preparing a discussion for a community group about how to prevent accidental poisoning. The nursing diagnosis identified for this group is Risk for poisoning related to lack of knowledge of safeguards.

    a. What are three interventions or areas for teaching that the nurse will incorporate into the presentation? *(926-928)*

    _____

    _____

    b. What strategies will the nurse share that will help participants prevent accidental poisoning? *(927, 928)*

    _____

    _____

20. Explain the factors that contribute to tobacco use among adolescents and suggest interventions that the nurse can use to help teens stop or never start using tobacco. *(921, 922)*

    _____

    _____

    _____

    _____

    _____

    _____

    _____

Basic Pediatric Nursing Care

Answer Key: Textbook page references are provided as a guide for answering these questions. A complete Answer Key is provided in your Additional Learning Resources on Evolve.

FILL-IN-THE-BLANK SENTENCES

Directions: Complete each sentence by filling in the blank with the correct word or phrase.

1. The crusade for _____ resulted in improved sanitation, the pasteurization of milk, and increased interest in infant care. *(932)*

2. _____ offers assistance with food and nutrition counseling for low-income pregnant, breastfeeding, and nonbreastfeeding postpartum women and infants and children under the age of 5 years. *(932)*

3. Three key components of family-centered care are _____, _____, and _____. *(934)*

4. A developmental approach considers children's individuality and personalities and builds on what they _____ to do rather than concentrating on what they _____ to do. *(936)*

5. When suctioning a child, the nurse should suction for _____ seconds. *(964)*

TRUE OR FALSE

Directions: Write T for true or F for false in the blanks provided.

_____ 6. In the early 1900s, children with contagious disease were isolated from adult patients. *(932)*

_____ 7. Despite the ability to regulate their temperatures, infants and toddlers are prone to wide variations, especially after crying for extended periods or after active play. *(939)*

_____ 8. After 2 or 3 months, the American Academy of Pediatrics states that the discontinuation of breastfeeding is a personal choice. *(944)*

_____ 9. Young children become very adept at understanding nonverbal communication. They sense anxiety or fear by the rise in pitch of the parent's voice. *(947)*

_____ 10. When young children play, this demonstrates that they are not having any pain. *(953)*

_____ 11. Compared to other age groups, newborns have the longest healing periods for fractures due to immature body systems. *(946)*

_____ 12. Generally, the extent of parental involvement is a good measure of the nurse's effectiveness as a teacher. *(956)*

SHORT ANSWER

Directions: Using your own words, answer each question in the space provided.

13. Identify three goals of pediatric nursing. *(933)*

    a. _____

    b. _____

    c. _____

14. Identify six stress points that are common for children undergoing surgery. *(953)*

    a. _____

    b. _____

    c. _____

    d. _____

    e. _____

    f. _____

15. Identify five things that the nurse can do to gain the trust of the parents. *(955)*

    a. _____

    b. _____

    c. _____

    d. _____

    e. _____

FIGURE LABELING

16. Directions: Look at the Wong-Baker FACES Pain Rating Scale below and label each face with the appropriate description of each face; then write an explanation that the nurse would give to a child about the scale, so that he or she could assess the child's pain. *(955)*

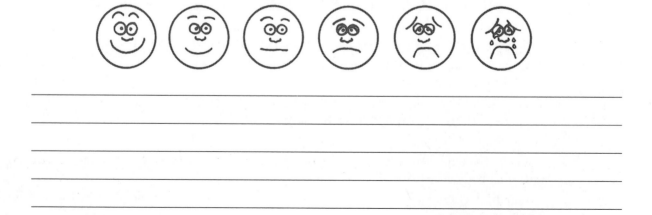

_____

_____

_____

_____

TABLE ACTIVITY

17. Directions: Complete the table below with the average vital signs for each age. *(940)*

Vital Signs (Averages)

Age	Heart Rate/Min	Respirations/Min	Blood Pressure
Newborn			
1-11 months			
2 years			
4 years			
6 years			
10 years			
12 years			
16 years			

CLINICAL APPLICATION OF MATH AND EQUIVALENTS

Directions: Calculate or make the necessary conversions for math problems encountered in pediatrics.

18. The mother reports that her 4-year-old has grown 3 inches in that last year. How many centimeters has he grown? _____ Is this growth within the normal range? _____ *(952)*

19. A 12-year-old is voiding 35 mL/hr. Over a period of 8 hours, how many mL of urine will he void? _____ *(965)*

20. Determine the expected systolic blood pressure of a 5-year-old using the quick formula to calculate normal systolic blood pressure. What is the calculated systolic blood pressure? _____ mm Hg *(941)*

21. The nurse is measuring the urine output for an infant. The wet diaper weighs 20 grams more than the dry diaper. How many mL does the nurse record as urine output? _____ mL *(965)*

22. A 6-year-old proudly hands the nurse an 8-ounce plastic cup full of urine, because he knows that "nurses like you to pee in a cup." Convert this to mL, so that the total can be added to the intake and output for the day. _____ mL *(965)*

23. The mother tells the nurse that she gave the child 4 cc (cubic centimeters) of liquid acetaminophen according to the instructions on the package. How many mL did the mother administer? _____ mL *(966)*

MULTIPLE CHOICE

Directions: Select the best answer(s) for each of the following questions.

24. There is a cry for help; a child is having a grand mal seizure and the mother is cradling his head and sobbing. The child recovers quickly, but the mother repeatedly sobs, "I didn't know what to do." What can the nurse do to empower the mother? *(934)*
    1. Stay with the family and observe for complications.
    2. Reinforce the fact that the child is going to be fine.
    3. Tell her that managing the head was the correct action.
    4. Ask her if this was the first time she witnessed a seizure.

25. Which nursing action best exemplifies partnering with the parent of a toddler who has been admitted for an exacerbation of asthma? *(934)*
    1. Suggests that the mother take the toddler to the play area
    2. Instructs the mother on how to hold the nebulizer
    3. Asks the mother for advice about the child's preferred rituals
    4. Maintains a cheerful and warm attitude toward the toddler

26. What factor(s) does the nurse consider when deciding which method to use to take a temperature measurement on a pediatric patient? (Select all that apply.) *(940)*
    1. Child's ability to cooperate
    2. Parent's preference for route
    3. Child's developmental age
    4. Parent's familiarity with route
    5. Child's need for precise temperature
    6. Child's psychological response to method

27. Which set of vital signs is closest to the average findings for a 2-year-old? *(940)*
    1. P 110, R 25, BP 94/66
    2. P 100, R 20, BP 110/80
    3. P 90, R 22, BP 108/70
    4. P 70, R 24, BP 120/76

28. Which vocalization exemplifies the vocabulary of a typical 1-year-old? *(946)*
    1. Mama, me; dada, me
    2. Burrr, ahhh, eeeehhhh
    3. Give me cookie cup.
    4. When is daddy coming?

29. Which set of vital signs for a 12-year-old requires a follow-up intervention? *(940)*
    1. P 124, R 32, BP 126/66
    2. P 90, R 20, BP 100/80
    3. P 88, R 20, BP 110/70
    4. P 74, R 22, BP 110/76

30. The nurse is reviewing infant development and recognizes that an expected finding for this age group is: *(936)*
    1. having a visual acuity of 20/100 at birth.
    2. enjoying "peek-a-boo" games.
    3. controlling bladder elimination by 18 months.
    4. tripling of birth weight by 6 months.

31. The nurse is preparing to administer an immunization to a 4-year-old child in the pediatric clinic. What is the best way to communicate this event to the child? *(957)*
    1. "This may feel like a pinch."
    2. "Don't move when I give you this."
    3. "Do you want to take this medicine now?"
    4. "I will be coming back to give you a shot."

32. The nurse has to administer a liquid medicine that has a bitter taste to a 5-year-old. Which strategy would be the best to use? *(966)*
    1. Use a syringe to squirt the liquid along the side of the mouth.
    2. Give the child an ice pop to suck on beforehand to numb the tongue.
    3. Give the child a glass of sweetened juice immediately after medicine.
    4. Hand the child the medication cup and allow independent sipping.

33. The nurse is evaluating the bath given to the infant by the adult caregiver. Identify what action(s) indicate(s) a need for additional teaching. (Select all that apply.) *(957)*
    1. Using soap around the eyes
    2. Using a cotton-tipped swab to clean the ear canal
    3. Supporting the head while bathing the infant in a tub
    4. Washing the extremities after washing the face
    5. Washing the perineum in an anterior to posterior direction
    6. Retracting the foreskin of the male infant

34. An older school-age child will be having surgery with anesthesia. The nurse intervenes to reduce anxiety by: *(955)*
    1. showing the child the mask that will be used for the anesthesia.
    2. introducing the child to a peer and having them discuss the procedure.
    3. reassuring the child that the procedure is safe and necessary for health.
    4. explaining the special type of sleep that will occur with the anesthetic.

35. The mother of a toddler asks the nurse how to get him to eat right. What advice should the nurse give? *(945)*
    1. "Food should be left out, so the child can eat when he feels like it."
    2. "The child should be restrained in the high chair for meals."
    3. "The child should sit at the table for scheduled meals."
    4. "Meals should be arranged about every 5 hours for the child."

36. The nurse is confident that health promotion teaching has been successful when the mother of a 3-month-old states: (Select all that apply.) *(946)*
    1. "My baby's birth weight should be doubled at the age of 6 months."
    2. "My baby should be actively exploring his environment."
    3. "My baby should enjoy parallel play by the age of 8 months."
    4. "My baby should enjoy toys that bang, shake, or can be pulled."
    5. "My baby should start eating rice cereals just before bedtime."

37. The nurse prepares to give an injection to an infant in the vastus lateralis muscle. Why does the nurse select this site? *(965)*
    1. This is the easiest area to expose on the baby.
    2. No blood vessels or nerves are near this site.
    3. This site is the least painful site for injections.
    4. The leg muscle is the least developed in an infant.

38. Which child is exhibiting behavior that warrants additional assessment? *(949)*
    1. 6-month-old infant coos and babbles to himself
    2. 2-year-old refuses to eat as much as he used to
    3. 10-year-old exhibits apprehension when another child cries
    4. 17-year-old is resistant to any parental suggestions

39. Which question best demonstrates the nurse's use of anticipatory guidance in helping the parents of an 8-month-old child? *(937, 970)*
    1. "Has your child been eating and drinking like he should?"
    2. "Have you looked at floor space from his perspective?"
    3. "Would you like to have a brochure on infant growth?"
    4. "Have you talked to the pediatrician about immunizations?"

40. The nurse is trying to auscultate the bowel sounds of a 4-year-old, but the child is resisting the placement of the stethoscope. What should the nurse do first? *(951)*
    1. Document the attempt as "deferred by patient."
    2. Let the child handle the stethoscope.
    3. Obtain the assistance of a helper.
    4. Ask the parent if the child has been eating.

41. Which vital sign should be performed first on an infant? *(939)*
    1. Temperature
    2. Pulse
    3. Respirations
    4. Blood pressure

42. Which assessment finding(s) would be reported to the health care provider for follow-up? (Select all that apply.) *(941, 942, 946)*
    1. Two palmar flexion creases in a newborn
    2. Tufts of hair along the spine of a newborn
    3. Preference for en face position in newborn
    4. Bumping into obstacles by 1 year old
    5. Lack of babbling by a 9-month-old
    6. Tongue protrusion by a toddler

43. The mother who is breastfeeding her infant tells the nurse that the infant's bowel movements, "look terrible." What should the nurse say to the mother? *(944)*
    1. "Infant stool is supposed to look different from ours because of immaturity."
    2. "The stool of breastfed babies is a light mustard color with seedlike particles."
    3. "The stool should be soft and formed with a pale greenish-yellow color."
    4. "As long as the baby does not have runny diarrhea, you should not worry."

44. What is the best rationale for advising the parent to withhold whole cow's milk until the child passes the 12-month mark? *(944)*
    1. Breast milk is cheaper and a better source of high-quality protein.
    2. The child is more likely to develop allergies to milk later in life.
    3. The protein and minerals in whole milk place stress on immature kidneys.
    4. Whole milk is more likely to cause vomiting, diarrhea, and flatus.

45. The aunt of an 11-month-old infant is making homemade baby food using materials that she has on hand. The mother would intervene if the aunt used: *(945)*
    1. white sugar.
    2. a blender.
    3. honey.
    4. frozen peaches.

46. What is the best indicator of readiness to wean in a 9-month-old breastfed infant? *(945)*
    1. The health care provider says that most children wean around 9 or 10 months.
    2. The infant reaches for his siblings' or parents' cup or drinking glass.
    3. The father remembers that the sibling was weaned at 8 months.
    4. The mother has to return to work, so breastfeeding is increasingly difficult.

47. Which child needs cholesterol testing somewhere between the age of 2 and 10 years? *(945)*
    1. Mother has a total cholesterol level of 200 mg/dL.
    2. Father has a total cholesterol level of 300 mg/dL.
    3. Grandparent died of a heart attack at age 65.
    4. Grandmother had a coronary bypass at age 70.

48. While examining a child, the nurse finds human bite marks, linear ecchymosis patterns, and round red sores. According to the parent, "he frequently gets into fights at school." What should the nurse do first? *(948)*
    1. Assist the health care provider to examine for occult injuries.
    2. Contact Child Protective Services and report suspected abuse.
    3. Ask the child to give details about how he sustained specific injuries.
    4. Assess the parent for signs of hostility toward the child.

49. How does the nurse use knowledge of body position and space to engage the preschooler and begin the nurse-patient relationship? *(950)*
    1. Stands in the doorway and greets the child by making a funny face.
    2. Directs the child to sit on mother's lap; then nurse holds child's hand.
    3. Puts chairs in a small circle and invites everyone to sit down.
    4. Allows the child to get comfortable; then nurse gets to child's eye level.

50. The nurse is placing the electrodes on the chest of a 4-year-old. What should the nurse say to the child? *(957)*
    1. Feel this; like little round band-aids with a bit of cold jelly.
    2. These snaps will hook you to the machine, so we can watch you.
    3. The electrodes allow us to watch your heart beat all the time.
    4. This won't hurt. It's just a way for us to see your heart.

CRITICAL THINKING ACTIVITIES

51. A child is being admitted to the hospital for surgical repair of a hernia. The nurse knows that the procedure should have an uncomplicated outcome, but the parents appear very nervous. The child is carefully watching his parents' reactions and the nurse sees that he is also fearful and distrustful of this new experience.

    a. What should the nurse do to reduce anxiety for the child and the parents? *(951)* _____

    _____

    _____

    _____

    _____

    _____

    b. What strategies can the nurse use when communicating with the child? *(938, 952)* _____

    _____

    _____

    _____

    _____

52. a. Identify the guidelines for performing a physical assessment on a child. *(938)* _____

    _____

    _____

    _____

    _____

    _____

    b. Describe methods that can be used to have the child assist while you auscultate his/her lungs. *(943)*

    _____

    _____

    _____

    _____

    _____

53. Identify characteristics in yourself that would make you a good pediatric nurse. *(933)* _____

_____

_____

_____

_____

_____

_____

_____

Care of the Child with a Physical and Mental or Cognitive Disorder

chapter
31

Answer Key: Textbook page references are provided as a guide for answering these questions. A complete Answer Key is provided in your Additional Learning Resources on Evolve.

MATCHING

Directions: Match the disorder with the clinical manifestations. Indicate your answer in the space provided.

Physical Disorder

_____ 1. hypertrophic pyloric stenosis *(1012)*

_____ 2. nephrotic syndrome *(1017)*

_____ 3. pneumonia *(996)*

_____ 4. septic arthritis *(1030)*

_____ 5. cerebral palsy *(1034)*

_____ 6. hyperthyroidism *(1021)*

_____ 7. diarrhea *(1009)*

_____ 8. otitis media *(1049)*

_____ 9. hypothyroidism *(1020)*

_____ 10. Duchenne's muscular dystrophy *(1029)*

Clinical Manifestations

a. Cough, wheeze or crackles, respiratory distress, chest pain, fever, malaise, myalgia, nasal discharge

b. Cool, pale skin; sunken eyes and fontanelles; poor skin turgor; lethargy; rapid pulse and respirations; weight loss

c. Projectile vomiting, hungry, weight loss, peristaltic waves from left to right, palpable olive-shaped mass

d. Delayed growth, dry skin, constipation, lethargy, mental slowness, cold intolerance

e. Nervous, irritable, hyperactivity, tremors, excessive appetite, exophthalmos, palpable thyroid gland, tachycardia

f. Involuntary movement, hypertonic movements, arching of back, delayed gross motor development, drooling

g. Increased body weight, decreased urine output, ascites, periorbital edema, vomiting, anorexia, diarrhea, irritability

h. Clumsy, frequent falls, a waddling gait, experiences difficulty running or climbing, Gowers' sign

i. Limited ROM to affected joint with erythema, edema, warmth, and exquisite pain; fever; limps or refuses to walk

j. Pulling, tugging, or rubbing the affected ear; fever; rhinitis; fussiness; irritability; decreased appetite

FILL-IN-THE-BLANK SENTENCES

Directions: Complete each sentence by filling in the blank with the correct word or phrase.

11. In coarctation of the aorta, the blood pressure in the arms will be _____ higher than that in the legs. *(983)*

12. American Academy of Pediatrics recommends that all infants be screened for iron deficiency anemia at _____ months of age. *(984)*

13. In aplastic anemia, red blood cells, white blood cells, and platelets are _____, and the red bone marrow becomes yellow, fatty marrow. *(986)*

14. The survival for children with acute lymphoid leukemia is more than _____. *(988)*

15. Performance of lymph node biopsy serves to determine the presence of _____ cells, an abnormal type of B lymphocyte, which is the main diagnostic feature of Hodgkin's lymphoma. *(990)*

16. The common indicator in all immunodeficiency disorders is the development of unusual or recurrent severe _____. *(990)*

17. A normal CD4+ lymphocyte count is _____ per microliter (μL) of blood. *(991)*

18. Successful treatment outcome for pulmonary tuberculosis depends on compliance with the _____ regimen. *(1001)*

TRUE OR FALSE

Directions: Write T for true or F for false in the blanks provided.

_____ 19.   In caring for a child with Hirschsprung's disease, the nurse anticipates that the parents will need teaching about how to care for a colostomy. *(1015)*

_____ 20.   Wilms' tumor (or nephroblastoma) is the most common renal and intraabdominal malignant tumor of childhood. *(1019)*

_____ 21.   The nurse expects that the treatment for a child with cryptorchidism will include circumcision. *(1020)*

_____ 22.   The nutritional needs of children with diabetes are very different from those of unaffected children and food intake is closely monitored to meet those needs. *(1023)*

_____ 23.   Children with Duchenne's muscular dystrophy (DMD) rarely live past age 20, with death resulting from respiratory or cardiac complications. *(1029)*

_____ 24.   Suicide is the third leading cause of death among 10- to 19-year-olds in the United States. *(1062)*

SHORT ANSWER

Directions: Using your own words, answer each question in the space provided.

25. The most current congenital heart disease categories are related to which four physiologic characteristics? *(978)*

    a. _____

    b. _____

    c. _____

    d. _____

26. Tetralogy of Fallot (TOF) involves a combination of four defects: *(982)*

    a. _____

    b. _____

    c. _____

    d. _____

27. What are three pathophysiologic changes of blood components and the associated effects that develop during leukemia? *(989)*

    a. _____

    b. _____

    c. _____

28. Identify the four classifications by causative agent for pneumonia. *(996)*

    a. _____

    b. _____

    c. _____

    d. _____

29. The ESSR feeding technique works especially well for infants with cleft lip/palate prior to corrective surgery. What does ESSR stand for? *(1007)*

    E _____

    S _____

    S _____

    R _____

TABLE ACTIVITY

30. Directions: Complete the table below by filling in the signs and symptoms for each assessment that indicates the clinical manifestations of dehydration. *(1008)*

Clinical Manifestations of Dehydration

Assessment	Signs and Symptoms
Skin	
Mucous membranes	
Eyes	
Fontanelles	
Behavior	
Pulse	
Blood pressure	
Respirations	

FIGURE LABELING

31. Directions: On the figure below, identify the assessment findings for the infant. *(1025)*

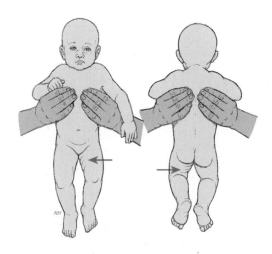

CLINICAL APPLICATION OF MATH AND CONVERSIONS

32. The nurse is performing a physical examination on a 9-month-old infant. At birth, the infant weighed 7 pounds. The current weight is 15 pounds. How much weight has the child gained in kilograms? _____ kg (979)

33. Toddlers require 7 mg/day of iron. The mother has purchased a bottle of liquid iron and the label indicates that there are 40 mg/15 mL. The mother is unable to determine how much to give. How many mLs does the nurse tell her to give the child to achieve the correct dose? _____ mL (983)

34. The nurse must calculate an infant's urine output by weighing the wet diaper. The wet diaper weighs 35 grams more than the dry diaper. What does the nurse record for urine output? _____ mL (965)

MULTIPLE CHOICE

Directions: Select the best answer(s) for each of the following questions.

35. The child has a hemoglobin (Hgb) value of 8 g/dL. Which symptom would the nurse expect to see at this hemoglobin level? (984)
    1. Fatigue
    2. Pallor
    3. Glossitis
    4. "Spoon" fingernails

36. A common sign or symptom of patent ductus arteriosus and septal defects is: (980)
    1. murmur.
    2. chest pain.
    3. hypotension.
    4. headache.

37. The nurse recognizes that the majority of congenital heart defects are treated with: (981, 982)
    1. diet.
    2. exercise.
    3. surgery.
    4. medication.

38. Screenings are being conducted on children for blood disorders. The nurse is aware that the most prevalent blood disorder is: (983)
    1. hemophilia.
    2. sickle cell anemia.
    3. iron deficiency anemia.
    4. idiopathic thrombocytopenic purpura.

39. The nurse instructs the parents of a child with iron deficiency anemia that iron absorption may be enhanced by: (984)
    1. giving the supplement with milk.
    2. giving the supplement with citrus juice or fruits.
    3. offering a chewable form once each day.
    4. waiting until the child has a full stomach to administer.

40. Which child(ren) need(s) an iron supplement? (Select all that apply.) (983, 984)
    1. A 5-month-old infant who is exclusively breastfed
    2. A healthy toddler with age-appropriate eating habits
    3. A 16-year-old girl who is trying to lose weight
    4. A preterm infant with low birth weight
    5. A 10-month-old infant who eats commercial infant cereal

41. A young woman with sickle cell disease wants to take a vacation with friends. Which trip would be the best choice to avoid the precipitating factors of a sickle cell crisis? (984, 985)
    1. Cross-country ski trip
    2. Hiking in the mountains
    3. Road trip to the beach
    4. Flying to Europe

42. The nurse is talking to a mother of a 10-year-old boy who has hemophilia. Which toy would be the best to recommend for this child? (987)
    1. Skateboard
    2. Football
    3. Swim fins
    4. Bicycle

43. Which blood disorder places a child at greatest risk for intracranial bleeding if head injury occurs? *(987, 988)*
    1. Sickle cell anemia
    2. Sickle cell trait
    3. Iron deficiency anemia
    4. Idiopathic thrombocytopenia purpura

44. The child with leukemia has been placed in reverse isolation. Which person should not enter the room? *(988, 989)*
    1. A 5-month-old sibling who was born prematurely
    2. A 3-year-old sibling who is coughing and sneezing
    3. A nursing student who is 5 months pregnant
    4. A parent who works at a waste management plant

45. In HIV testing for a child who is younger than 18 months of age, what is the physiologic explanation for not using the standardized testing procedures [Western blot test and enzyme-linked immunosorbent assay (ELISA)]? *(991)*
    1. Infant's immune system is too immature to produce antibodies.
    2. It is unclear whether antibodies are the mother's or the infant's.
    3. The polymerase chain reaction (PCR) test is safer for infants.
    4. Standardized tests yield too many false negatives for infants.

46. The nurse is talking to a 17-year-old who recently found out that he is HIV positive. He says, "I guess I really blew it. I'm so screwed." What is the most therapeutic response? *(992)*
    1. "Yes, you made a serious mistake, but you can take the medications."
    2. "You are very young and you shouldn't blame yourself for making a mistake."
    3. "You are thinking about your future and how to live with being HIV positive."
    4. "You sound really scared. Well, don't worry; with treatments, you'll be okay."

47. The child has recently been diagnosed with juvenile idiopathic arthritis. The nurse will prepare an educational brochure for which type of drugs? *(993)*
    1. Nonsteroidal antiinflammatory drugs (NSAIDs)
    2. Slower-acting antirheumatic drugs (SAARDs)
    3. Disease-modifying antirheumatic drugs (DMARDs)
    4. Tumor necrosis factor (TNF) blockers

48. In caring for a neonate who was intubated for respiratory distress syndrome (RDS), when does the nurse perform endotracheal tube suctioning? *(995)*
    1. Routinely every 2 hours or according to facility policy
    2. According to the health care provider's written orders
    3. After auscultation of lungs and noting moisture in the tube
    4. When the neonate begins to secrete and cough up mucus

49. In the acute phase of RDS, which route of feeding is most likely to be used for the neonate? *(995)*
    1. Bottle feeding
    2. Breastfeeding
    3. Parenteral nutrition
    4. Gavage feeding

50. The nurse is reinforcing the instructions to treat the child's viral pharyngitis with lozenges, gargles, and acetaminophen. The mother tells the nurse that she wants a prescription for antibiotics. What is the best response? *(998)*
    1. "The health care provider didn't order any antibiotics."
    2. "Viral pharyngitis is always treated conservatively."
    3. "Let me call the health care provider so that you can talk to him."
    4. "The throat culture showed no evidence of bacterial infection."

51. Which two conditions can develop if streptococcal infections are inadequately treated? *(998)*
    1. Heart failure and nephrotic syndrome
    2. Rheumatic fever and acute glomerulonephritis
    3. Iron deficiency anemia and gastroenteritis
    4. Bronchopulmonary dysplasia and pneumonia

52. The nurse is caring for a child who had a tonsillectomy. Which report from the UAP is the greatest concern? *(999)*
    1. "I put the bed flat, because he wanted to go to sleep."
    2. "His pulse is 140/min and earlier in the shift it was 90/min."
    3. "I gave him a cup of red soda, because that's what he wanted."
    4. "He got out of bed and has been running up and down the hall."

53. The nurse is assisting an inexperienced health care provider to examine a child who appears acutely ill with high fever, muffled voice, drooling, and progressive respiratory distress. The nurse would intervene if the provider started to perform which action? *(1000)*
    1. Suggested that the mother hold the child on her lap
    2. Called the operating room to alert them about the child
    3. Examined the back of the throat using a tongue blade
    4. Took a history of prior upper respiratory infection

54. The child presents with a nonproductive, hacking cough that worsens at night. The health care provider makes the diagnosis of bronchitis. Which instruction will the nurse give to the parent? *(1000)*
    1. "Complete all antibiotics as prescribed."
    2. "Cough suppressants will cause drowsiness."
    3. "Use a cool-mist humidifier to relieve cough."
    4. "Withhold fluids at night to decrease secretions."

55. The nurse is working on the pediatric unit and five patients have bronchiolitis caused by respiratory syncytial virus. What infection-control measure could be considered in making care assignments? *(1001)*
    1. Health care personnel with minor infections should not be assigned to these patients.
    2. Each patient is placed in a negative pressure room and care is more time-consuming.
    3. All of these patients should be placed in the same room with one nurse to give care.
    4. Nurses who care for these patients should not be assigned to other high-risk patients.

56. For patients with cystic fibrosis, which body system is targeted to prevent the most likely complications? *(1002)*
    1. Cardiac
    2. Renal
    3. Gastrointestinal
    4. Respiratory

57. Immediately following cleft palate surgery, the infant is NPO. After the nurse determines that the effects of the anesthesia have disappeared, what is the first thing to feed the infant? *(1007)*
    1. Breast milk
    2. Regular formula
    3. Dextrose water
    4. Whole milk

58. For the child experiencing gastroenteritis with diarrhea, the nurse anticipates that treatment will include: *(1009)*
    1. nothing-by-mouth status (NPO).
    2. oral rehydration.
    3. no solid foods for 48 hours.
    4. traditional BRAT diet.

59. There are several different types of hernias that children may experience. The type of hernia that usually has spontaneous closure by the time the child is 2 years old is: *(1016)*
    1. hiatal.
    2. inguinal.
    3. umbilical.
    4. diaphragmatic.

60. The most severe type of hernia that is found within hours of delivery and requires immediate surgical repair is: *(1016)*
    1. hiatal.
    2. inguinal.
    3. umbilical.
    4. diaphragmatic.

61. The nurse anticipates that a child who is receiving pharmacologic treatment for gastroesophageal reflux will receive: *(1011)*
    1. Compazine (prochlorperazine).
    2. Mylanta (calcium chloride).
    3. Tagamet (cimetidine).
    4. Cerebyx (fosphenytoin).

62. The nurse is caring for an 8-year-old child who has severe diarrhea. IV fluid is ordered and potassium has been added by the pharmacy as ordered by the health care provider. Before the nurse hangs the IV solution, which function must be verified? *(1009)*
    1. Auscultate the lungs for the presence of crackles or wheezes.
    2. Check the urine output to ensure that output is at least 30 mL/hour.
    3. Auscultate for bowel sounds to determine presence of peristalsis.
    4. Check blood sugar for evidence of hypoglycemia.

63. A mother brings the 5-year-old child to the clinic for constipation. The mother reports that the child eats what the family eats, takes no medication, has no known health problems, and is very active. What question(s) will the nurse ask the child? (Select all that apply.) *(1010)*
    1. "What does it feel like when you try to go to the bathroom?"
    2. "When you feel like you have to go, do you go right then or wait?"
    3. "Do you take time to use the bathroom when you are at school?"
    4. "What do you think is making you so constipated?"
    5. "Would you like to eat more fruit or would you rather take medicine?"

64. The nurse is caring for a child who had hydrostatic reduction for intussusception. Which outcome statement indicates that the goal of the therapy was met? *(1014)*
    1. "Barium enema procedure was well-tolerated."
    2. "Parents understand the criteria for surgery if needed."
    3. "Bowel sounds are present; passing stool with barium."
    4. "NG tube in place attached to low wall suction as ordered."

65. The nurse is aware of the disease process and treatment for nephrotic syndrome. It is anticipated that treatment for the child will include: *(1017, 1018)*
    1. frequent ambulation.
    2. increased sodium.
    3. decreased protein.
    4. adrenocortical steroids.

66. An infant is diagnosed with hypothyroidism. Which teaching point should be stressed? *(1021)*
    1. Prompt treatment is needed to avoid permanent cognitive impairment.
    2. A delay in treatment could result in damage to the heart and great vessels.
    3. Noncompliance with therapy will result in unusually short stature.
    4. Hypothyroidism will contribute to psychological disorders if untreated.

67. The nurse recognizes that hyperthyroidism is most common in which one of the following age groups? *(1021)*
    1. Neonates
    2. Toddlers
    3. Preschoolers
    4. Adolescents

68. For a child with talipes equinovarus, the nurse explains to the parents that treatment usually includes: *(1028)*
    1. oxygen administration.
    2. medication therapy.
    3. skeletal traction.
    4. cast applications.

69. A possible etiology associated with atopic dermatitis (eczema) is: *(1043)*
    1. food allergies.
    2. bacterial infection.
    3. exposure to poison ivy.
    4. sebaceous gland activity.

70. The nurse determines that the child has varicella as a result of observing: *(1051)*
    1. pinpoint red spots with white specks in the buccal cavity.
    2. a pinkish-red maculopapular rash that began on the face.
    3. a rose-pink macular rash on the trunk.
    4. vesicles on an erythematous base.

71. The nurse is assessing a school-age child for signs of scoliosis. Clinical manifestation(s) for this disease include(s): (Select all that apply.) *(1027)*
    1. unequal hip and shoulder height.
    2. scapular and rib prominence.
    3. protrusion of the spine in the lumbar region.
    4. posterior rib hump that is visible when bending forward.
    5. taller-than-expected for age group.

72. The parent of a child with strabismus demonstrates an understanding of the disorder by stating, "If we don't get treatment for this problem, my child may develop _____." *(1054)*
    1. myopia
    2. hyperopia
    3. presbyopia
    4. amblyopia

73. The nurse notices that a patient is constantly scratching the skin as a result of atopic dermatitis. The nurse knows that the scratching may lead to: *(1043)*
    1. subluxation.
    2. lichenification.
    3. pica.
    4. priapism.

74. Which intervention(s) would the nurse use during a child's seizure? (Select all that apply.) *(1037)*
    1. Keeping the side rails padded
    2. Moving the child to the bed when the seizure begins
    3. Loosening restrictive clothing
    4. Turning the child's head to the side
    5. Pushing a tongue blade between the teeth
    6. Staying with the child throughout the seizure

75. What is the most important assessment that nurses who work in well-baby clinics should perform in order to contribute to the early detection of hydrocephalus? *(1033)*
    1. Weigh the infant at every visit and compare to the previous weights.
    2. Routinely measure head circumference and compare for rapid changes.
    3. Check the infant's pupillary response and accommodation.
    4. Ask parents about subtle changes in mental status or behavior.

76. The mother is quite frustrated because the child has attention-deficit/hyperactivity disorder (ADHD), and it is taking several hours each night to help the child finish his homework. What would the nurse suggest for the mother to try first? *(1055)*
    1. Use a large variety of brightly colored shapes to hold the child's attention.
    2. Create an interactive approach that stimulates all of the senses.
    3. Have the child run and do very active play to tire him out before studying.
    4. Create a calm and quiet space with limited objects and fewer distractions.

77. The nurse anticipates that the child who is depressed will receive which one of the following medications? *(1062)*
    1. Prozac (fluoxetine)
    2. Ritalin (methylphenidate)
    3. Benadryl (diphenhydramine)
    4. Dexedrine (dextroamphetamine)

78. The parents of a child with an IQ of 40 demonstrate an understanding of the child's capabilities by stating: *(1056)*
    1. "Our child can go to school, but he may have difficulties with abstract concepts."
    2. "Our child can be taught activities of daily living and perform them on his own."
    3. "Our child is likely to have trouble with tasks like swallowing or sitting upright on his own."
    4. "Our child will never be able to perform self-care tasks like bathing on his own."

79. How can the nurse assist and support the parents if the child is experiencing school avoidance? *(1059, 1060)*
    1. Reassure parents that the behavior is normal and related to stress.
    2. Tell the parents to allow the child to stay home if he is too stressed.
    3. Tell the child that no one will pressure him if he doesn't want to go.
    4. Suggest getting the homework assignments when he misses school.

80. Appropriate intervention(s) for a child with autism is/are: (Select all that apply.) *(1059)*
    1. bring favorite possessions during hospitalization.
    2. teach the parents about the cure for the disease.
    3. vary routine and schedule from day to day.
    4. provide brief, concrete communication with the child.
    5. promote increased auditory and visual stimulation.

CRITICAL THINKING ACTIVITIES

81. a. Discuss information that the nurse can share with parents about preventing sudden infant death syndrome (SIDS). *(997)*

    _____

    _____

    _____

    _____

    _____

    _____

    _____

    _____

    b. Identify risk factors for SIDS and explain how the nurse would use these factors in helping parents prevent SIDS. *(997)*

    _____

    _____

    _____

    _____

    _____

    _____

    _____

    _____

    _____

    _____

82. For bronchial asthma, identify the following. *(1004, 1005)*

   a. Signs and symptoms: _____

   _____

   b. Diagnostic tests: _____

   _____

   c. Medical treatment: _____

   _____

   d. Nursing interventions: _____

   _____

83. For meningitis, identify the following. *(1031, 1032)*

   a. Most common cause: _____

   _____

   b. Classic signs and symptoms: _____

   _____

   c. Diagnostic test: _____

   _____

   d. Medical treatment: _____

   _____

   e. Preventive measure: _____

   _____

84. For lead poisoning, identify the following. *(1040, 1041)*

   a. Sources of lead: _____

   _____

   b. Prevention: _____

   _____

   c. Screening: _____

   _____

   d. Parent guidelines to reduce lead levels: _____

   _____

85. The school nurse is talking to a 15-year-old girl. The girl tells the nurse that one of the teachers accused her of using drugs because she thought "I was acting weird." The nurse asks her to describe the "weird behavior" and the girl talks about being withdrawn, with less interest in school work, school activities, or socializing with her friends. Further assessment reveals that the girl often feels sad, down, and empty and has fantasized about committing suicide.

a. What questions would the nurse ask? *(1062)* _____

_____

_____

b. How would the nurse determine whether to contact others, such as parents, health care provider, or school administrators? *(1063)*

_____

_____

_____

Health Promotion and Care of the Older Adult

chapter
32

Answer Key: Textbook page references are provided as a guide for answering these questions. A complete Answer Key is provided in your Additional Learning Resources on Evolve.

SHORT ANSWER

Directions: Using your own words, answer each question in the space provided.

1. What changes in the integumentary system occur with aging? *(1075)*_____

   _____

2. What changes in the gastrointestinal system occur with aging? *(1077)* _____

   _____

   _____

3. What changes in the urinary system occur with aging? *(1081)* _____

   _____

   _____

4. What changes in the cardiovascular system occur with aging? *(1083)*_____

   _____

   _____

5. What changes in the respiratory system occur with aging? *(1085)* _____

   _____

   _____

6. What changes in the musculoskeletal system occur with aging? *(1087)* _____

   _____

   _____

7. What changes in the endocrine system occur with aging? *(1090)* _____

_____

_____

8. What changes in the reproductive system occur with aging? *(1091)* _____

_____

_____

9. What changes occur with the aging process in the following sensory areas? *(1092)*

   a. Vision: _____

   _____

   b. Hearing: _____

   _____

   c. Taste and smell: _____

   _____

10. What changes in neurologic function occur with aging? *(1095)* _____

_____

_____

TABLE ACTIVITY

11. Directions: Fill in the blank boxes to complete the table for comparison of characteristics associated with delirium, dementia, and depression. *(1097)*

	Delirium	Dementia	Depression
Onset	Sudden		
Cognitive impairment		Minimal cognitive impairment initially; progresses to impaired abstract thinking, judgment, memory, thought patterns, calculations, agnosia	
Activity	Increased or decreased; may fluctuate		
Speech and language		Disordered, rambling, or incoherent; struggles to find words	
Reversibility			Can be treated

MULTIPLE CHOICE

Directions: Select the best answer(s) for each of the following questions.

12. The patient retired years ago. He was very involved with community, family, and friends, but now appears content to spend more time alone and others support his privacy. Which theory of aging most directly explains his behavior? *(1072)*
    1. Disengagement theory
    2. Exchange theory
    3. Continuity theory
    4. Activity theory

13. The patient, aged 80 years, weighs 130 pounds. In order to maintain this weight, the patient needs to take in approximately 30 calories per kilogram of body weight. How many calories per day should the patient consume? _____ *(1077)*

14. The patient has a history of peripheral vascular disease. Which symptom is the cause for greatest concern? *(1084)*
    1. Gradual and progressive edema going up both legs
    2. Excessive warmth of the lower leg on dominant side
    3. Sudden onset of cold foot on nondominant side
    4. Cramping of the calf muscles after exertion

15. The patient is recovering from a stroke, but some residual symptoms continue. Which statement by a family member demonstrates an understanding that precautions need to be taken during meals? *(1100)*
    1. "We hope the aphasia will improve as the condition improves."
    2. "The dysphagia creates a risk for developing pneumonia."
    3. "Presbyopia can be resolved with the proper corrective devices."
    4. "We will encourage the appropriate exercises to counteract akinesia."

16. The patient reports that typically nocturia occurs once each night, but recently the urge occurs 4-5 times at night. What should the nurse suggest as the first measure? *(1081)*
    1. Assess the environment for fall hazards.
    2. Take diuretic medication in the morning.
    3. Contact health care provider for medical evaluation.
    4. Limit fluids and semisolid foods at bedtime.

17. The UAP is assigned to assist an older adult who is experiencing pruritus with bathing and hygiene. The nurse would intervene if the UAP performs which action? *(1075)*
    1. Uses tepid water for washing and rinsing the body.
    2. Uses an antibacterial soap to reduce potential for infection.
    3. Gives a partial bath of face, hands, axillary, and perineal areas.
    4. Applies a water-based lotion with gentle even strokes.

18. For the older adult patient with dysphagia, which intervention is appropriate to use during mealtimes? *(1079)*
    1. Add thickeners to liquids.
    2. Feed the patient quickly to reduce fatigue.
    3. Place the patient in low Fowler's position.
    4. Provide opportunities for socialization while eating.

19. The patient is taking alendronate (Fosamax). Based on knowledge of this medication, which intervention will the nurse use when caring for the patient? *(1089)*
    1. Handle gently when assisting to move or change position.
    2. Encourage pursed-lip breathing to control breathlessness.
    3. Frequently note the rate, regularity, and strength of the pulse.
    4. Teach the patient how to perform Kegel exercises.

20. The nurse notes that the patient has kyphosis. Which symptom is cause for the greatest concern because of the kyphosis? *(1085)*
    1. Heartburn sensation after eating large meal
    2. Weak stream when urinating
    3. Swelling of ankles with prolonged sitting
    4. Difficulty coughing up secretions

21. The nurse is giving a health promotion presentation to a community group of older people. What would be included as primary prevention strategy(ies)? (Select all that apply.) *(1069)*
    1. Quit smoking to reduce the risk of heart disease.
    2. Eat a well-balanced diet without excess sugar, fat, or alcohol.
    3. Receive the recommended vaccinations.
    4. Take prescribed medications according to instructions.
    5. Do 20-30 minutes of moderate exercise three to five times a week.

22. Which statement by a senior citizen best indicates an understanding of the "donut hole" in her Medicaid prescription plan? *(1073)*
    1. "My dental bills are covered if my dentist prescribes any medication."
    2. "I don't have any money to pay for extra nongeneric medications."
    3. "A percentage of the cost of medications is paid to a certain amount."
    4. "The Affordable Care Act is going to take care of all my medical expenses."

23. The nurse is talking to the daughter of a patient who has dementia. Which comment by the daughter most strongly indicates the nursing diagnosis of Caregiver role strain? *(1100)*
    1. "Would you think I was a horrible person if I asked about respite care?"
    2. "Dealing with Dad is pretty exhausting, but I try to focus on happier times."
    3. "Well, I had to decrease my hours at work, but they do let me telecommute."
    4. "My sister says that I am too impatient with Dad, but she doesn't offer to help."

24. The patient reports feelings of grief related to multiple losses and recent death of her spouse. She appears sad and withdrawn. What is the best intervention to help this patient deal with grief and loss? *(1074)*
    1. Role-model cheerful and optimistic behavior.
    2. Encourage alone time and introspection.
    3. Help to set realistic short-term goals.
    4. Suggest temporarily moving in with an adult child.

25. The nurse is caring for a very thin patient who is bedridden. Which intervention is the best method to prevent damage to the skin at pressure points? *(1076)*
    1. Gently massage fragile skin with water-based lotion.
    2. Reposition the patient at least every 2 hours.
    3. Use a mechanical lifting device to prevent shearing forces.
    4. Place pressure-reducing pads and aids over bony prominences.

26. The nursing student is caring for a patient with fragile skin. The nurse would intervene if the student performed which action(s)? (Select all that apply.) *(1076)*
    1. Asks the patient to grab side rail and slide across the bed to change wet linens
    2. Secures the patient's IV with several pieces of tape to prevent dislodgement
    3. Washes dried fecal material from rectal area and rubs to dry moisture
    4. Asks for lifting help when trying to move patient from bed to stretcher
    5. Firmly grasps the patient on the forearm when moving from bed to chair

27. The nurse hears during handover report that the patient has a diminished gag reflex. Which morning assessment would be particularly important? *(1077)*
    1. Checking other reflexes
    2. Auscultating lung fields
    3. Assessing for pain in the neck area
    4. Assessing nutritional status

28. The nurse is encouraging the older adult to reduce calories and consume quality foods. Which breakfast choice is the best to supply vitamins, minerals, and fiber? *(1077)*
    1. Biscuits and gravy with coffee and artificial sweetener
    2. Orange juice and a low-fat banana-nut muffin
    3. Bacon with white toast and skim milk
    4. Oatmeal with fresh berries and hot tea

29. The patient reports controlling incontinence by limiting fluid intake. In order to encourage the patient to meet the minimum daily intake of 1500 mL of fluid, which intervention would be the most helpful? *(1078)*
    1. Suggest the use of an adapted cup with a double handle.
    2. Propose voiding every 2 hours during the day and every 4 hours at night.
    3. Divide the 1500 mL of fluid into portions to be taken during waking hours.
    4. Emphasize the importance of adequate fluid for body function.

30. The patient reports sensation of abdominal distention and early satiety. Based on knowledge of how aging affects gastric motility, which intervention would the nurse suggest? *(1078, 1079)*
    1. Walking for short distances several times a day
    2. Providing food that has a variety of different seasonings
    3. Preparing homemade frozen dinners with extra portions
    4. Performing oral hygiene to remove offensive tastes and odors

31. Which patient statement is most relevant to the medical diagnosis of gastric reflux? *(1077, 1078)*
    1. "I have never really liked the taste of milk."
    2. "I have gained a lot of weight within the last year."
    3. "Lately, my stool seems to be a very dark brown color."
    4. "Recently, I noticed a sore in mouth that won't heal."

32. The patient requests a laxative because "I feel constipated." What should the nurse do first? *(1080)*
    1. Find out when the last laxative was administered.
    2. Assist the patient to the bathroom and observe afterward.
    3. Ask the patient to describe the typical bowel pattern.
    4. Offer a high-fiber snack of prune juice and bran muffin.

33. The nurse is teaching the patient about self-care measures for modifiable cardiac risk factors. Which point(s) would be included? (Select all that apply.) *(1083, 1084)*
    1. Take blood pressure medications as prescribed.
    2. Decrease intake of complex carbohydrates and vegetable proteins.
    3. Perform moderate exercise 30 minutes/day at least twice a week.
    4. Aim for body mass index of 18.5-24.9 kg/m².
    5. Get adequate sleep and rest.
    6. Avoid exposure to secondhand smoke.

34. The patient with COPD states, "I can't cough up this phlegm in the back of my throat." Which intervention is the best to address this problem? *(1086)*
    1. Teach purse-lipped breathing.
    2. Promote moderate exercise 3-5 days/week.
    3. Use oxygen therapy as prescribed.
    4. Encourage plenty of fluids to liquefy secretions.

35. A normally cheerful and alert resident in a long-term facility demonstrates lethargy, disorientation, and a low-grade fever. What action should the nurse take first? *(1086)*
    1. Allow the patient to rest for several hours and then reassess mental status.
    2. Give a PRN dose of acetaminophen to relieve the fever and discomfort.
    3. Assess for the presence of other signs or symptoms.
    4. Use reality orientation and give simple, brief commands.

36. The nurse walks into a room and finds the patient on the floor. The patient reports severe pain in the hip area and the affected leg appears shorter than the other side. What should the nurse do first? *(1101)*
    1. Assist the patient back into bed.
    2. Assess for other injuries.
    3. Immobilize the affected side.
    4. Report the findings to the health care provider.

37. The nurse is interviewing a 56-year-old woman who reports that over the past year she has had frequent minor infections, minor wounds that seem slow to heal, blurred vision, and weight gain. Which laboratory finding is most likely to be observed? *(1084, 1090, 1108)*
    1. Elevated thyroid-stimulating hormone level
    2. Elevated blood glucose level
    3. Elevated estrogen level
    4. Elevated serum cholesterol level

38. The nurse notes that the patient's total cholesterol level is 130 g/dL. Which dietary information is the most relevant to this laboratory finding? *(1084)*
    1. Value is within normal limits, maintain current diet.
    2. Consumption of fluid and fiber should be increased.
    3. Amount of saturated fat in diet should be decreased.
    4. Reduce caloric intake to achieve a body mass index of 18.5-24.9 kg/m².

39. Patient reports "running out of my levothyroxine several weeks ago." What sign/symptom would the nurse expect because the patient has not been taking the medication? *(1091)*
    1. Apathy
    2. Heat intolerance
    3. Diarrhea
    4. Weight loss

40. A newly graduated nurse, age 22, is starting an interview with a 68-year-old gentleman who presents himself as very proper and conservative. The nurse feels that she will have trouble asking questions related to sexuality. What is the best strategy for this situation? *(1092)*
    1. Get another nurse to complete the interview.
    2. Have the patient wait and quickly assess own discomfort.
    3. Ask the patient for permission to initiate the discussion about sex.
    4. Defer the questions until after rapport is established.

41. The nurse is making a home visit and notices that the patient is squinting while reading the newspaper. There is no eye chart available to test the patient's vision. What should the nurse do first? *(1093)*
    1. Ask the patient to read the newspaper out loud.
    2. Suggest an appointment with an eye doctor.
    3. Assess the eyes for yellowing of the lens.
    4. Use a small flashlight to check pupil reaction.

42. Which symptom is an early sign of primary open-angle glaucoma? *(1093)*
    1. Severe eye pain
    2. Rainbow halo surrounding lights
    3. Pupil dilation
    4. Deteriorating peripheral vision

43. The patient watches the speaker's lips and tilts head towards the person who is speaking. Which position should the nurse assume when interviewing the patient? *(1094)*
    1. Stand near the window, so that there is bright light behind the nurse.
    2. Sit at the patient's eye level and directly face the patient.
    3. Sit beside the patient with mouth at the level of best ear.
    4. Stand over the patient, but lean into eye level when speaking.

44. The nurse is caring for several elderly patients in a long-term care center. Which patient is the most likely candidate for restraints? *(1099)*
    1. An 83-year-old woman who has suddenly become combative, aggressive, and hostile.
    2. A 76-year-old man who frequently falls, but refuses to ask for help or stay seated.
    3. An 85-year-old woman with dementia who keeps wandering off the unit and into the street.
    4. A 65-year-old man with depression who has suicidal ideation and thoughts of death.

45. A patient has Parkinson's disease. Which long-term outcome is considered the most important? *(1099)*
    1. Adapting to long-term memory loss through reminiscence
    2. Maintaining mobility through exercise and activity
    3. Decreasing confusion by using reality orientation
    4. Managing pain with pharmacologic and nonpharmacologic intervention

46. The patient is slowly recovering from a cerebrovascular accident, but hemianopia has not resolved. Which reminder will the nurse give during mealtimes? *(1100)*
    1. Sit upright before attempting to swallow.
    2. Ask for help if having trouble with utensils or opening wrapped items.
    3. Move head to the right and left when looking at the food tray.
    4. Minimize distractions and focus on chewing and swallowing.

47. Which factor(s) contribute(s) to polypharmacy where the risk for the patient outweighs the benefits? (Select all that apply.) *(1101)*
    1. Takes five or more prescription medications
    2. Sometimes borrows medication
    3. Uses a pill box with pockets for each day of the week
    4. Uses over-the-counter medications including vitamins and herbal preparations
    5. Sees primary health care provider on a regular basis
    6. Fills prescriptions at local pharmacies and through the mail

48. The nurse is discharging an elderly woman to return home to the care of her daughter. Which patient response would prompt the nurse to gather more information about possible elder abuse? *(1104)*
    1. "My daughter leaves me alone when she goes to work."
    2. "You are nice. Would you come and visit me sometime?"
    3. "Could I have a lunch tray before I go home?"
    4. "When you are old, family can do whatever they want with you."

49. The patient had minor surgery 8 hours ago. He refuses to walk to the bathroom. "I'm old and I just had surgery. You should bring me the urinal. That's what you get paid for." What is the best response? *(1105)*
    1. "I'll bring you the urinal, but you have to promise to get up soon."
    2. "Actually, I get paid to make sure that you recover from your surgery."
    3. "Getting up helps prevent constipation, pneumonia, and blood clots."
    4. "Sir, your doctor has ordered that you get up and walk around."

50. Which nursing action helps to meet goals for older adults according to *Healthy People 2020*? *(1011)*
    1. Checks the patient's blood pressure every 4 hours while in the hospital
    2. Reminds female patients that breast self-examination should be done annually
    3. Teaches fall prevention tips to community-dwelling elders
    4. Reports onset of new symptoms promptly to the primary care provider

51. The nurse works in a long-term care facility and is concerned about the quality of care. Which concern would be supported by the Omnibus Budget Reconciliation Act of 1987? *(1099)*
    1. A resident cannot file a complaint because there is no assigned ombudsman.
    2. A resident's chronic health condition was never assessed or documented.
    3. A resident is treated disrespectfully and there are no consequences for the offender.
    4. A resident dies and the room is immediately assigned to a new resident.

CRITICAL THINKING ACTIVITIES

52. For the following systems, describe the nursing assessment of the older adult.

    a. Integumentary: *(1075)* _____

    _____

    b. Cardiovascular: *(1083)* _____

    _____

    c. Respiratory: *(1085)* _____

    _____

    d. Gastrointestinal: *(1077)* _____

    _____

    e. Urinary: *(1081)* _____

    _____

    f. Musculoskeletal: *(1087)* _____

    _____

    g. Neurologic: *(1096)* _____

    _____

    h. Vision and hearing: *(1094, 1095)* _____

    _____

53. The nurse is caring for a 78-year-old woman who comes to the clinic with reports of "problems with my stomach and bowels."

    a. What questions would the nurse use to obtain data about the patient's concerns? *(1077)* _____

    _____

    _____

    _____

    _____

    b. The health care provider examines the patient and informs the nurse that the patient is likely to be having gastric reflux and constipation. What nursing interventions may be implemented for the older adult who is experiencing gastric reflux and constipation? *(1079, 1080)*

    _____

    _____

    _____

    _____

54. At the beginning of her new job, the nurse is open to any suggestions from others and makes an effort to get along with everyone. As time goes by, she feels comfortable and likes working with a group of younger nurses. There are several older staff members who are nice, but working with them is less stimulating and interesting. In fact, she finds the older staff members to be rigid in their outlook and slow to complete assigned tasks. When the nurse is assigned to precept an older nursing student, she hesitates, because her impression of older people is that they don't make the best nurses.

   a. Do you think that this nurse is guilty of ageism? Why or why not? *(1073)* _____

   _____

   _____

   b. How could the nurse create a better situation for herself and others? *(1073)* _____

   _____

   _____

   _____

55. The nurse is making a home visit to a 75-year-old woman who lives with her 80-year-old husband. Both the wife and husband are alert and oriented. Both are taking medication to treat hypertension. The wife has recently returned from a rehabilitation center following a hip fracture that she sustained during a fall. The nurse notes that the home is full of items that reflect a lifetime of living. Many of the rooms in the house tend to be poorly lighted. The house has an upstairs and downstairs bathroom. Identify the factors that are fall risks and make suggestions about how this elderly couple can prevent future falls. *(1101)*

   _____

   _____

   _____

   _____

   _____

   _____

   _____

   _____

   _____

   _____

Concepts of Mental Health

chapter

33

Answer Key: Textbook page references are provided as a guide for answering these questions. A complete Answer Key is provided in your Additional Learning Resources on Evolve.

FILL-IN-THE-BLANK SENTENCES

Directions: Complete each sentence by filling in the blank with the correct word or phrase.

1. _____ often consists of a pattern of behaviors that is conspicuous, threatening, and disruptive of relationships or that deviates significantly from behavior that is considered socially and culturally acceptable. *(1111)*

2. An astounding _____% of people in the U.S. will develop a mental health disorder in their lifetime. *(1111)*

3. During the 1930s, mental health practitioners developed electroconvulsive therapy (ECT) and insulin shock therapy and used them to treat _____. *(1112)*

4. In the 1950s, the introduction of _____ drugs allowed the individual to control his or her behavior and thus spend more time in the community. *(1112)*

5. The reduction in funding has resulted in reduced availability of _____; access to care providers; and limited access to psychotropic medications, therapy, and _____ services. *(1113)*

MULTIPLE CHOICE

Directions: Select the best answer(s) for each of the following questions.

6. The nurse is assessing an individual's use of defense mechanisms. A parent had a bad day at work and comes home and shouts at the children. This is an example of: *(1117)*
    1. projection.
    2. displacement.
    3. identification.
    4. reaction formation.

7. Which person is demonstrating regressive behavior? *(1117)*
    1. Victim of sexual abuse laughs while telling about the incident.
    2. Aggressive adolescent participates in a lot of competitive sports.
    3. An 80-year-old acts as if an incident of incontinence did not occur.
    4. An 8-year-old sucks his thumb when hospitalized for the first time.

8. An adolescent female patient tells the nurse that she often feels very "uneasy," but can't identify any specific reasons for this feeling. This patient is experiencing: *(1115)*
   1. stress.
   2. anxiety.
   3. crisis.
   4. mental illness.

9. Based on factors that possibly affect mental health, which adolescent is most likely to have the best mental health later in life? *(1110)*
   1. Participates in several school activities and has reasonably good grades
   2. Very competitive in sports and especially eager to be better than older brother
   3. Has a successful father, but mother died shortly after adolescent was born
   4. Has exceptional academic record and parents expect superior performance in all areas

10. A nurse is talking to people who are in a substance abuse support group. Which statement is evidence of the best level of mental health? *(1110)*
    1. "I don't have any problems with drinking anymore."
    2. "I just try to avoid drinking, one day at a time."
    3. "As long as my wife doesn't drink, then I won't drink either."
    4. "I have had a really hard time in life and I don't like being judged."

11. What is the best rationale for all nurses to study and be familiar with the concepts of basic mental health? *(1110)*
    1. Every nurse must study mental health concepts that are tested for licensure.
    2. Nurses need excellent mental health in order to help their patients.
    3. Nurses have daily contact with patients who are at risk for mental health problems.
    4. Younger nurses may lack personal experience in dealing with loss or mental illness.

12. Based on Freud's theory of personality development, the superego would cause the nurse to perform which action? *(1114)*
    1. Focuses on own duties and ignores extraneous requests to perform additional tasks
    2. Disagrees with patient's decision to refuse treatment, but shows respect and support
    3. Minimizes the importance of a medication error to facilitate patient care
    4. Obtains the continuing education units required to maintain licensure

13. The nurse suffered a terrible traumatic event during childhood, but now appears happy and satisfied with her life and career. According to Freud's theory on preconsciousness, the nurse would: *(1114)*
    1. be unable to recall any memory of the traumatic event.
    2. frequently think about the event and experience growth in reflection.
    3. remember the event, but generally repress the unpleasant aspects.
    4. attempt to experience pleasure and avoid pain at all costs.

14. There is a fire in the facility and the nurse is attempting to instruct patients to go to a safe area. Which patient is least likely to be able to understand and appropriately respond to a simple command? *(1116)*
    1. Using a wheelchair to assist bedbound roommate to safe area
    2. Frantically searching through belongings to find her wedding ring
    3. Standing in the corner, crying, and clinging to the bedrail
    4. Walking towards safe area, but arguing about the need to leave

15. Which nursing student is most likely to experience stress during the final examination for a course? *(1115)*
    1. Has done well throughout the semester, but didn't get much sleep the night before the exam
    2. Knows that the test is important, but believes that test is just another hurdle to get over
    3. Is smart and a good student, has children, works full-time, and spouse has chronic illness
    4. Has studied hard for final examination, but graduating is contingent on test results

16. A newly admitted patient appears upset. She says, "I'm going to wear my own clothes. I'm not going to answer any more questions and I'm not giving anyone any blood or pee or anything else!" How should the nurse respond? *(1118)*
    1. "You can wear your own nightgown if you would prefer."
    2. "Let me call your health care provider, so you can talk to him."
    3. "Coming into the hospital is really difficult. What can I do to help?"
    4. "Looks like you are having a bad time. I'll come back later."

17. The home health nurse is visiting an older patient who is socially isolated. The patient is very resistant to talking and rejects all suggestions related to social activities. Based on knowledge of how aging affects mental health, what should the nurse do first? *(1118)*
    1. Conclude that the resistance to socialization is an exaggeration of younger behavior.
    2. Assess for physical, financial, or relationship limitations that exist for the patient.
    3. Assist the patient to reminisce about happier times with friends and family.
    4. Locate and contact family members and suggest that they visit the patient.

18. A parent reports that her 8-year-old child has complained of feeling sick on school days, although there is no fever, pain, change in behavior, or any other physical symptoms. Which question should the nurse ask to determine if the child is using the sick role as a coping strategy related to a problem at school? *(1118, 1119)*
    1. "Don't you like your school and your teachers anymore?"
    2. "Did something happen at school that made you feel uncomfortable?"
    3. "What will happen if you keep missing school all the time?"
    4. "What do you and your friends like to do during recess and lunch break?"

19. The son of an elderly woman who lives in a long-term care facility reports that his mother seems to get sick whenever he tries to take vacation time with his wife. He feels frustrated, but also guilty, so he doesn't leave. What should the nurse do first? *(1120)*
    1. Validate the son's feelings of frustration and guilt and offer emotional support.
    2. Reassure the elderly mother that she will be well cared for while her son is gone.
    3. Suggest that the son take an overnight trip as a trial run for everyone.
    4. Tell the son that the mother is manifesting a secondary gain by being sick.

20. The health care provider has just informed a woman that her husband, who is in a coma, is likely to die during the night. The woman is sitting at the husband's bedside and silently weeping. Which action would be the most therapeutic? *(1119, 1129)*
    1. Silently step outside and call other family members to come and support the wife.
    2. Ask the health care provider for an order for an antianxiety medication for the wife.
    3. Make the patient as comfortable as possible and reassure the wife that he is pain-free.
    4. Quietly stand nearby and watch for the wife's receptiveness to touching or hugging.

CRITICAL THINKING ACTIVITIES

21. Think about times in the past where you have witnessed (or personally experienced) various levels of anxiety. Briefly describe the behaviors that you observed (or feelings that you personally experienced) in each case. *(1116)*

    a. Mild anxiety:_____

    _____

    b. Moderate anxiety: _____

    _____

    c. Severe anxiety: _____

    _____

    d. Panic: _____

    _____

    e. Refer back to the situation of mild anxiety that you just described. What coping responses were used by the individual to deal with stress? *(1116)*

    _____

    _____

    _____

    f. What would you do to strengthen the healthy coping mechanisms and alter or adapt the unhealthy or overused coping mechanism for that person? *(1116-1120)*

    _____

    _____

    _____

22. The nurse is making a home visit with 70-year-old woman who was recently discharged from the hospital. Her husband, who is also in his 70s, confides to the nurse that "Martha just doesn't seem to be herself. The doctor said she is okay to be at home, but she just seems so helpless."

    a. How would the nurse go about assessing the wife's emotional state? *(1120)* _____

    _____

    _____

    _____

    b. What considerations should be made for the older adult in regard to mental health? *(1118)* _____

    _____

    _____

    _____

23. Based on the characteristics of a mentally healthy individual, select characteristics that currently apply to yourself and give an example of an action, behavior, or event that illustrates your good mental health. *(1110)*

_____

_____

_____

_____

_____

_____

24. Discuss the advantages and disadvantages of the movement to "deinstitutionalize" from the point of view of an individual with a chronic mental illness. *(1113)*

_____

_____

_____

_____

_____

_____

_____

_____

_____

_____

_____

Care of the Patient with a Psychiatric Disorder

Answer Key: Textbook page references are provided as a guide for answering these questions. A complete Answer Key is provided in your Additional Learning Resources on Evolve.

MATCHING

Directions: Match the therapy to the correct description of therapy. Indicate your answers in the spaces provided.

Therapy

_____ 1. therapeutic communication *(1136)*

_____ 2. behavioral therapy *(1136)*

_____ 3. cognitive therapy *(1136)*

_____ 4. group therapy *(1136)*

_____ 5. play therapy *(1136)*

_____ 6. hypnosis *(1136)*

_____ 7. psychoanalysis *(1136)*

_____ 8. adjunctive therapies *(1136)*

_____ 9. electroconvulsive therapy *(1137)*

_____ 10. psychopharmacology *(1138)*

Description of Therapy

a. Breaking negative thought patterns and developing positive feelings about memories
b. Using toys, such as a puppet, to be a "spokesperson" for feelings
c. Helps to recover deeply repressed emotions
d. A very small amount of electrical current used to trigger a tonic-clonic seizure
e. Share meaning and interact in the interests of problem-solving and growth
f. Includes occupational, recreational, music, magnetic, and art therapies, and hydrotherapy
g. Medications that help modify an individual's behavior
h. Conditioning and retraining of behavioral responses by repetition
i. Intense therapy that brings unconscious thoughts to the surface
j. Group of patients with similar problems gain insight through discussion

FILL-IN-THE-BLANK SENTENCES

Directions: Complete each sentence by filling in the blank with the correct word or phrase.

11. In schizophrenia, the ventricles of the brain are larger, with the left ventricle larger than the right, and the cerebral cortex is smaller than normal; theoretically, this may account for the _____. *(1128)*

12. The inability to experience happiness or joy is known as _____. *(1128)*

13. Patients with schizophrenia often experience _____, which is a reduced content of speech. *(1128)*

14. The patient with schizophrenia shows little or no nonverbal expression of emotions. The nurse documents that the patient displays a(n) _____. *(1128)*

15. _____ is exhibited by a person showing a lack of caring or a state of indifference to the world around him or her. *(1128)*

16. *DSM-V* is a(n) _____ system used to diagnose psychiatric disorders; it includes the physical, psychiatric, and social factors affecting the individual. *(1142)*

TRUE OR FALSE

Directions: Write T for true or F for false in the blanks provided.

_____ 17.   People with neurosis often have no insight that they have a psychiatric problem. *(1123)*

_____ 18.   Behavior that indicates a persistent desire to be the opposite sex is termed *transgender*. *(1135)*

_____ 19.   Depression affects 1 in every 100 people every year. *(1129)*

_____ 20.   Hereditary factors account for 60% to 80% of mood disorders. *(1129)*

MULTIPLE CHOICE

Directions: Select the best answer(s) for each of the following questions.

21. The patient is in the manic phase of a bipolar affective disorder. What is primary aim of the nurse's therapeutic communication? *(1130)*
    1. To reinforce assertive behaviors
    2. To provide focus and consistency
    3. To orient to surroundings and time
    4. To encourage expression of feelings

22. The nurse anticipates that the patient with an obsessive-compulsive disorder (OCD) will receive: *(1127)*
    1. Lithobid (lithium carbonate).
    2. Haldol (haloperidol).
    3. Thorazine (chlorpromazine).
    4. Anafranil (clomipramine).

23. The nurse is aware that a patient who is receiving lithium therapy needs to have an adequate intake of: *(1139)*
    1. calcium.
    2. sodium.
    3. magnesium.
    4. potassium.

24. A patient tells you that he is hearing voices right now that are telling him not to eat. What is the best response? *(1125)*
    1. "What specifically did the voices tell you not to eat?"
    2. "Did the voices say why they didn't want you to eat?"
    3. "Just ignore the voices. Lunch is served at 1:00 PM."
    4. "I don't hear any voices. What you are experiencing now?"

25. Based on the information provided in the change-of-shift report, which patient will the nurse see first? *(1130)*
    1. Patient had ECT therapy 30 minutes ago.
    2. Patient has refused to take the morning medication.
    3. Patient has said, "I am going to meet my [dead] wife."
    4. Patient identified "voices" with a message from God.

26. The patient was admitted to the acute care facility for drug-induced psychosis. He tells the nurse that he has smelled his own flesh rotting for the past 2 days. Which positive symptoms is the patient is experiencing? *(1128)*
    1. Delusion
    2. Avolition
    3. Akathisia
    4. Hallucination

27. Signs and symptoms of schizophrenia typically include: (Select all that apply.) *(1128)*
    1. phobias.
    2. delusions.
    3. mania.
    4. paranoia.
    5. redoing.

28. Which patient statement would indicate a compulsion? *(1133)*
    1. "I can't stop thinking about my hand towels being out of place on the towel rack."
    2. "I had to drive back home 8 times this morning to be sure I locked my front door."
    3. "Those voices in my head are driving me crazy. Can you make them stop?"
    4. "It terrifies me to think about going fishing; I know there may be spiders in the boat."

29. A woman has bipolar disorder and is currently displaying an outgoing personality, productivity in her work, and great optimism. What phase of bipolar disorder is she experiencing? *(1126)*
    1. Manic
    2. Depressive
    3. Cyclothymic
    4. Hypomanic

30. A wife complains that her husband must be neurotic. What signs and symptoms would the nurse expect the husband to display? (Select all that apply.) *(1123)*
    1. Nervousness
    2. Low self-esteem
    3. Out of touch with reality
    4. Phobias
    5. Impaired judgment

31. The patient asks the nurse not to tell anyone that he wants to end his life. What should the nurse tell the patient? *(1130)*
    1. "Information must be shared with the rest of the health care team."
    2. "All disclosures from patient to nurse are always confidential."
    3. "Consider talking to a spiritual advisor before acting impulsively."
    4. "Information is documented in writing, but not verbally discussed."

32. The UAP reports that an elderly patient said, "You have been kind and I want you to remember me," and then she gave the UAP her grandmother's necklace. What should the nurse do first? *(1130)*
    1. Investigate the relationship between the patient and the UAP.
    2. Instruct the UAP to return the necklace to the patient.
    3. Talk to the patient about the gesture of gift-giving to employees.
    4. Praise the UAP for having trust and rapport with the patient.

33. Which person is likely to have the lowest Global Assessment of Functioning (GAF) score? *(1124)*
    1. Nursing student who just failed an important examination
    2. Person who was just released from long-term imprisonment
    3. Working mother who just delivered her first new baby
    4. Teenager who broke his arm during football practice

34. It's lunchtime and a staff member walks into the dayroom of an acute psychiatric unit and announces, "It's chow time folks! Hop on down." Which patient is most likely to start physically hopping? *(1128)*
    1. Major depression with apathy and flat affect
    2. Disorganized schizophrenia with concreteness
    3. Panic disorder with agoraphobia and anxiety
    4. Dysthymic disorder with suicidal ideations

35. The nurse's neighbor has a teenage son who displays poor hygiene and odd excessive religious beliefs. Before referral to the health care provider, what could the nurse do to try to differentiate between prodromal phase schizophrenia and normal adolescent behavior? *(1129)*
    1. Help the neighbor compare current behavior to previous behavior.
    2. Talk directly to the teenager and ask about his beliefs and interests.
    3. Assess and compare the parent's religious beliefs to the teen's.
    4. Ask the neighbor if there is a family history of mental illness.

36. The patient reports nausea, vomiting, and stomach pain. She has a new job with a lot of responsibilities, many people to supervise, and two projects that are due within the month. If physical causes are ruled out, these symptoms are consistent with which mental health disorder? *(1135)*
    1. Psychophysiologic reaction
    2. Posttraumatic stress disorder
    3. Generalized anxiety disorder
    4. Bulimia nervosa

37. The nurse is trying to assess a patient who is newly diagnosed with schizophrenia. The patient refuses to speak, but whispers, "They are listening to my conversations through the intercom." What should the nurse do? *(1125)*
    1. Conduct the interview in whispers or by writing.
    2. Walk over to the intercom and turn it off.
    3. Suggest that they move to the garden area.
    4. Acknowledge his feelings of fear and anxiety.

38. The patient says, "The man on the television is telling me to buy that motorcycle." What is the most therapeutic response? *(1125)*
    1. "It's just a television program; he wasn't really talking to you."
    2. "You can't buy a motorcycle right now; you are in the hospital."
    3. "Have you been thinking about buying a motorcycle?"
    4. "Television advertisements try to persuade us to buy products."

39. The nurse is caring for a patient who is scheduled to have surgery in the morning, but she also happens to have an anxiety disorder. What should the nurse do first to decrease stimuli for this anxious patient? *(1126)*
    1. Close the door and give the patient some privacy.
    2. Ask if sounds, light, or movement are disturbing.
    3. Turn off the lights so that the patient can sleep.
    4. Limit the number of visitors to decrease noise.

40. Which information is appropriate when preparing a patient for electroconvulsive therapy (ECT)? (Select all that apply.) *(1131)*
    1. "Pain will be experienced, but it only lasts a few seconds."
    2. "Confusion may last for a few hours."
    3. "A grand mal seizure occurs, but it is very brief."
    4. "Temporary memory loss is experienced after treatment."
    5. "Most patients are kept in the hospital for 2-3 days afterward."

CRITICAL THINKING ACTIVITIES

41. The nurse is working in a long-term care facility. There are two residents who have been living there for several years. Both are showing signs of new-onset mental health change. A resident with quadriplegia was recently admitted to the hospital for treatment of decubitus ulcers. He returned to the long-term care facility several weeks ago, but now he seems sullen and withdrawn and frequently talks about death. The other resident is an elderly gentleman with no family. He has a history of chronic depression. He is ambulatory and able to independently perform most ADLs. He has been talking about the loss of friends and family and his desire to join them. He mentions feeling "lonely, old, and useless." He asked the nurse if she would "give him a few extra pills."

    a. What warning signs of suicide are these two patients currently showing? What are other signs to watch for? *(1130)*

    _____

    _____

    _____

    _____

    b. Compare and contrast precautions that should be taken for these two residents who are suicidal. *(1130)*

    _____

    _____

    _____

    _____

    _____

    _____

    _____

    _____

42. The nurse is caring for a patient with chronic pain who displays sadness, loss of interest in activities, and pessimistic thoughts. The nurse reports these findings. A consulting psychiatrist makes the medical diagnosis of depression.

    a. Identify possible patient outcomes for this patient who is experiencing depression. *(1132)* _____

    _____

    _____

    _____

    _____

    _____

b. What specific treatments for depression should the nurse anticipate? *(1126)* _____

_____

_____

_____

_____

_____

_____

_____

c. What medications are typically used for depression? *(1130-1138)* _____

_____

_____

_____

d. For antidepressant medications, what side effects could the patient experience, and what are the nursing actions to address these effects? *(1140)*

_____

_____

_____

_____

_____

_____

_____

Student Name_____ Date_____

Care of the Patient with an Addictive Personality

chapter

35

Answer Key: Textbook page references are provided as a guide for answering these questions. A complete Answer Key is provided in your Additional Learning Resources on Evolve.

MATCHING

Directions: Match the substances that can potentially be abused to their defining characteristics. Indicate your answers in the spaces provided.

Substances with Potential for Abuse

_____ 1. caffeine *(1155)*

_____ 2. cocaine *(1156)*

_____ 3. amphetamine *(1156)*

_____ 4. alcohol *(1147)*

_____ 5. ecstasy *(1157)*

_____ 6. heroin *(1154)*

_____ 7. nicotine *(1155)*

_____ 8. lysergic acid diethylamide (LSD) *(1156)*

_____ 9. marijuana *(1157)*

_____ 10. inhalants *(1158)*

Defining Characteristics

a. Central nervous system (CNS) depressant
b. Most widely abused opioid
c. Present in some foods, cold and sinus medications, and appetite suppressants
d. Treatments include gum, transdermal patches, nasal spray, or bupropion
e. Chronic abuse erodes the nasal septum and often causes sinusitis and rhinitis
f. Weight loss and malnutrition from the anorexia effect are sometimes severe
g. Associated with flashbacks and "bad trip"
h. Includes solvents, glues, aerosols, refrigerants, and anesthetic gases
i. Baby pacifier is used to relieve bruxism
j. Medicinal use legal in some states

TRUE OR FALSE

Directions: Write T for true or F for false in the blanks provided.

_____ 11. It is impossible to suffer from more than one addiction at the same time. *(1145)*

_____ 12. The older adult sometimes turns to alcohol, prescription and nonprescription drugs, caffeine, and nicotine to cope with the physiologic and sociologic changes of aging. *(1145)*

_____ 13. Despite education of the public and laws set forth to limit availability to minors, there is an increased use of alcohol across all age groups. *(1146)*

_____ 14. The first areas that alcohol affects are the higher centers of the brain, including the frontal cortex, which governs self-control. *(1148)*

_____ 15. As many as 70% of people who quit smoking relapse within 1 year. *(1155)*

_____ 16. Heroin is the most commonly used illicit drug in the United States. *(1158)*

_____ 17. The National Council of State Boards of Nursing mandates that suspected drug abuse by a nurse must be reported. *(1158)*

SHORT ANSWER

Directions: Using your own words, answer each question in the space provided.

18. Identify the four elements that are included in the definition of addiction. *(1145)*

a. _____

b. _____

c. _____

d. _____

19. Identify five personality traits that are associated with an addictive personality. *(1146)*

a. _____

b. _____

c. _____

d. _____

e. _____

TABLE ACTIVITY

20. Directions: On the table below, indicate at least one or two disorders that are associated with chronic alcohol use for each body system. *(1149)*

Disorders Associated with Alcoholism

System	Disorders
Gastrointestinal	
Hepatic	
Cardiovascular and blood disorders	
Respiratory	
Uroreproductive	
Musculoskeletal	
Neurologic	

MULTIPLE CHOICE

Directions: Select the best answer(s) for each of the following questions.

21. A patient has a blood alcohol level of >500 mg/ dL (>0.50%). Which action is the nurse most likely to use first? *(434, 1159)*
    1. Assess for changes in mental status.
    2. Assist with ambulation because of clumsiness.
    3. Set limits for loosening of inhibitions.
    4. Assist health care provider with intubation.

22. A coworker states that he has had too much caffeine and wants to eliminate it from his diet. Which question would the nurse ask first? *(1149)*
    1. "Are you aware that you will have withdrawal symptoms?"
    2. "Do you take any supplements or over-the-counter medications?"
    3. "Have you ever tried to give up or cut down on your consumption?"
    4. "What would you typically eat and drink during a 24-hour period?"

23. The patient is quitting smoking cigarettes. The withdrawal from nicotine may result in the patient having: *(1155)*
    1. lethargy.
    2. improved concentration.
    3. decreased heart rate.
    4. decreased appetite.

24. The nurse is working at a facility that assists patients who have substance abuse problems. Which substance is unlikely to produce withdrawal signs and symptoms? *(1159)*
    1. Cannabis
    2. Amphetamine
    3. Heroin
    4. Hallucinogen

25. A college student who has used marijuana since early high school is diagnosed with amotivational cannabis syndrome. Which behavioral characteristic(s) is he likely to display? (Select all that apply.) *(1158)*
    1. Unusual irritability
    2. Frequent mood swings
    3. Physical aggression
    4. Psychosis
    5. Depression

26. A patient was prescribed an opiate analgesic for a fractured femur. He states that he has noticed that he doesn't seem to get the relief that he used to, despite the fact that his leg is healing. What should the nurse tell the patient? *(1155)*
    1. "Tolerance to opioids develops rapidly, but abstinence reverses tolerance."
    2. "You should switch to nonsteroidal antiinflammatory medications (NSAIDs)."
    3. "Addiction to opioid medications is common for those who have chronic pain."
    4. "This is an expected effect; I will contact the provider to increase your dosage."

27. The nurse's friend tells her that she thinks her boyfriend may have an alcohol problem. Which question will elicit indicators of the early stage of alcoholism? *(1147)*
    1. "What form of alcohol does he drink?"
    2. "Is the drinking controlling him?"
    3. "What makes you think there's a problem?"
    4. "Have you talked to him about this?"

28. The nurse is caring for a teenager who crashed his parents' car while he was intoxicated. The mother, wracked with guilt, confides that she knew he had a drinking problem, but didn't do anything about it. What is the most therapeutic response? *(1150)*
    1. "You can't watch your kids all of the time, especially when they are teenagers."
    2. "The accident may be a blessing; now you can get help for his drinking."
    3. "You feel like you are to blame, but it was his choice to drink and drive."
    4. "It's hard for parents to really believe that their child has a drinking problem."

29. The nurse is a assessing a patient who has been in the middle stage of substance abuse for years. Which factor is likely to hasten the progression from the middle stage to the late stage? *(1147)*
    1. Poor family relationships
    2. Multiple substance abuse
    3. Gastrointestinal problems
    4. Substance abuse on the job

30. From a cultural standpoint, which patient is the least likely to develop alcoholism? *(1147)*
    1. Asian
    2. Irishman
    3. Mormon
    4. Inuit

31. Which patient represents the leading national health problems in the United States? *(1147)*
    1. An infant who has birth defects and fetal alcohol syndrome
    2. An adolescent with cancer who smokes medicinal cannabis
    3. An executive who uses cocaine to counteract his depression
    4. An elderly patient who is an alcoholic with heart disease

32. What is the physiologic reason for the vitamin B_1, folic acid, and vitamin B_{12} deficiencies that occur in alcoholism? *(1148)*
    1. Alcohol affects the intestinal mucosa and results in decreased absorption.
    2. One ounce of alcohol provides 200 kcal but has no other nutritional value.
    3. Alcohol has a diuretic effect, so most nutrients are excreted in the urine.
    4. The liver metabolizes most of the alcohol; thus the liver is damaged.

33. The nurse is caring for a postoperative patient who demonstrates restlessness, tachycardia, and mild diaphoresis. How could the nurse differentiate between suspected alcohol withdrawal and postoperative complications, such as bleeding or infection? *(1149)*
    1. Call the provider and obtain an order for blood alcohol level.
    2. Monitor vital signs and assess for pain related to the surgery.
    3. Explain concerns and then ask the patient about alcohol use.
    4. This differentiation is beyond the nurse's scope of practice.

34. Which substance has the most potential for danger during withdrawal? *(1148)*
    1. Alcohol
    2. Heroin
    3. Amphetamine
    4. Nicotine

35. The nurse is interviewing a patient who has an alcohol problem and his wife has decided to file for divorce. Which patient statement typifies the most common defense mechanism used by substance abusers? *(1149)*
    1. "My wife is the one who has a drinking problem. I am glad she is gone."
    2. "I don't have a drinking problem. My wife just used that as an excuse."
    3. "Have you ever been married? I wouldn't recommend it to anyone."
    4. "My wife got on my nerves, so sometimes I would have a few drinks."

36. Which laboratory finding(s) is/are likely to be seen for a patient who has chronic alcoholism? (Select all that apply.) *(1149)*
    1. Elevated liver enzymes
    2. Decreased hemoglobin
    3. Electrolyte imbalances
    4. Abnormal blood proteins
    5. Hyperglycemia
    6. Abnormal clotting times

37. A person is brought to the hospital for an acute opioid overdose, which is most likely a suicide attempt. The patient is difficult to arouse and the family is hysterical. What is the priority action? *(1155)*
    1. Assess for time of ingestion.
    2. Check airway and respirations.
    3. Calm the family to obtain a history.
    4. Administer naloxone (Narcan).

CRITICAL THINKING ACTIVITIES

38. A daughter of a home health patient very hesitantly approaches the nurse and asks for information about alcohol abuse. At first, the daughter is very vague and claims to be asking out of general interest. As rapport develops between the nurse and the daughter, the daughter discloses that her mother (home health patient) and her stepfather seem to be drinking more alcohol. The daughter is not sure if they are true "alcoholics," but is worried about the long-term health effects.

   a. The nurse decides to collect data to determine if the family members have risk factors that could contribute to alcoholism. What are some contributing factors? *(1147)*

   _____

   _____

   _____

   _____

   b. Explain how the CAGE questionnaire can be used to help determine alcohol abuse. *(1149)*

   _____

   _____

   _____

   _____

   c. What can the nurse tell the daughter about the effect that alcoholism can have on relationships between family members who abuse alcohol and family members who do not? *(1147)*

   _____

   _____

   _____

   _____

   _____

   _____

39. The nurse suspects that something unusual is happening during the night shift. The patients frequently complain that the pain medication that they receive at night seems ineffective. These complaints seem to occur when the same two nurses are working together; however, the nurse hesitates to report these complaints because he recognizes that subjective reports of pain could be influenced by a number of factors.

   a. What should the nurse do? *(1158, 1160, 1161)* _____

   _____

   _____

   _____

   _____

b. What are the specific role-related signs or behaviors that may be seen if nurses are chemically impaired? *(1160)*

_____

_____

c. The nurse recognizes that reporting a chemically impaired nurse may be a way for that nurse to get assistance in overcoming the problem and prevent possible dangers to patients. What assistance is available? *(1161)*

_____

_____

_____

_____

_____

_____

d. What is the Healthcare Integrity and Protection Data Bank (HIPDB) and how does it impact the chemically impaired nurse? *(1161)*

_____

_____

_____

_____

_____

e. How would you feel about reporting a friend/coworker for stealing opioid medication?_____

_____

_____

_____

_____

_____

Home Health Nursing

Answer Key: Textbook page references are provided as a guide for answering these questions. A complete Answer Key is provided in your Additional Learning Resources on Evolve.

FILL-IN-THE-BLANK SENTENCES

Directions: Complete each sentence by filling in the blank with the correct word or phrase.

1. Home health care is not a new concept; however, _____, _____, and current _____ trends have changed the way it is provided. *(1178)*

2. Patients older than 65 years account for over _____% of all home health patients. *(1164)*

3. For the older adult, modifications to the home environment are made with consideration of the older adult's _____ and remaining _____. *(1165)*

4. _____ continued to reduce the payments to home care agencies for the year 2013. *(1166)*

TRUE OR FALSE

Directions: Write T for true or F for false in the blanks provided.

_____ 5. All home health agencies must be licensed by the state. *(1166)*

_____ 6. Anyone who needs assistance at home can receive home health services. *(1166)*

_____ 7. Early discharge from the hospital has increased the number of patients who need home health services. *(1165)*

_____ 8. Medicare provides federal monies for the care of the poor and indigent of all ages. *(1165)*

_____ 9. The purpose of diagnosis-related groups (DRGs) is to help clinicians to standardize diagnosis of patients. *(1165)*

_____ 10. The prospective payment system has not led to a decline in quality of care or negative outcomes in patient care. *(1166)*

MULTIPLE CHOICE

Directions: Select the best answer(s) for each of the following questions.

11. The nurse observes that the home health patient has trouble with tasks that require fine motor skills, such as writing or manipulating eating utensils. Which member of the health care team is best able to assist the patient with these problems? *(1171)*
    1. Health care provider
    2. Physical therapist
    3. Home health aide
    4. Occupational therapist

12. The home health nurse is reviewing use of home oxygen with the patient and family. Which information should be included? *(1171)*
    1. Use petrolatum-based lubricant on the lips.
    2. Place "No Smoking" signs where they are clearly visible.
    3. Change disposable equipment once a month.
    4. Use wool blankets to provide warmth and static control.

13. Which home health patient would be the best candidate for a telehealth program? *(1173)*
    1. Lacks fine motor control to perform ostomy care
    2. Needs infusion of total parenteral nutrition every morning
    3. Recently prescribed insulin and blood glucose measurement
    4. Requires assessment of home environment for safety

14. What do Medicare and Medicaid require for the patient to enter into the formalized system? *(1173)*
    1. An evidence-based clinical pathway that relates to the primary medical diagnosis
    2. A standardized nursing care plan that is linked to the hospital discharge diagnosis
    3. An individualized nursing care plan that is developed by the RN and LPN/LVN
    4. An interdisciplinary treatment plan that is signed by the health care provider

15. Which evaluative statement indicates that the "restorative" goal of service is being met? *(1169)*
    1. Patient who had a stroke 4 weeks ago is now able to feed self without signs of choking.
    2. Patient who had smoking cessation classes reports no smoking for past 2 months.
    3. Patient who had bariatric surgery reports exercising routinely with no weight gain.
    4. Patient who has hypertension reports compliance with low-cholesterol, low-sodium diet.

16. The LPN/LVN who is working under the supervision of the RN has been assigned to do home care for an elderly patient with diabetes and hypertension. Which nursing action(s) is the LPN/LVN allowed to perform? (Select all that apply.) *(1170)*
    1. Conduct the admission assessment in the home environment.
    2. Prefill insulin syringes.
    3. Perform fingersticks for blood glucose readings.
    4. Monitor blood pressure and weight.
    5. Reinforce therapeutic diabetic diet information.
    6. Evaluate the patient at the end of the 60-day period.

17. The daughter of an elderly patient with emphysema is trying to determine if her father can continue to live independently in his own home. The nurse advises the daughter that Medicare home health will not cover a visit solely for assistance with: *(1172)*
    1. bathing and oral hygiene.
    2. walking and transfers.
    3. shopping and cooking.
    4. eating and toileting.

18. A home health aide has been assigned to assist a patient with a bath several times a week. Which instruction is appropriate for the nurse to give to the aide? *(1172)*
    1. "Try to do everything for the patient, so he feels nurtured."
    2. "Ask the patient if he prefers a shower, tub bath, or a partial bath."
    3. "If you or the patient has any problems, just let me know."
    4. "Watch for redness of the skin, particularly on the buttocks and back."

19. A nurse is spending 3 or more hours with each patient for home visits. The supervisor sees this as a problem. What should the supervisor do first? *(1173)*
    1. Explain that clinical efficiency is critical within the industry.
    2. Describe how the current Medicare prospective payment system works.
    3. Ask the nurse to describe what happens on a typical home visit.
    4. Review the nurse's documentation for evidence of how the time is spent.

20. For home health care, what is/are the purpose(s) of documentation? (Select all that apply.) *(1173)*
    1. Provides an accurate picture of the type and quality of care
    2. Replaces verbal nursing reports that are used in facilities
    3. Allows the health care team to make internal evaluations as needed
    4. Provides evidence required for reimbursement and payments
    5. Serves as a legal document that is subject to close scrutiny
    6. Allows family to have access to all patient information

CRITICAL THINKING ACTIVITIES

21. A 63-year-old woman had several toes amputated because of complications of diabetes. The patient also takes medication for high blood pressure. She was recently discharged from the hospital and needs home health care. The home health care team includes an RN, LPN/LVN, physical therapist, and a home health aide. The patient is having trouble with balance and ambulation and currently needs some assistance with hygiene.

    a. What is the role of the LPN/LVN in home health care of this patient? *(1170, 1175)* _____

    _____

    _____

    b. What activities may be delegated to a home health aide? *(1172)* _____

    _____

    _____

    c. What are the Medicare requirements for the following services? *(1171, 1172)*

        i. Physical therapy: _____

        _____

        ii. Home health aide: _____

        _____

22. Identify qualities/attributes in yourself that would indicate that a career in home health would either be suitable or not suitable for you. *(1169, 1170)*

    _____

    _____

    _____

    _____

    _____

23. Compare and contrast the admission process to home health service to the admission process to an acute care facility. *(1172, 1173)*

_____

_____

_____

_____

_____

_____

_____

_____

_____

Long-Term Care

Answer Key: Textbook page references are provided as a guide for answering these questions. A complete Answer Key is provided in your Additional Learning Resources on Evolve.

TABLE ACTIVITY

Directions: Complete the table below by adding the correct term for each definition of the service to support older adults. (1182)

Terminology	Definition of Services to Support Older Adults
1.	Scheduled stays for the older adult to give the caregiver a break from the responsibility of providing care.
2.	Facilities are frequently used by family members and caregivers who work during the day.
3.	Includes homemakers, shoppers, respite care workers, personal care attendants, home health aides, and nursing care staff.
4.	Senior centers serve meals or home delivery of one hot meal per day.
5.	Centers that provide recreational activities, lunch, health screening, exercises classes, educational classes, and transportation to and from the site if needed.
6.	Service for grocery shopping or medical appointments.

TRUE OR FALSE

Directions: Write T for true or F for false in the blanks provided.

_____ 7. The need for long-term care arises when an individual has a chronic illness. *(1180)*

_____ 8. By 2050, 42% of the population will be of older age. *(1181)*

_____ 9. It costs approximately half as much to care for an older adult at home as it would cost in a long-term care facility, unless there are significant physical impairments. *(1182)*

_____ 10. In the United States, Program of All-Inclusive Care for the Elderly (PACE) is available to any patient 55 years of age or older. *(1183)*

MULTIPLE CHOICE

Directions: Select the best answer(s) for each of the following questions.

11. The nurse is assisting in training a new certified nurse assistant (CNA) at a long-term care facility. The nurse would be correct in describing activities of daily living (ADLs) as: (Select all that apply.) *(1182)*
    1. bathing.
    2. brushing teeth.
    3. socializing.
    4. ambulating.
    5. shopping.
    6. toileting.

12. A patient requires extensive wound care and intravenous antibiotics due to an infection of the surgical wound. Which type of care will best meet his needs? *(1185)*
    1. Long-term care facility
    2. Subacute unit
    3. Residential care facility
    4. Hospice unit

13. Which nursing action reflects the positive influence of the Omnibus Budget Reconciliation Act (OBRA) on long-term care? *(1188)*
    1. Instructs CNAs on the use of restraints for confused patients
    2. Reviews and updates the residents' advance directives
    3. Reviews the qualifications of a CNA who applied for a job
    4. Ensures that each resident qualifies for Medicaid or Medicare

14. An elderly couple needs assistance with bathing, dressing, and taking their medication. Both are alert and oriented at all times. They are mobile, but suffer from arthritis. Which setting would be the most beneficial for this elderly couple? *(1184)*
    1. Skilled nursing facility
    2. Subacute unit
    3. Adult daycare facility
    4. Assisted-living community

15. The interdisciplinary team at a long-term care facility is meeting to discuss the care plan of one of the residents. Who should attend this meeting? (Select all that apply.) *(1186)*
    1. Physical therapist
    2. Activities director
    3. Certified nursing assistant
    4. Nursing unit manager
    5. Other interested residents
    6. Resident

16. The nurse is talking to a nursing student who is doing a clinical rotation in a nursing home facility. What is the priority concept that the nurse will emphasize during the student's orientation to the facility? *(1181)*
    1. Respectful communication
    2. Complete documentation
    3. Residents' safety and security
    4. Assistance with ADLs

17. What is the purpose of a resident assessment instrument (RAI)? *(1189)*
    1. Facilitates assessment of functional, medical, mental, and psychosocial status
    2. Allows residents to self-assess and report on what they can do for themselves
    3. Identifies the problems that residents will have in communicating needs
    4. Used by surveyors during unannounced visits to assess residents' quality of life

18. How does documentation in a long-term care facility differ from that in a hospital setting? *(1189)*
    1. Documentation occurs at the beginning and ending of each 24-hour period.
    2. The CNAs do most of the physical care, so they do most of the documentation.
    3. Summaries of resident status over a longer time, usually monthly, are recorded.
    4. Documentation occurs only if there is a sudden change in a resident's status.

19. An older gentleman is alert, ambulatory, and can independently perform ADLs. Recently, he has wandered off and the police had to bring him back home. Which question would the nurse use first to help the family determine if long-term care is needed? *(1186)*
    1. "Who has the power of attorney for health care?"
    2. "What are the current living arrangements for family members?"
    3. "What kinds of options have you considered for your dad?"
    4. "Is there any way to plan 24-hour care among the family?"

20. An interdisciplinary team meeting is planned to discuss the needs and goals of a resident who is very hostile about being in the long-term care facility. The CNA who has the best relationship with the resident is not invited to attend. What should the nurse do? *(1187)*
    1. Ask the resident to invite the CNA.
    2. Advocate for the CNA to attend.
    3. Ask the CNA to do a written statement.
    4. Inform the CNA of the outcomes.

CRITICAL THINKING ACTIVITIES

21. You are considering applying for a job in a long-term care facility. You have had clinical experiences in nursing school in acute care facilities and in long-term care. You recognize that part of selecting a job is to match your interests and experiences with the setting, patients, other caregivers, and philosophy of the institution.

    a. What is the profile of the patient who requires long-term care in an institutional setting? Envision yourself working with this type of patient. Is it a good fit for you? *(1186)*

    _____

    _____

    _____

    _____

    _____

    _____

    b. The administration of medications can differ in long-term care facilities. Describe the differences and state your comfort level with this process. *(1187, 1188)*

    _____

    _____

    _____

    _____

    _____

    _____

    _____

22. Your grandmother has reached a stage where the family has decided that she requires more care than the family is able to give her at home.

    a. Discuss points about choosing a nursing home. *(1187)* _____

    _____

    _____

    _____

    _____

    _____

    _____

    b. How will your family finance the nursing home care for your grandmother? *(1188)* _____

    _____

    _____

    _____

23. Why would a nurse who works in long-term care actually need a better understanding of legal aspects, such as advance directives and power of attorney or guardianship, compared to a nurse who works in an acute care facility? *(1188, 1189)*

    _____

    _____

    _____

    _____

    _____

    _____

    _____

    _____

    _____

    _____

Rehabilitation Nursing

chapter

38

Answer Key: Textbook page references are provided as a guide for answering these questions. A complete Answer Key is provided in your Additional Learning Resources on Evolve.

MATCHING

Directions: Match the terms on the left to the correct definition on the right. (1194)

Term		**Definition**
_____	1. impairment	a. Loss of the ability to function physically or psychologically in normal activities in work, school, home, community, or social activities
_____	2. disability	
_____	3. handicap	b. Irreversible lifelong disease state or impairment
_____	4. functional limitation	c. Loss or abnormality of psychological, physical, or anatomic structure or function
		d. Physical, mental, or emotional impairment or disability that interferes with one's normal functioning
_____	5. chronic illness	e. Loss of ability to perform tasks or activities of daily living

FILL-IN-THE-BLANK SENTENCES

Directions: Complete each sentence by filling in the blank with the correct word or phrase.

6. Emphasis on acute care persists, despite the fact that people with _____ constitute the largest group of health consumers. *(1194)*

7. Rehabilitation services for the older person are built around maintaining _____ abilities, ensuring safety, promoting effective coping, preventing _____, and modifying the _____ for maximum independence. *(1194, 1195)*

8. A disability has a number of potential effects on both the patient and the family, including _____ and emotional changes and changes in roles, body _____, self-concept, and family _____. *(1194)*

9. Rehabilitation is a(n) _____ process. *(1194)*

10. Individuals with disabilities do not always accept their disability; learning to _____ to the circumstances is a positive method of coping. *(1195)*

11. The role of a rehabilitation nurse is to put the individual in _____ of his or her own care rather than taking charge. *(1197)*

12. Rehabilitation nursing roles include those of 1) _____, 2) _____, 3) _____, 4) _____, 5) _____, 6) _____, 7) _____, 8) _____, 9) _____, 10) _____, and expert witness. *(1197)*

13. It is important to recognize that having a disability is just one of many _____ of the normal human experience. *(1201)*

14. The primary difference between rehabilitation of children and rehabilitation of adults is the _____ of the child. *(1206)*

15. Studies of resource allocation show that _____ rehabilitation saves thousands of dollars and increases the chance of the individual being able to live independently. *(1199)*

MULTIPLE CHOICE

Directions: Select the best answer(s) for each of the following questions.

16. The patient experienced a spinal cord injury at the T1–T5 level. The nurse anticipates that the patient should be able to: *(1202)*
    1. assist with activities of daily living (ADLs).
    2. ambulate with the use of assistive devices.
    3. resume normal sexual activities.
    4. control bowel and bladder function.

17. The construction worker sustained an injury to C3 after a fall at a work site. The nurse anticipates that this patient will have: *(1201)*
    1. use of the arms, but not the legs.
    2. control of bladder, but not bowels.
    3. potential for respiratory failure and infections.
    4. problems understanding and following instructions.

18. The spouse reports that the patient tripped and bumped his head. He never lost consciousness, but seemed confused for a few minutes after the accident. Which assessment finding does the nurse expect? *(1204)*
    1. Headache and vertigo
    2. Difficulty with judgment and reasoning
    3. Posttrauma amnesia and aggressiveness
    4. Appears awake, but does not respond

19. The patient has a spinal cord injury above the level of T5. While assisting with hygiene care, the nurse notices that the patient is diaphoretic and shivering, and he states that he has a headache. Upon assessment, it is found that his blood pressure is elevated. The nurse's next action should be to: *(1204)*
    1. reposition to a position of comfort.
    2. inform the health care provider.
    3. check for bladder distention.
    4. give an antihypertensive medication.

20. The nurse anticipates that the patient with a spinal cord injury is at risk for deep vein thrombosis (DVT). Which intervention(s) will be used? (Select all that apply.) *(1204)*
    1. Fluid restriction
    2. Passive and active range-of-motion exercises
    3. Application of heat
    4. Administration of anticoagulants
    5. Application of elastic stockings
    6. Assessment for swelling, redness, and heat in extremities

21. The nurse is assessing a patient who had a stroke and was recently admitted to the rehabilitation unit. What is the best method to determine how much assistance is required for hygienic care? *(1198)*
    1. Ask the UAP to go with the patient and assist as needed.
    2. Ask the patient how much he feels like he can do for himself.
    3. Read the documentation from the transferring facility.
    4. Observe the patient as he performs tasks such as eating.

22. The elderly patient with a hip fracture has a self-care deficit related to bathing due to problems with ambulation and balance. Which action would the nurse use to foster independence, while ensuring safety? *(1205, 1206)*
    1. Help the patient sit in the bathtub and bathe self, rather than attempt to stand and balance in the shower.
    2. Have the UAP stay with the patient for the whole time it takes for showering, but tell the UAP to let the patient wash herself.
    3. Have the patient remain in bed and bring her a basin of water and towels and allow her to wash her own hands and face.
    4. Assist the patient to sit in a stable chair in the shower stall and adjust the water temperature of the handheld shower spray.

23. Which patient is most likely to need minimization of distractions that would prevent participation in therapy? *(1204)*
    1. Patient who has been depressed for several months
    2. Patient who had a myocardial infarction
    3. Patient who had a traumatic brain injury
    4. Patient who has chronic obstructive pulmonary disease

24. A patient had cardiac surgery. He is slowly improving, but it seems unlikely that he will be able to return to his job. The spouse expresses fears that her husband will die if she doesn't quit her job and stay home to take care of him. In this case, what would be considered a successful outcome? *(1199)*
    1. Patient continuously works toward resuming his old job.
    2. Spouse acknowledges patient's ability to independently stay at home.
    3. Spouse quits her job, and fears about husband's death are alleviated.
    4. Patient acknowledges spouse's fears, and encourages her to stop worrying.

25. A patient was involved in an explosion at a chemical factory and sustained polytrauma/blast-related injury (PT/BRI). What type(s) of injuries would the health care team expect to find? (Select all that apply.) *(1200)*
    1. Burns
    2. Fractures of extremities
    3. Chemical pneumonitis
    4. Brain injury
    5. Myocardial infarction
    6. Hearing loss

CRITICAL THINKING ACTIVITIES

26. The nurse is caring for a patient who sustained a traumatic brain injury in a motor vehicle accident. The patient was admitted to an acute care facility immediately after the accident. Now that the patient is stable, he has been transferred to a rehabilitation facility. The patient is alert and ambulatory, but suffers residual effects from the brain injury.

    a. In the rehabilitative assessment of this patient, what may the nurse expect to find? *(1204, 1205)*

    _____

    _____

    _____

    _____

    _____

b.   What type of interventions does the nurse anticipate for the patient with a traumatic brain injury? *(1204, 1205)*

_____

_____

_____

_____

_____

_____

c.   The patient with a traumatic brain injury has nursing diagnoses of Self-care deficit related to grooming and Risk for Injury related to poor judgment. Write outcomes for these two diagnoses. *(1205, 1206)*

_____

_____

_____

_____

_____

_____

Hospice Care

chapter
39

Answer Key: Textbook page references are provided as a guide for answering these questions. A complete Answer Key is provided in your Additional Learning Resources on Evolve.

FILL-IN-THE-BLANK SENTENCES

Directions: Complete each sentence by filling in the blank with the correct word or phrase.

1. Hospices serve patients with various primary disease processes, the most common being _____, comprising 37.7% of the patient population. *(1210)*

2. _____ is aggressive care in which the goal is curing the disease and prolonging life at all costs. *(1211)*

3. The Hospice Medicare Benefit covers all expenses for palliative care related to the terminal illness, including _____, _____, _____, and _____ and _____ care. *(1223)*

4. _____ is appropriate when a cure is not possible, but care is still necessary. *(1223)*

5. It is possible to begin palliative care earlier in the dying process, whereas hospice is usually available only _____ of life. *(1210)*

TABLE ACTIVITY

6. Directions: Complete the table below with the functions or responsibilities of the Core Interdisciplinary Hospice Team. *(1213, 1214)*

Core Interdisciplinary Hospice Team

Team Member	Function or Responsibility
a. Medical director	
b. Nurse coordinator	
c. Social worker	
d. Spiritual coordinator	

MULTIPLE CHOICE

Directions: Select the best answer(s) for each of the following questions.

7. The patient asks the nurse what the criteria are for admission to a hospice. What is the best response? *(1212)*
   1. "Hospice care is available to everyone regardless of sex, race, age, religion, diagnosis, or ability to pay."
   2. "There must be a medical diagnosis of terminal cancer with poor prognosis for curative treatment."
   3. "You and your primary caregiver must understand and be willing to participate in the planning of care."
   4. "The whole family must be informed about life support measures and be willing to be involved in the decision-making."

8. The family of a dying patient is feeling physically and emotionally exhausted while taking shifts to care for their loved one 24 hours a day. This family could best benefit from the hospice service of: *(1214)*
   1. respite care.
   2. palliative care consultation.
   3. bereavement counseling.
   4. the hospice ethics committee.

9. The health care provider orders oral opioid medication for the terminally ill patient for pain control. What other medication(s) would the nurse expect the provider to order? (Select all that apply.) *(1216-1219)*
   1. Anticholinergics
   2. Anticonvulsants
   3. Anticoagulants
   4. Antiemetics
   5. Antihypertensives
   6. Anxiolytics

10. The wife of a terminally ill patient asks the hospice nurse why she gives different amounts of pain medication to her husband rather than the same dose each time. What is the best response? *(1217)*
    1. "Determining the right dose of medication is difficult. We must try different amounts to determine a safe dose."
    2. "It is difficult to determine how much pain medication is a safe dose for someone who is dying. I want to be sure we get the right dose."
    3. "Finding the correct dose for pain medication is by trial and error. Every patient is different in how he or she responds to the medication."
    4. "I am titrating his medication amount so that we can best manage his pain while keeping him alert enough to interact with you and your family."

11. Which nursing intervention would help the patient/family to meet the hospice goals? *(1212)*
    1. Encourage the family to consider putting the patient into long-term care.
    2. Remind the cancer patient that hoping for remission is therapeutic and beneficial.
    3. Reassure the primary caregiver that going out to a movie is not being selfish.
    4. Reinforce that eating and drinking as much as possible facilitates healing and recovery.

12. The hospice nurse is working with a patient and family who are from a different culture than the nurse's own. The family insists on performing some rituals that seem to be making the patient physically uncomfortable and emotionally distraught. What should the nurse do first? *(1214)*
    1. Graciously respect the patient's and family's cultural beliefs and allow them to continue.
    2. Politely ask the patient if he wants to continue or if he would like the family to stop.
    3. Humbly attempt to understand the benefit of the rituals from a cultural point of view.
    4. Respectfully inquire if there is a way to modify the rituals to make them less traumatic.

13. The hospice volunteer tells the nurse that he is thinking about quitting. "I like the patient, but the wife has me doing the shopping, the yardwork, and walking the dog. Now she wants me to paint the house." What should the nurse do? *(1214)*
    1. Talk to the wife and explain the role and responsibilities of the volunteer.
    2. Call the volunteer coordinator and ask for additional help to paint the house.
    3. Ask the patient how he has been getting along with the volunteer.
    4. Instruct the volunteer to explain the situation to the volunteer coordinator.

14. The hospice nurse notices that the patient and hospice aide joke and talk and seem to have a close relationship. The nurse suspects that the patient is disclosing more feelings and concerns to the aide than he is to the rest of the staff. What is the most important thing that the nurse should do? *(1215)*
    1. Praise the hospice aide for having a supportive rapport with the patient.
    2. Have frequent contact with the aide to get updates on the patient's concerns.
    3. Remind the aide about scope of practice and staff-patient boundaries.
    4. Try to spend more time with the patient to develop a better rapport and trust.

15. The patient is a large man who needs assistance to move and transfer to a wheelchair. His wife, the caregiver, is a relatively small woman. Who would be contacted first to address this problem? *(1213)*
    1. Interdisciplinary team
    2. Hospice aide
    3. Physical therapist
    4. Nurse coordinator

16. The nurse reads in the documentation that the Edmonton Symptom Assessment System (ESAS) was used when the patient was first admitted into hospice. Which current assessment findings could be compared to the baseline established by ESAS? *(1216)*
    1. Patient's satisfaction with plan of care and recommendations for improvement
    2. Patient's subjective feeling of pain, tiredness, and overall feeling of well-being
    3. Patient's cognitive, intellectual, and perceptual status and ability to make judgments
    4. Patient's ability to perform activities of daily living and home maintenance

17. The patient is having significant pain, but refuses to take oral morphine that the nurse offers. "Because it makes me feel confused and I hallucinate." What should the nurse do first? *(1216)*
    1. Encourage taking the medication for now, but promise to call health care provider.
    2. Offer a prescribed nonopioid drug and try several nonpharmacologic options.
    3. Call the pharmacist to see if alternative routes of administration cause fewer side effects.
    4. Give the patient a lower dose and observe for confusion or other side effects.

18. Patient has nausea that is likely to be related to a mechanical obstruction caused by the progressive growth of a tumor and her nausea is exacerbated by anxiety. Which medication, if ordered, would the nurse question? *(1219)*
    1. Promethazine (Phenergan) suppository 30 minutes before meals
    2. Prochlorperazine (Compazine) oral dose as needed for nausea
    3. Lorazepam (Ativan) oral dose PRN every 6-8 hours for anxiety
    4. Metoclopramide (Reglan) oral dose 30 minutes before meals

19. The patient is having nausea and vomiting, so the nurse gives the patient an antiemetic and the vomiting subsides. What should the nurse offer the patient first? *(1219)*
    1. Diluted bouillon
    2. Plain white rice
    3. Vanilla pudding
    4. Favorite food

20. The patient has not had a bowel movement. What is the initial nursing action? *(121)*
    1. Explain to the patient that a decreased oral intake decreases the amount of stool.
    2. Assess the amount and frequency of opioid usage.
    3. Advise the patient to increase fiber and fluids in the diet.
    4. Assess discomfort, bowel sounds, and firmness of the abdomen.

21. The nurse notes that the patient is weak and emaciated and determines that stomatitis is contributing to the problem. Which intervention would be the most helpful? *(1219)*
    1. Administer an antiemetic medication 30 minutes before meals.
    2. Weigh the patient after meals and point out small improvements.
    3. Assist with oral hygiene and use water-soaked swabs before and after meals.
    4. Have family bring in meals, rather than cook at home.

22. The health care provider has informed the hospice patient, family, and nurse that there is an invasive untreatable tumor that is contributing to the patient's anorexia. Which intervention is the best for the patient at this time? *(1220)*
    1. Emotional support
    2. Artificial hydration
    3. Total parental nutrition
    4. Tube feedings

23. The nurse gets a phone call from the caregiver who reports hearing the "death rattle." What instructions should the nurse give to the caregiver? *(1220)*
    1. "I will get an order for a bronchodilator medication and bring it to the house."
    2. "Apply oxygen and stay with him. I will come to the house right now."
    3. "Sit the patient upright in bed, apply oxygen, and call 911."
    4. "This is expected: mucus and fluids will pool in the back of his throat."

24. The caregiver reports that the patient is having a hard time managing excessive secretions especially at night, which causes a lot of coughing and choking. He is unable to sit up by himself. What is the best intervention to suggest for this problem? *(1220)*
    1. Teach the patient to cough and deep-breathe.
    2. Obtain an order for droperidol (Inapsine).
    3. Teach the caregiver to perform oral-tracheal suctioning.
    4. Obtain an order for transdermal scopolamine.

25. The hospice aide was devastated when the patient died and the nurse discovers that the aide has been visiting the caregiver on daily basis for the past 12 months. What should the nurse do? *(1222)*
    1. Assess the caregiver's feelings about the frequent visits from the aide.
    2. Report the hospice aide's behavior to the nurse coordinator.
    3. Assess the hospice aide's feelings and motivations for behavior.
    4. Suggest that the hospice aide contact the bereavement counselor.

26. The nurse makes a home visit and the caregiver, who is normally calm and eager to participate in the plan of care, is very angry and insists that the plan needs to be changed because "nothing is working!" What should the nurse do first? *(1216)*
    1. Contact the interdisciplinary team so that the plan can be reevaluated.
    2. Call the nurse coordinator to come and assess the situation.
    3. Check the patient for changes in physical, emotional, or behavioral status.
    4. Use therapeutic communication and encourage the caregiver to express concerns.

CRITICAL THINKING ACTIVITIES

27. The family of a patient with terminal cancer has requested information about hospice care. The patient has severe pain and potential curative treatments have been exhausted.

    a. How would the nurse assess the patient's pain? *(1216)* _____

          _____

          _____

          _____

    b. In addition to assessment, what are the other nursing responsibilities for management of a hospice patient's pain? *(1217)*

          _____

          _____

          _____

    c. For pain relief or reduction, identify the types of medications that may be used for the following. *(1215, 1217)*

        i. Mild to moderate pain: _____

            _____

        ii. Severe pain: _____

            _____

        iii. Long-lasting results:_____

            _____

    d. In addition to pharmacologic therapy, the nurse recognizes that the following measures may also be implemented to relieve or reduce pain. *(1217)*

          _____

          _____

          _____

          _____

          _____

          _____

28. The patient is an 86-year-old who has Alzheimer's disease. His 80-year-old wife has been taking care of him at home for the past 10 years. He was recently diagnosed with an aggressive and inoperable cancer. His family agrees that he should be in hospice, but they are unable to agree on who should be the primary caregiver. The wife insists that she has been taking care of her husband for 10 years and is capable. The eldest son has been responsible for paying the bills and overseeing his parents' finances; he thinks that his sister, who is a nurse but lives in a different state, should move back and be the caregiver. The sister thinks that the grandson who is living with his grandparents and attends the university should be the caregiver. The grandson agrees that he is at the house most often, but is reluctant to take the responsibility. Discuss how the hospice team can assist this family in the decision-making process. *(1213, 1214)*

_____

_____

_____

_____

_____

_____

_____

_____

_____

Introduction to Anatomy and Physiology

Answer Key: Textbook page references are provided as a guide for answering these questions. A complete Answer Key is provided in your Additional Learning Resources on Evolve.

CROSSWORD PUZZLE

1. Directions: Use the clues to complete the crossword puzzle.

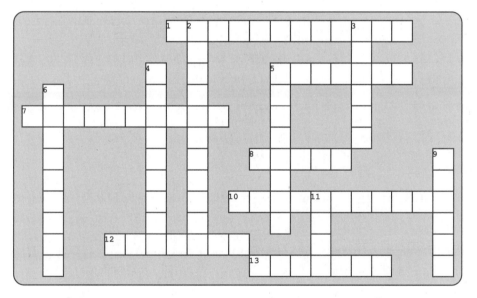

Across

1. Engulf and digest foreign material *(1233)*
5. Cell division *(1232)*
7. Movement of water and particles through a membrane by force from either pressure or gravity *(1234)*
8. Several kinds of tissues united to perform a more complex function *(1237)*
10. Extracellular fluid taken into the cell and digested *(1233)*
12. Diffusion of water through a selectively permeable membrane in the presence of at least one impermeant solute *(1234)*
13. Largest organelle within the cell *(1231)*

Down

2. Body's internal environment is relatively constant *(1231)*
3. Perform more complex functions than any one organ can perform alone *(1237)*
4. Internal living material of cells *(1231)*
5. Thin sheets of tissue that serve many functions in the body *(1231)*
6. Solid particles in a fluid move from an area of higher concentration to an area of lower concentration *(1233)*
9. Groups of similar cells that work together to perform a specific function *(1235)*
11. Smallest living unit of structure and function in the body *(1230)*

FILL-IN-THE-BLANK SENTENCES

Directions: Complete each sentence by filling in the blank with the correct terminology that the nurse uses to document and identify location on the human body.

2. The patient reports, "I ran into the coffeetable and bruised my shin." Nurse documents: 4-cm area of ecchymosis noted on the mid-_____ of right lower extremity. *(1227)*

3. The patient reports, "I was laying on my stomach, so my entire back got sunburned." Nurse documents: Superficial sunburn sustained on _____ body surface. *(1227)*

4. The patient states, "I have small lump just above my collarbone." Nurse documents: 3-cm nontender nodule _____ to the midclavicular area. *(1227)*

5. After being in an automobile accident, the patient has many abrasions on the surface of the skin. Nurse documents: Multiple _____ lacerations. *(1228)*

6. The patient states, "I noticed a patch of dry, itchy skin just underneath my bellybutton." Nurse documents: 4-cm dry, scaly skin _____ to umbilicus. *(1227)*

7. The patient reports, "Occasionally I have a mild pain in the middle of my chest." The nurse documents: Occasional mild pain in the _____ chest area. *(1227)*

8. The patient asks for assistance to turn onto the right side. The nurse documents: Assisted into a right _____ side-lying position. *(1227)*

9. The patient reports, "I have lost sensation in the tip of my right ring finger. The nurse documents: Paresthesia in the _____ tip of the fourth phalanx. *(1228)*

10. The patient reports, "My forearm is tender right below the bend of my elbow." Nurse documents: Tenderness anterior _____ forearm. *(1228)*

TABLE ACTIVITY

11. The table below lists one part of each of the major systems of the body. Identify the major system and then identify at least one function. *(1238)*

One Body Part of Major System	Major System	Function
Lungs		
Heart		
Brain		
Stomach		
Kidneys		
Bones		
Voluntary muscles		
Skin		
Thyroid gland		
Lymph nodes		
Gonads		

FIGURE LABELING

Planes of the Body

12. Directions: Label the figure below with the correct names of the body planes and anatomical directionality of the body: sagittal; coronal, ventral, dorsal, transverse, caudal, and cranial. *(1228)*

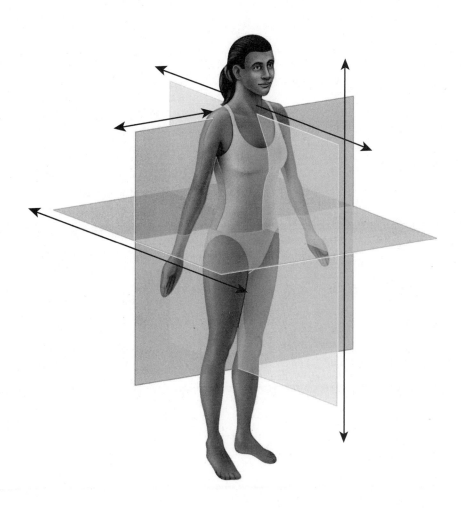

MULTIPLE CHOICE

Directions: Select the best answer(s) for each of the following questions.

13. The patient reports pain in the right upper abdomen just inferior to the ribs. Based on the nurse's knowledge of anatomy, which organ is most likely to be contributing to the patient's discomfort? *(1229)*
    1. Small intestine
    2. Spleen
    3. Gallbladder
    4. Cecum

14. The nurse suspects that the patient has urinary retention and must assess for bladder distention. Which region of the patient's abdomen will the nurse palpate? *(1229)*
    1. Umbilical region
    2. Hypogastric region
    3. Right hypochondriac region
    4. Left iliac region

15. The patient has a stomach ulcer. Based on knowledge of anatomy, the nurse recognizes that the patient is likely to report pain or discomfort in which region of the abdomen? *(1229)*
    1. Epigastric region
    2. Right iliac region
    3. Left lumbar region
    4. Hypogastric region

16. The patient is diagnosed with appendicitis. The health care provider orders ice to abdomen pending emergency surgery. Where will the nurse place the prepared icebag? *(1229)*
    1. Left lower quadrant
    2. Right lower quadrant
    3. Left upper quadrant
    4. Right upper quadrant

17. In the case of bowel obstruction, which condition is most likely to cause the first episodes of vomiting if the patient is allowed to consume solid foods? *(1227)*
    1. Distal large intestine obstruction
    2. Proximal large intestine obstruction
    3. Distal small intestine obstruction
    4. Proximal small intestine obstruction

18. The patient sustains injury to the epidermis. Which problem will the nurse anticipate and try to prevent? *(1236)*
    1. Risk for infection
    2. Loss of strength
    3. Decreased secretion of mucus
    4. Loss of insulation

19. The patient is in a coma and has continuous open-mouthed breathing, which causes dry mucous membranes of the mouth. What is the most important rationale for the nurse to perform good oral hygiene for this patient? *(1237)*
    1. Preserve patient's dignity
    2. Lubricate food for digestion
    3. Prevent respiratory infection
    4. Maintain condition of teeth

20. The patient tells the nurse that he has a history of bursitis. Which focused assessment is the nurse most likely to perform that relates to this information? *(1237)*
    1. Auscultate the bowel sounds and palpate the abdomen
    2. Auscultate the lung sounds and watch respiratory effort
    3. Put joints through range of motion and ask about discomfort
    4. Ask patient to balance on right leg and then on left leg

CRITICAL THINKING ACTIVITIES

Activity 1

21. Why is it important for the nurse to have knowledge of anatomy and physiology? *(1227)*

_____

_____

_____

Activity 2

22. The patient says, "I have a bruise on the tip of my right big toe." Document the patient's report using anatomical terminology. *(1227)*

_____

Activity 3

23. Discuss how the accurate usage and correct spelling of anatomical terminology enhances the credibility of your nursing documentation. *(1227)*

_____

_____

_____

Care of the Surgical Patient

Answer Key: Textbook page references are provided as a guide for answering these questions. A complete Answer Key is provided in your Additional Learning Resources on Evolve.

MATCHING

Directions: Match the term or suffix on the left with the meaning on the right. (1242)

		Term		**Meaning**
_____	1.	anastomosis	a.	Surgical removal of
_____	2.	-ectomy	b.	Direct visualization by a scope
			c.	Opening into
_____	3.	-lysis	d.	Surgical joining of two ducts or blood vessels to allow flow from one to another; to bypass an area
_____	4.	-orrhaphy	e.	Surgical repair of
_____	5.	-oscopy	f.	Destruction or dissolution of
_____	6.	-ostomy	g.	Opening made to allow the passage of drainage
			h.	Plastic surgery
_____	7.	-otomy	i.	Fixation of
_____	8.	-pexy		
_____	9.	-plasty		

TRUE OR FALSE

Directions: Write T for true or F for false in the blanks provided. (1242)

_____	10.	A rhinoplasty could be performed for cosmetic reasons.
_____	11.	Removal of the appendix is an ablative type of surgery.
_____	12.	A breast biopsy is a palliative surgery.
_____	13.	The surgeon may perform an exploratory laparotomy to confirm a diagnosis.
_____	14.	A carotid endarterectomy could be performed under same-day admit conditions.
_____	15.	Total hip replacement is a type of transplant surgery.
_____	16.	Closure of an atrial septal defect in the heart is constructive surgery.
_____	17.	Internal fixation of a right fibula is reconstructive surgery.
_____	18.	Coronary artery bypass is one example of major surgery.
_____	19.	Cataract extraction is usually considered an urgent surgery.

TABLE ACTIVITY

20. Directions: The patient has just returned from gastric surgery. Next to each assessment, list what normal findings the nurse would expect and how frequently the data collection would be performed. *(1270-1277)*

Assessment	Normal Findings	Frequency
a. Vital signs		
b. Incision		
c. Ventilation		
d. Pain		
e. Urinary function		
f. Venous status		
g. Activity		
h. Gastrointestinal function		

MULTIPLE CHOICE

Directions: Select the best answer(s) for each of the following questions.

21. The patient is in the induction stage of anesthesia. Which activity will most likely be taking place? *(1263)*
    1. Positioning the patient to perform the surgical procedure
    2. Decreasing the dosage(s) of anesthetic agent(s)
    3. Cleaning, shaving, and preparing the skin
    4. Establishing and verifying placement of the endotracheal tube

22. During the preoperative teaching session, a patient voices concerns about waking up during surgery. Which response should the nurse give to the patient? *(1263)*
    1. "The anesthesia given during surgery will not wear off and allow you to wake up."
    2. "The anesthesiologist is able to monitor for this and will provide medications as needed."
    3. "Waking up is a risk you will face during the surgical procedure."
    4. "Emergence from anesthesia is a rare complication of surgery."

23. The patient is scheduled to undergo a urologic procedure in the surgical suite. The patient will be conscious during the procedure. What type of anesthesia will most likely be used? *(1263)*
    1. Nerve block
    2. Epidural anesthesia
    3. Spinal anesthesia
    4. Local anesthesia

24. The patient is scheduled to undergo the removal of a benign cyst from his hand in the health care provider's office. The nurse is aware that the health care provider will most likely use which type of anesthesia? *(1264)*
    1. Regional anesthesia
    2. Local anesthesia
    3. Conscious sedation
    4. Intrathecal anesthesia

25. The nurse is preparing to assist the health care provider who is performing a procedure using conscious sedation. Which nursing action is the most important during the procedure? *(1264)*
    1. Monitoring intake and output
    2. Administering the medication
    3. Reassuring the patient
    4. Assessment of vital signs

26. The nurse is preparing an in-service for nursing staff on conscious sedation. What should be emphasized in the presentation? *(1265)*
    1. The recovery from the procedure is often risky.
    2. The patient should not be prematurely extubated.
    3. Resuscitation equipment should be readily available.
    4. Nurses should not administer central nervous system depressants.

27. When developing the plan of care for an Arab American undergoing surgery, what cultural consideration may be of concern? *(1245)*
    1. Stoicism during pain and discomfort
    2. Expected submissive role of women
    3. Need for a written consent for surgery
    4. Avoidance of sustained eye contact

28. Preoperative teaching is ideally provided: *(1248)*
    1. 1 to 2 days before surgery.
    2. the morning of surgery.
    3. at least 2 weeks preoperatively.
    4. when the nurse has extra time.

29. Before surgery of the bowel, neomycin, sulfonamides, or erythromycin may be given to: *(1250)*
    1. decrease likelihood of bowel perforation.
    2. prevent urinary tract infections.
    3. detoxify the gastrointestinal tract.
    4. reduce the risk of pneumonia.

30. The nurse is providing care for a patient in the PACU who had an unexpected surgical procedure performed. The patient has been on antihypertensive medications for a long time. What side effects related to use of antihypertensive medications should the nurse monitor for? (Select all that apply.) *(1262)*
    1. Tachycardia
    2. Hypotension
    3. Bradycardia
    4. Impaired circulation
    5. Diaphoresis

31. The patient is instructed to discontinue taking nonsteroidal antiinflammatory drugs (NSAIDs) for several days before surgery. What is the best explanation for the need to hold this medication? *(1262)*
    1. "NSAIDs increase susceptibility to postoperative bleeding."
    2. "NSAIDs impair healing during the postoperative period."
    3. "NSAIDs interact with the medications used for anesthesia."
    4. "NSAIDs are associated with an increase in postoperative infections."

32. A mastectomy is scheduled for an 81-year-old patient. What is the highest priority during the immediate postoperative recovery period? *(1270)*
    1. Assessing for confusion
    2. Airway management
    3. Pain management
    4. Monitoring bleeding

33. The patient is being prepared to go to the operating room. With proper instructions, which task(s) can be delegated to the UAP? (Select all that apply.) *(1244)*
    1. Compare current vital signs to baseline measurements.
    2. Assist the patient to remove personal clothing and don a hospital gown.
    3. Check the IV pump rate and the IV insertion site.
    4. Assist the patient to move from the bed to the stretcher.
    5. Ensure that the preoperative checklist is complete.
    6. Apply antiembolic stockings.

34. The nurse is performing preoperative teaching for a patient who must undergo a breast biopsy. The patient begins to cry softly and says, "I can't believe this is happening to me." What response should the nurse use first? *(1246)*
    1. "Do you need more information about the procedure?"
    2. "The biopsy is a minor procedure, there are very few risks."
    3. "Don't cry, everything will be okay; we'll take care of you."
    4. "You seem scared; tell me what you are thinking about."

35. Which patient is most likely to have problems related to medications that are given in the perioperative setting? *(1245)*
    1. A 23-year-old woman who believes in alternative and complementary medicines
    2. A 73-year-old woman who takes multiple medications for several chronic conditions
    3. A 56-year-old man who has recently started an oral antidiabetic medication
    4. A 7-year-old child who occasionally uses a rescue inhaler for asthma

36. The patient tells the nurse that he has been smoking for years and is likely to continue to smoke before and after his surgery. Which piece of equipment will the nurse emphasize during the preoperative teaching? *(1252)*
    1. Normal range for pulse oximeter
    2. Use of incentive spirometer
    3. Use of patient-controlled analgesia pump
    4. Operation of the call bell

37. The nurse is evaluating the patient's understanding of the preoperative teaching. Which question should the nurse ask? *(1278)*
    1. Do you have any questions about postoperative care?
    2. Would you like written information about the care plan?
    3. Did you understand everything I told you about the care?
    4. What questions do you have about the postoperative care?

38. The health care provider is preparing to explain a procedure to the patient and obtain informed consent. Which information is the most vital to relate to the provider before he/she enters the patient's room? *(1249)*
    1. Patient has been talking about refusing the surgery.
    2. Patient had a hypoglycemic episode 3 hours ago.
    3. Patient's laboratory reports are not available yet.
    4. Patient received morphine and a sedative 1 hour ago.

39. The patient is on NPO status starting at midnight the night before surgery. Which task can be delegated to the UAP? *(1249)*
    1. Give the patient small sips of water if he reports thirst.
    2. Assist with oral care, but instruct the patient not to swallow fluids.
    3. Obtain small hard candy for the patient to suck on.
    4. Check the patient's intravenous fluids every 2 hours.

40. Which patient would not be instructed to cough after surgery? *(1254)*
    1. The patient who had abdominal surgery
    2. The patient who had pneumonia before surgery
    3. The patient who had intracranial surgery
    4. The patient who had thoracic surgery

41. The patient had surgery at 10:00 AM. At 6:00 PM the nurse notes that the patient has not voided since returning from surgery. What should the nurse do first? *(1257)*
    1. Help the patient to the toilet and open the faucet so that water runs.
    2. Palpate the symphysis pubis to determine if the bladder is distended.
    3. Call the health care provider and obtain an order for catheterization.
    4. Help the patient to get up and ambulate to stimulate urination.

42. The patient is undergoing spinal anesthesia and the patient's position has to be slightly adjusted during the procedure. Which occurrence is cause for greatest concern? *(1263)*
    1. Slight decrease in blood pressure
    2. Loss of sensation in both feet
    3. Slowing of respiratory rate
    4. Inability to freely move the legs

43. A patient who had surgery on the left hip tells the nurse, "You might think I am crazy, but my right arm kind of hurts since I had my surgery." What should the nurse do first? *(1271)*
    1. Check the operating records for the position the patient was in during the operation.
    2. Call the health care provider and inform him/her of the new onset arm pain.
    3. Assess the arm for pulse, sensation, movement, pain, and temperature of skin.
    4. Give the patient a mild PRN pain medication and elevate the arm on a pillow.

44. Which instruction is the nurse most likely to give to the patient before administering the preoperative medication? *(1260)*
    1. "Please go to the bathroom and void."
    2. "Let me mark the operative site."
    3. "I am going to take your vital signs."
    4. "Please sign the consent form."

45. The patient will soon be transferred from the PACU to the nursing unit. Which task(s) can be delegated to the UAP? (Select all that apply.) *(1244)*
    1. Place the bed in a high position with side rails in appropriate position.
    2. Obtain a clean gown and extra pillows for positioning.
    3. Set up suction equipment and test function.
    4. Get stethoscope, thermometer, and sphygmomanometer.
    5. Check the function of the IV pump.
    6. Place bed pads to protect linens from drainage.

46. The anesthesia provider has written the order to transfer the patient from PACU to the nursing unit. Which assessment finding would delay the transfer? *(1268-1270)*
    1. Patient is awake, but nausea and some vomiting continue.
    2. Patient is breathing normally, but reports a sore throat and cough.
    3. Patient is crying and reports pain related to the surgical incision.
    4. Patient has a decreased blood pressure and pulse is increasing.

47. The patient had surgery 10 hours ago. The UAP tells the nurse that the blood pressure (BP) is 96/60 mm Hg and the patient says, "My blood pressure is usually 120/78." What should the nurse do first? *(1271)*
    1. Check the patient for signs and symptoms of hypovolemic shock.
    2. Tell the UAP to go back and repeat the BP and report back.
    3. Tell the UAP to take and report BP and pulse every 5 minutes for 15 minutes.
    4. Call the health care provider and report the low reading of 96/60.

48. Which task is the responsibility of the scrub nurse? *(1269)*
    1. Sends for the patient at the proper time
    2. Checks medical record for completeness
    3. Performs and confirms patient assessment
    4. Assists with surgical draping of patient

49. The nurse is preparing to discharge a patient from an ambulatory surgery setting. How does the nurse determine when the patient is ready to be discharged? *(1280)*
    1. Patient states he is ready to drive himself home.
    2. Patient is groggy, but readily arouses to normal stimuli.
    3. Patient reports that pain is controlled and nausea has ceased.
    4. Family is available and willing to take responsibility.

50. The nurse is caring for a postoperative patient
    who has preexisting type 2 diabetes. Which
    assessment is most relevant to a complication
    associated with diabetes? *(1244)*
    1. Impaired communication
    2. Bloody emesis
    3. Poor wound healing
    4. Hypoventilation

CRITICAL THINKING ACTIVITIES

Activity 1

A 35-year-old woman reports to the health care provider's office with complaints of itching; hives on her
arms, neck, and chest; and sore throat. She further reports that these symptoms occur when she is at work.
Further assessment reveals she works in a local nursing home in the housekeeping department. Her health
history is uneventful. She is diagnosed with a latex allergy.

51. Discuss latex allergies. Include types, influencing factors, risk factors, and methods of prevention. *(1250)*

_____

_____

_____

_____

_____

_____

Activity 2

The health care provider informs the nurse that the patient has an unexpected problem that requires urgent
surgery, which is likely to occur within the next several days.

52. Describe how the nurse can use the ABCDEF mnemonic device to ascertain serious illness or trauma in
    the preoperative patient. *(1244)*

_____

_____

_____

_____

_____

_____

Activity 3

53. Discuss four or five considerations for older adults who require surgery. *(1243)*

_____

_____

_____

_____

_____

Care of the Patient with an Integumentary Disorder

Answer Key: Textbook page references are provided as a guide for answering these questions. A complete Answer Key is provided in your Additional Learning Resources on Evolve.

MATCHING

Primary Skin Lesions

Directions: Match the type of lesion on the left to the example and description on the right, and in the blank space provided indicate the letter of the correct description and example. (1286-1291)

Type of Lesion		**Description and Example**
_____ 1. macule	a.	Elevated irregularly shaped area of cutaneous edema; solid, transient; variable diameter (e.g., insect bite)
_____ 2. papule	b.	Flat, nonpalpable, irregularly shaped macule; >1 cm in diameter (e.g., port-wine stains)
_____ 3. patch	c.	Elevated and solid lesion; deeper in dermis; >2 cm in diameter (e.g., neoplasm)
_____ 4. plaque		
_____ 5. wheal	d.	Elevated, circumscribed, superficial, not into dermis; filled with serous fluid; <1 cm in diameter (e.g., chickenpox)
_____ 6. nodule	e.	Elevated, firm, and rough lesion with flat top surface; >1 cm in diameter (e.g., psoriasis)
_____ 7. tumor		
_____ 8. vesicle	f.	Elevated, circumscribed, encapsulated lesion; filled with liquid or semisolid material (e.g., sebaceous cyst)
_____ 9. bulla	g.	Dried serum, blood, or purulent exudate; slightly elevated; brown, red, black, or tan (e.g., eczema)
_____ 10. pustule		
_____ 11. cyst	h.	Elevated, firm, circumscribed area; <1 cm in diameter [e.g., wart (verruca)]
_____ 12. lichenification	i.	Elevated, firm, circumscribed lesion; deeper in dermis than a papule; 1-2 cm in diameter (e.g., lipomas)
_____ 13. scale		
_____ 14. keloid	j.	Flat, circumscribed area with a change in color; < 1 cm in diameter (e.g., freckles)
_____ 15. scar	k.	Irregularly shaped, progressively enlarging scar; excessive collagen (e.g., keloid formation after surgery)
_____ 16. excoriation		
_____ 17. fissure	l.	Linear crack or break from the epidermis to the dermis; may be moist or dry (e.g., athlete's foot)
_____ 18. erosion	m.	Elevated, superficial lesion; similar to a vesicle but filled with purulent fluid (e.g., acne)
_____ 19. ulcer		
_____ 20. crust	n.	Vesicle >1 cm in diameter (e.g.. blister)
_____ 21. atrophy		

(Continued next page)

(Continued)

o. Heaped-up keratinized cells; flaky skin; irregular; thick or thin; dry or oily (e.g., flaking of skin)

p. Partial loss of the epidermis; depressed, moist, glistening; follows rupture of a vesicle (e.g., variola after rupture)

q. Loss of epidermis and dermis; concave; varies in size (e.g., pressure sore)

r. Thin to thick fibrous tissue that replaces normal skin after injury to the dermis (e.g., healed surgical incision)

s. Loss of the epidermis; linear, hollowed-out, crusted area (e.g., abrasion)

t. Rough, thickened epidermis secondary to persistent rubbing, itching (e.g., chronic dermatitis)

u. Thinning of skin surface and loss of skin markings; skin translucent and paperlike (e.g., aged skin)

SHORT ANSWER

Directions: Using your own words, answer each question in the space provided.

22. What are the functions of the skin? *(1283, 1284)*

_____

_____

_____

_____

_____

23. When performing an assessment of an integumentary problem, what should be included using "PQRST"? *(1292)*

_____

_____

_____

_____

24. When performing an assessment of a mole, what characteristics should be included using "ABCDE" for assessment of skin lesions? *(1292)*

_____

_____

_____

_____

FIGURE LABELING

Rule of Nines

25. Directions: Label the body according to the rule of nines. *(1324)*

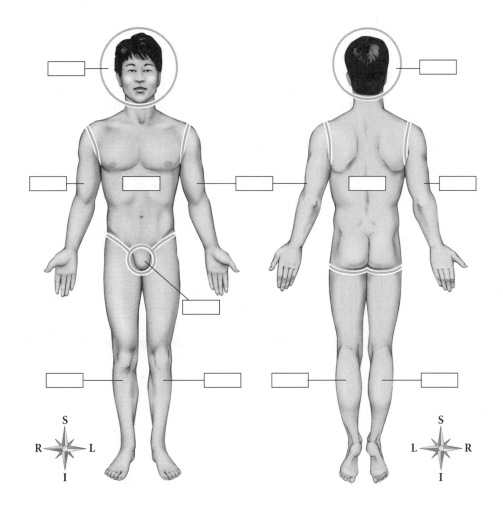

26. Calculate the percentage of burns for each of the situations listed below using the rule of nines. *(1323, 1324)*

    a. A 19-year-old was burned while playing with fireworks. He has burns on both of his arms (anterior and posterior) and his anterior chest. _____%

    b. A 70-year-old man was burned when he backed up into an open-flame heater. He has burns on the posterior of his body from his ankles to his neck. He also has burns on the anterior portion of his legs. _____%

    c. The patient, who has diabetes mellitus, stepped into a hot shower and has burns on his back and buttocks. _____%

MULTIPLE CHOICE

Directions: Select the best answer(s) for each of the following questions

27. The nurse hears in report that a young female patient is very upset because of alopecia; she cannot focus on the overall cancer treatment plan. In addition to therapeutic communication, which nursing intervention could the nurse use? *(1314)*
    1. Suggest therapeutic baths using colloid solution.
    2. Teach the patient about use of scarves or wigs.
    3. Suggest shaving, tweezing, or rubbing with pumice.
    4. Advise the patient to use lotion immediately after bathing.

28. The health care provider has diagnosed a patient with paronychia. Which assessment is the nurse most likely to perform before administering the ordered therapy? *(1322)*
    1. History of allergies to antibiotics
    2. Rating of pain on a pain scale
    3. Baseline range of motion
    4. Feelings about body image

29. A patient reports hair loss (hypotrichosis). Which assessment is the nurse mostly likely to conduct to assist the health care provider in determining the etiology of hypotrichosis? *(1322)*
    1. Type of hair-care products
    2. Use of herbal supplements
    3. Smoking history
    4. Dietary assessment

30. A patient is admitted for pain and tenderness in his lower right leg. The nurse's assessment reveals that the extremity is warm, swollen, and has a slightly pitted appearance. Which measure would the nurse use to relieve the discomfort? *(1302)*
    1. Assist the patient to ambulate as much as possible.
    2. Administer cool compresses or a covered icebag.
    3. Elevate the leg with pillows to reduce edema.
    4. Assist with a therapeutic bath and gently pat skin to dry.

31. When assisting a mother to plan meals for a child recently diagnosed with eczema, the nurse should advise her that common allergies for a patient with this diagnosis may include: *(1309)*
    1. strawberries and cured meats.
    2. eggs, rye, and preservatives.
    3. orange juice, wheat, and eggs.
    4. wheat, sugar, and bananas

32. The nurse knows that the health care provider frequently prescribes isotretinoin (Accutane) for patients with acne. Which question is the most important to routinely ask? *(1296)*
    1. Are you pregnant or contemplating a pregnancy in the near future?
    2. Do you have a history of kidney problems or frequent urinary tract infections?
    3. How often do you sunbathe? Are you willing to abstain during treatment?
    4. Do you have any problems with your liver or a history of hepatitis?

33. The nurse is interviewing an older adult. Which statement is cause for the greatest concern? *(1319)*
    1. "My toenails are tough and thick."
    2. "This black mole on my neck is itching."
    3. "My hair thinning and I have a bald spot."
    4. "I have a lot of 'age spots' on my hands."

34. The nurse notes that the patient has clubbing of the fingertips. Based on this finding, which question would the nurse ask? *(1286)*
    1. Have you been diagnosed with a respiratory disorder?
    2. Do you take medication for high blood pressure?
    3. Do you have a family history of diabetes mellitus?
    4. Are you taking medication for osteoporosis?

35. To assess the temperature and texture of the patient's skin, which technique would the nurse use? *(1286)*
    1. Use the fingertips and gently palpate the affected area.
    2. Use the palms of the hands and compare opposite body areas.
    3. Use a cotton-tipped applicator and apply gentle pressure.
    4. Use a gloved finger to touch skin and ask about sensations.

36. The school nurse is assessing a 15-year-old girl and notices multiple linear superficial cuts over the girl's anterior forearms. What should the nurse do first? *(1292)*
    1. Call child protective services to report possible abuse.
    2. Notify the girl's parents about the finding.
    3. Ask the girl directly what happened to her arms.
    4. Initiate protective measures to prevent self-harm.

37. The nurse is assessing a patient who was recently transferred from home to a skilled nursing facility. The nurse sees a pressure ulcer with full-thickness tissue loss, which is covered by a thick, black layer of eschar. What should the nurse do first? *(1293)*
    1. Gently remove the eschar and check for tunneling and depth.
    2. Document the size and location of this stage IV ulcer.
    3. Contact the wound care specialist for wound management.
    4. Leave eschar intact; collaborate with RN to develop care plan.

38. The home health aide phones the nurse and says, "I helped the patient bathe. I wore gloves during the bath, but then afterwards he said that he was just diagnosed with herpes zoster." Which question would the nurse ask first? *(1299)*
    1. "Are you having a painful burning rash with itching?"
    2. "Do you have fluid-filled vesicles on your back or trunk?"
    3. "Have you received two doses of varicella vaccine?"
    4. "How long were you in contact with the patient?"

39. The nurse hears during shift report that the patient was admitted for penicillin-induced dermatitis medicamentosa. Which question is the most important to ask? *(1307)*
    1. Was the affected area immediately washed and rinsed?
    2. Has the patient been medicated for pain and itching?
    3. Has the patient had any respiratory distress?
    4. Does the patient have any fever or other signs of infection?

40. The nurse would be prepared to administer epinephrine as needed for which patient? *(1308)*
    1. Has burning sensation and a dry crusty lesion on the lip
    2. Has a single pink, scaly patch that resembles a large ringworm
    3. Has skin maceration, fissures, and vesicles around the toes
    4. Has raised red wheals and hives and an expiratory wheeze

CRITICAL THINKING ACTIVITIES

Activity 1

41. Discuss the nursing care of a patient who has sustained a major burn through the emergent phase, acute phase, and rehabilitation phase. *(1325, 1326, 1330)*

    a. Emergent phase _____

    _____

    _____

b. Acute phase _____

_____

_____

c. Rehabilitation phase _____

_____

_____

Activity 2

42. a. The nurse is assessing the skin of several patients. What are the physiologic factors that influence skin color? *(1285, 1286)*

_____

_____

_____

_____

b. Based on the patient's low hemoglobin and hematocrit, the nurse would assess for pallor. The patient is a very dark-skinned individual. How would the nurse assess this patient for pallor? *(1292)*

_____

_____

_____

_____

c. The darker-skinned patient reports an itching sensation, but the nurse cannot detect a rash with visual inspection. What technique can the nurse use? *(1292)*

_____

_____

_____

_____

Care of the Patient with a Musculoskeletal Disorder

Answer Key: Textbook page references are provided as a guide for answering these questions. A complete Answer Key is provided in your Additional Learning Resources on Evolve.

FIGURE LABELING

1. Directions: Label the figure of the anterior view of skeleton below with the correct names of the bones of the body. *(1338)*

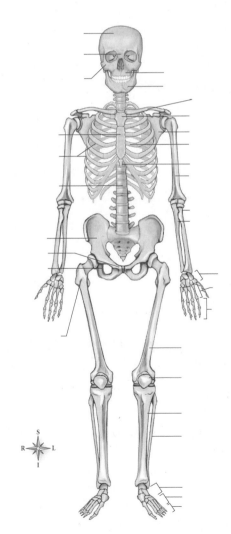

SHORT ANSWER

Directions: Using your own words, answer each question in the space provided.

2. List five functions of the skeletal system. *(1336, 1337)*

a. _____

b. _____

c. _____

d. _____

e. _____

3. List three functions that muscles perform when they contract. *(1337, 1338)*

a. _____

b. _____

c. _____

4. Discuss neurovascular assessment and include the seven Ps of orthopedic assessment. *(1372)*

_____

_____

_____

_____

_____

_____

_____

5. What does "RICE" mean in relation to the treatment for sprains? *(1388)* _____

_____

TRUE OR FALSE

Directions: Write T for true or F for false in the blanks provided.

_____ 6. Following hip surgery, the nurse uses a wedge-shaped foam bolster or pillow for 7-10 days to ensure postoperative maintenance of leg adduction and to prevent dislocation of the prosthesis. *(1368)*

_____ 7. A common posture deformity is kyphosis, which is a lateral (or S) curvature of the spine. *(1397)*

_____ 8. Buck's traction is used as a temporary measure to provide support and comfort to a fractured extremity while waiting for more definitive treatment. *(1367)*

_____ 9. Approximately 50% of patients with fibromyalgia report the condition impairs their ability to successfully complete activities of daily living. *(1361)*

_____ 10. An erythrocyte sedimentation rate (ESR) is the most objective laboratory test for determining the severity of rheumatoid arthritis. *(1344)*

MULTIPLE CHOICE

Directions: Select the best answer(s) for each of the following questions.

11. A patient is prescribed colchicine to treat gout. For which potential side effects associated with the medication should the nurse be assessing? *(1355)*
    1. Diarrhea, nausea, and vomiting
    2. Seizures and dysrhythmias
    3. Fluid retention and sodium retention
    4. Hypercalcemia and orthostatic hypotension

12. When assisting in planning meals for a 59-year-old woman who is concerned about her risk of osteoporosis, which food should the nurse recommend as a good source of calcium? (Select all that apply.) *(1358)*
    1. Milk
    2. Spinach
    3. Potatoes
    4. Sardines
    5. Organ meats

13. The nurse is interviewing a young woman who injured her ankle while playing soccer. With regards to the diagnostic testing that is mostly likely to be ordered, which question is the most important to ask? *(1341)*
    1. Do you have allergies to seafood or iodine?
    2. Is there any chance you could be pregnant?
    3. Are you currently taking any medications?
    4. Do you have a history of radiation exposure?

14. The nurse is assessing a patient who had a myelogram 3 hours ago. Which patient comment causes the greatest concern? *(1341)*
    1. "My head hurts. Could I get an aspirin or a Tylenol tablet?"
    2. "I am thirsty. Would if be okay if I drank a soda or some juice?"
    3. "My foot feels numb and I can't move my toes very well."
    4. "I am not used to lying in bed all day long; I'd like to walk around."

15. The nurse hears in report that the patient has a medical diagnosis of ankylosing spondylitis (AKS). What will the nurse include in the focused assessment for this patient? *(1351)*
    1. The 7 Ps of orthopedic assessment
    2. Assessment of back pain and vision
    3. Frequent mental status checks
    4. Urinary retention and back stiffness

16. The patient says to the nurse, "I have excruciating pain in my big toe at night." Which assessment question is the nurse most likely to ask? *(1355)*
    1. Have you noticed a change in your bowel movements?
    2. How much exercise would you normally get in a week?
    3. Do you eat organ meats, yeast, herring, or mackerel?
    4. Do you notice jaw tension, excessive fatigue, or anxiety?

17. The patient is admitted for acute osteomyelitis of the left lower extremity. Which instruction should the nurse give to the UAP? *(1359)*
    1. Use drainage and secretion precautions when caring for the patient.
    2. Assist the patient to ambulate in the hall every 2-3 hours.
    3. Anticipate that movement is more difficult in the morning.
    4. Refresh the patient's ice pack every 2 hours or as needed.

18. The nurse is caring for a patient who had unicompartmental knee surgery. Which interventions will the nurse use in the postoperative period? (Select all that apply.) *(1363)*
    1. Encourage deep-breathing and coughing every 2 hours.
    2. Begin with a clear liquid diet and advance to regular as tolerated.
    3. Inspect the skin at the edge of the cast for erythema.
    4. Assess the patient's ability to use an assistive device such as a walker.
    5. Monitor IV fluids and effectiveness of antibiotics.
    6. Administer intraarticular injections of corticosteroids.

19. The nurse is assessing a patient following a hip arthroplasty and returned from surgery early in the shift. The patient is now restless and anxious. What is the nurse's first action? *(1375, 1376)*
    1. Decrease anxiety by reassuring the patient that everything is going as expected.
    2. Initiate vital signs q 15 minutes, compare to baseline and monitor trends.
    3. Look at the urinary output and compare the total to baseline.
    4. Call the patient's family and invite them to spend time at the bedside.

20. A fiberglass cast has been applied to the forearm of a 6-year-old child to treat and stabilize a greenstick fracture. Which teaching point is the most important to emphasize with the child? *(1376)*
    1. Instructing the child to keep the cast dry
    2. Teaching the child to report pain to the parents
    3. Showing the child how to test capillary refill
    4. Reminding the child to wiggle the fingers

21. The nurse is supervising a nursing student in the care of a patient who had internal fixation for a hip fracture. The nurse would intervene if the student performed which action? *(1368)*
    1. Assessed the amount of drainage in the Jackson-Pratt drain
    2. Encouraged coughing and the use of the incentive spirometer
    3. Removed the antiembolism stocking to assess the skin
    4. Placed the patient in high Fowler's position prior to eating

22. The nurse is providing care for a patient who has just had a hip replacement. Which comment from the patient indicates the need for further education? *(1363)*
    1. "I need to be on bedrest for the first 72 hours."
    2. "I need to obtain a seat riser for my toilet at home."
    3. "I should never sit with my legs crossed."
    4. "I'll have limitations in hip position for 2-3 months."

23. A nurse is checking on an elderly neighbor who just fell down. The man cheerfully tells the nurse, "I just tripped on the carpet and took a spill. No harm done!" Based on mechanism of injury, which assessment is the nurse most likely to perform if the neighbor will allow it? *(1371)*
    1. Head-to-toe to detect occult injury
    2. Palpation and range of motion for wrist injury
    3. Mental status examination for head injury
    4. Environmental assessment for other hazards

24. The patient was in a car accident and reports pain over the pelvic region with difficulty raising legs in a supine position. The nurse notes ecchymosis over the pelvic region. Which laboratory test is the primary concern in the immediate phase of care? *(1375)*
    1. Hemoglobin and hematocrit
    2. Blood type and Rh
    3. Urinalysis
    4. Stool for occult blood

25. The patient with a cast on the lower extremity reports pain at 7/10. What should the nurse do first? *(1367)*
    1. Reposition the leg so that elevation is maintained.
    2. Administer pain medication as ordered.
    3. Report potential compartment syndrome to RN.
    4. Perform the 7 Ps of orthopedic assessment.

26. The nurse hears in report that the patient has Volkmann's contracture of the dominant upper extremity. Which intervention would the nurse plan to use? *(1376)*
    1. Frequent assessment using the 7 Ps of orthopedic assessment
    2. Assess the patient's abilities to perform activities of daily living
    3. Teach the patient to report pain, loss of sensation, or swelling
    4. Instruct the UAP on how to maintain proper position and alignment

27. The nurse is caring for a patient with a long bone fracture. The laboratory reports the following arterial blood gas results. What should the nurse do first? (1378)

pH	7.4
Paco₂	40 mm Hg
Pao₂	95 mm Hg
HCO₃	26 mEq/L
Sao₂	98%

1. Assess the patient for signs of fat embolism and respiratory distress.
2. Report these normal results to the health care provider.
3. Place the patient in high Fowler's position to ease respirations.
4. Check the vital signs and continue to monitor the patient.

28. A computer data entry clerk reports paresthesia in the thumb, index finger, and middle finger and pain that increases during the night. The clerk has an appointment with a health care provider next week. In the meantime, what self-care measure would the nurse advise? (1391, 1392)
1. Use warm packs and sleep with hands on a pillow.
2. Frequently change position and stretch hands while working.
3. Use a mild analgesic such as ibuprofen or aspirin.
4. Wrap the wrist snugly with an elastic bandage.

29. The patient who had a laminectomy reports abdominal discomfort with a gaseous, bloated feeling and mild nausea. What should the nurse do first? (1393)
1. Offer clear liquids
2. Encourage ambulation
3. Listen for bowel sounds
4. Administer an antiemetic

30. The patient reports long bone pain that increases with weight-bearing. The health care provider tells the nurse that the patient has an elevated serum alkaline phosphatase. The nurse prepares to give emotional support because the health care provider must tell the patient that additional diagnostic testing is need to rule out: (1394)
1. phantom limb pain.
2. compartment syndrome.
3. fibromyalgia.
4. osteogenic sarcoma.

CRITICAL THINKING ACTIVITIES

Activity 1

31. Discuss factors that contribute to osteoporosis and the nurse's role in helping patients prevent bone loss and fractures. (1356)

_____

_____

_____

_____

_____

_____

Activity 2

32. A 32-year-old woman has been told that she might have fibromyalgia syndrome; however, the health care provider tells her that this is just a possibility and that additional diagnostic testing would be needed. The patient is angry at first and then she begins to cry and confides in the nurse, "I am just so frustrated with these doctors and I just want to be able to live a normal life." Discuss fibromyalgia syndrome from the patient's point of view. *(1358-1361)*

_____

_____

_____

_____

_____

Activity 3

33. The home health nurse is visiting a thin elderly woman who lives alone. The three-story house is a little cluttered with old belongings. Her bedroom and bathroom are on the second floor. The rugs are worn and the hallways are poorly lit. The woman cheerfully reports that she has a cane, a walker, and eyeglasses, but frequently misplaces "all of the 'old person' stuff." The woman has a small friendly dog; he jumps at her legs and she frequently bends down to pet him. Discuss the potential for hip fracture for this woman. *(1366)*

_____

_____

_____

_____

_____

Activity 4

34. A patient diagnosed with rheumatoid arthritis requests additional information. She states that she has heard of two types of arthritis. She asks about the differences between rheumatoid arthritis and osteoarthritis. Compare and contrast rheumatoid arthritis and osteoarthritis. Include cause, clinical manifestations, treatment options, and prognosis. *(1345-1354)*

_____

_____

_____

_____

_____

_____

Care of the Patient with a Gastrointestinal Disorder

Answer Key: Textbook page references are provided as a guide for answering these questions. A complete Answer Key is provided in your Additional Learning Resources on Evolve.

FIGURE LABELING

1. Directions: Label the digestive organs. *(1403)*

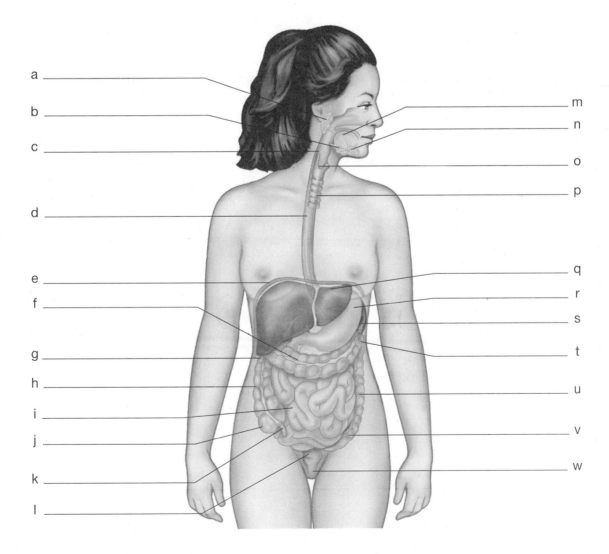

a _____

b _____

c _____

d _____

e _____

f _____

g _____

h _____

i _____

j _____

k _____

l _____

m _____

n _____

o _____

p _____

q _____

r _____

s _____

t _____

u _____

v _____

w _____

FILL-IN-THE-BLANK SENTENCES

Directions: Complete each sentence by filling in the blank with the correct word or phrase.

2. _____ is the coordinated, rhythmic, sequential contraction of smooth muscle that pushes food through the digestive tract, as well as bile through the bile duct. *(1402)*

3. Lysozyme is a salivary enzyme that destroys bacteria and thus protects the mucous membrane from _____ and the teeth from _____. *(1404)*

4. The cardiac sphincter contracts and prevents _____, which can be irritating to the esophagus. *(1404)*

5. Pancreatic juices are essential in breaking down _____ into their amino acid components, in reducing dietary _____ to glycerol and fatty acids, and in converting starch to _____. *(1405)*

6. The large intestine has four major functions: (1) absorption of _____, (2) manufacture of certain vitamins (such as vitamin K and B$_7$), (3) formation of _____, and (4) _____ of feces. *(1405)*

7. The bacteria in the large intestine are also responsible for the synthesis of vitamin K, which is needed for normal _____. *(1406)*

8. Bile, produced in the liver, is a yellow-brown or green-brown liquid necessary for the emulsification of _____. *(1406)*

9. (Trypsin), lipase (steapsin), and amylase (amylopsin), which are produced by the pancreas, are important because they digest the three major components of chyme: _____, _____, and _____. *(1417)*

10. The _____, a portion of the brain, contains one center that stimulates the individual to eat, and the other signals the individual to stop eating. *(1407)*

MULTIPLE CHOICE

Directions: Select the best answer(s) for each of the following questions.

11. The nurse caring for a patient with fecal incontinence recognizes that common causes of the disorder include which of the following? (Select all that apply.) *(1454)*
    1. Normal changes of aging
    2. Injury during anal intercourse
    3. Surgical trauma to anal sphincter
    4. Injury during childbirth
    5. Spinal cord lesions
    6. Voluntary inhibition of defecation

12. When planning care for a patient with a motor paralysis, which intervention is the most important as a long-term solution for the patient's defecation status? *(1454)*
    1. Teach the family and patient the log roll to clean fecal incontinence.
    2. Include the patient and family in planning a bowel training program.
    3. Contact social services to find funds for incontinence pads and briefs.
    4. Arrange for home health services for assistance with hygiene and toileting.

13. The most effective bowel training programs will include: *(1454)*
    1. biofeedback.
    2. surgery.
    3. enemas to prevent constipation.
    4. routine use of glycerin suppositories.

14. The patient is practicing a bowel training program. Which food will the nurse encourage the patient to eat? *(1454)*
    1. Lean chicken meat
    2. Low-fat milk
    3. Whole-grain cereal
    4. Red meat

15. A patient is being treated with sucralfate (Carafate) for gastroesophageal reflux disease (GERD). Which teaching point would the nurse emphasize? *(1422)*
    1. Oral anticoagulants, theophylline, and propranolol may require dosage reductions.
    2. Coating action may interfere with the absorption of other drugs—separate by 2 hours.
    3. Contraindicated during pregnancy; women of childbearing age must use reliable contraception.
    4. Avoid driving or other hazardous activities until accustomed to sedating effects.

16. A patient had a partial gastrectomy. Because this surgery creates an increased risk for pernicious anemia, which teaching point is important to emphasize? *(1428)*
    1. Blood serum vitamin B_{12} level should be measured every 1 to 2 years.
    2. Hemoglobin and hematocrit should be measured every 1 to 2 months.
    3. Injections of iron dextran (DexFerrum) are given because of intestinal ulceration.
    4. Increase fresh fruits and vegetables, and decrease intake of fat and red meat.

17. The risk of cancer of the stomach is associated with which factors? (Select all that apply.) *(1425)*
    1. Hyperkalemia
    2. Hypochlorhydria
    3. Chronic atrophic gastritis
    4. Diet high in smoked and preserved foods
    5. Gastric ulcers
    6. Diet high in fresh fruits and whole grains

18. When caring for a patient diagnosed with Crohn's disease, what signs and symptoms does the nurse expect to observe? (Select all that apply.) *(1438)*
    1. Nausea and vomiting
    2. Diarrhea and abdominal pain
    3. Weight gain and lactose intolerance
    4. Weight loss and malnutrition
    5. Fatigue and fever

19. The nurse is providing care to a patient suspected of having acute appendicitis. Which interventions may be included in care? (Select all that apply.) *(1440)*
    1. Apply heating pad to the abdomen.
    2. Maintain bedrest and nothing by mouth (NPO).
    3. Administer PRN antacids to decrease gastric acidity.
    4. Monitor vital signs including temperature.
    5. Administer antibiotics as ordered.
    6. Administer enemas until clear.

20. The patient had an esophagogastroduodenoscopy several hours ago and now reports abdominal pain and tenderness to the nurse. What should the nurse do first? *(1408)*
    1. Auscultate for bowel sounds
    2. Administer pain medication
    3. Assess the abdominal pain
    4. Check for melena

21. The patient had capsule endoscopy. Which discharge instruction should the nurse give to the patient? *(1408)*
    1. Return in 8 hours to have the monitoring device removed.
    2. Examine stool for several days to retrieve pill camera device.
    3. Use a mild laxative to facilitate expulsion of pill camera.
    4. Small amounts of blood and mucus in the stool are expected.

22. The nurse inserts a nasogastric tube (NG) so a patient can undergo the Bernstein test to determine the cause of esophageal pain. Which outcome is considered a positive test result? *(1408, 1409)*
    1. Administering nitrates relieves pain.
    2. Taking an antacid has no effect on pain.
    3. Decompressing the stomach relieves pain.
    4. Instilling hydrochloric acid causes pain.

23. The patient needs to have a series of tests for the gastrointestinal system. Which test must be scheduled last? *(1410)*
    1. Barium studies
    2. Stool sample for ova and parasites
    3. Colonoscopy
    4. Flat plate of the abdomen

24. The nursing student reports seeing a pearly, bluish-white "milk-curd" on the mucous membranes of the older patient's mouth. The nurse would intervene if the student performs which action? *(1411)*
    1. Checks for angular cheilitis at the corner of the mouth
    2. Removes the plaques with a soft toothbrush
    3. Observes the quantity and type of food consumed
    4. Offers the patient unsweetened yogurt

25. The nurse is talking to a neighbor who says that she has had a sore on her lip for about 3 weeks. What advice should the nurse give? *(1412)*
    1. Use lipstick or lip balm that has includes a sunscreen.
    2. Advise rinsing the mouth with diluted hydrogen peroxide.
    3. Consult the health care provider because of the duration of the sore.
    4. Increase intake of fresh fruits and vegetables for vitamin content.

26. The health care provider has recommended a conservative approach to manage the patient's gastroesophageal reflux disease (GERD). What would be included in the nurse's instructions to support the provider's recommendation? *(1414)*
    1. Give the patient a brochure about Nissen fundoplication.
    2. Suggest methods for elevating the head of the bed at home.
    3. Teach the signs and symptoms of Barrett's esophagus.
    4. Give the patient a reminder card for endoscopy and biopsy.

27. The nurse is caring for a patient who was admitted for peptic ulcer disease. Which diagnostic finding is greatest cause for concern? *(1408)*
    1. Fecal assay antigen test is positive for *H. pylori.*
    2. Stool for occult blood is positive.
    3. White blood cell count is elevated.
    4. Pain is present during the hydrochloric acid test.

28. The patient who had surgery for a peptic ulcer several weeks ago reports experiencing an episode of diaphoresis, nausea, vomiting, epigastric pain, explosive diarrhea, and dyspepsia. Which question is most relevant to the symptoms and the surgical history? *(1427)*
    1. Can you describe the pain? Where was it and how long did it last?
    2. Did you eat before the symptoms? And if so, what did you eat?
    3. Have you been taking your medications according to instructions?
    4. Did you ever experience these symptoms before the surgery?

29. The patient is admitted for hemorrhagic colitis caused by the *E. coli* pathogen. Which order would the nurse question? *(1429)*
    1. Encourage oral fluids as tolerated
    2. Dextrose 5% in normal saline at 150 mL/hour
    3. Loperamide (Imodium) 2 mg after unformed stool
    4. Initiate contact isolation

30. The elderly patient has been put into contact isolation because of watery diarrhea. Laboratory results are pending, but the *C. difficile* pathogen is suspected. What instruction should the nurse give to the UAP? *(1429)*
    1. Cluster care and limit the amount of time spent in the room.
    2. Use diluted bleach solution to clean the toilet bowl after each use.
    3. Wear a mask during patient care and discard upon exiting the room.
    4. Use soap and water to wash hands, rather than the antiseptic hand rub.

31. A patient who is diagnosed with celiac sprue must be taught to avoid which food? *(1431)*
    1. Fish
    2. Rice
    3. Meat
    4. Wheat

32. The patient confides in the nurse that she feels angry because the health care provider has hinted that irritable bowel syndrome (IBS) might be the problem, but offers no definitive diagnosis. What is the most therapeutic response? *(1433)*
    1. "IBS is hard to diagnose. It is more a process of excluding other disorders."
    2. "I'll ask the health care provider to talk to you about your concerns."
    3. "You seem really frustrated. What has the provider told you so far?"
    4. "I can get some literature about IBS; maybe additional information will help."

33. The patient is admitted for an exacerbation of ulcerative colitis and the nurse hears in report that the patient had 20 liquid stools within the past 24 hours. Which laboratory result is the most important to query? *(1435)*
    1. Electrolyte levels
    2. Liver function studies
    3. Hemoglobin and hematocrit
    4. Fecal occult blood

34. The nurse enters the room of a young woman and sees that she is crying. The patient states, "The doctor told me I need surgery and an ileostomy. I'll be pooping into a bag! I'm leaving the hospital right now!" What should the nurse do first? *(1436)*
    1. Obtain a Leaving Against Medical Advice form and contact the provider.
    2. Sit with the patient and help her verbalize her fears and concerns.
    3. Arrange for the patient to meet another person who has an ostomy.
    4. Contact the enterostomal therapist to talk with the patient.

35. Which medical diagnosis requires that the nurse be extra vigilant for concurrent urinary tract infections? *(1438)*
    1. Crohn's disease
    2. Appendicitis
    3. Ulcerative colitis
    4. Peptic ulcer disease

36. A parent says, "I think my son has appendicitis. He won't eat and he says he has pain just to the right of his belly button." If the nurse places the child on an examination table, which position is the child most likely to assume if the mother is correct about appendicitis? *(1440)*
    1. Prone with head supported by forearm
    2. Supine with arms and legs extended
    3. Sits upright, with chest extended
    4. Side-lying with knees flexed

37. The patient is admitted for acute diverticulitis. The nurse would intervene if a nursing student performed which action? *(1442)*
    1. Advises to avoid heavy lifting
    2. Assists with a meal tray
    3. Assesses bowel sounds
    4. Checks the white blood cell count

38. A patient sustained blunt trauma to the abdomen. Several hours after being admitted for observation, the patient reports severe abdominal pain with exquisite tenderness to light palpation. What should the nurse do first? *(1443)*
    1. Take vital signs and perform additional assessment of the abdomen.
    2. Place the patient in a semi-Fowler's position to localize purulent drainage.
    3. Call the health care provider and report possible peritonitis.
    4. Administer a PRN pain medication and reevaluate pain in 30 minutes.

39. The nurse is caring for a patient who had a right hemicolectomy for colorectal cancer. Which postoperative interventions will the nurse use in the care of this patient? (Select all that apply.) *(1451)*
    1. Monitor vital signs, pain level, and return of bowel sounds.
    2. Check dressings for drainage and bleeding and change as ordered.
    3. Discontinue the Foley catheter when the patient is discharged.
    4. Encourage the patient to cough, deep-breathe, and turn.
    5. Maintain bedrest while the nasogastric tube is on suction.
    6. Keep accurate intake and output records to monitor fluid balance.

40. An obese male truck driver reports to the clinic complaining of rectal itching. After the medical examination, a diagnosis of hemorrhoids is made. What nonsurgical approaches can the nurse teach the patient to help manage the condition? *(1452)*
   1. Suggest a low-fiber diet.
   2. Advise the use of a hydrocortisone cream.
   3. Increase fluid intake.
   4. Recommend rubber-band ligation.

CRITICAL THINKING ACTIVITIES

Activity 1

41. For each phase of the nursing process, indicate specifically how that phase relates to patients with esophageal disorders. *(1455)*

   a. Assessment: _____

   _____

   b. Nursing diagnoses and planning: _____

   _____

   c. Implementation: _____

   _____

   d. Evaluation: _____

   _____

Activity 2

42. For each topic, list the nursing interventions appropriate for a patient who is having gastric surgery. *(1428)*

   a. Preoperative

       i. Preparation: _____

   _____

       ii. Knowledge: _____

   _____

   b. Postoperative

       i. Knowledge: _____

   _____

       ii. Pain: _____

   _____

iii. Noncompliance: _____

_____

iv. Nutrition: _____

_____

Activity 3

43. The nurse is providing care to a patient suspected of having an intestinal obstruction. *(1446, 1447)*

a. When performing an assessment on the patient, what objective data should be included?

_____

_____

b. What diagnostic tests may be performed to confirm the presence of an intestinal obstruction?

_____

_____

c. What are the goals of treatment for an intestinal obstruction? _____

_____

_____

d. Compare and contrast mechanical and nonmechanical intestinal obstruction. _____

_____

_____

chapter
45

Care of the Patient with a Gallbladder, Liver, Biliary Tract, or Exocrine Pancreatic Disorder

Answer Key: Textbook page references are provided as a guide for answering these questions. A complete Answer Key is provided in your Additional Learning Resources on Evolve.

MATCHING

Directions: Match the word or prefix on the left with the definition on the right and indicate the correct answer in the space provided.

	Word or prefix	**Definitions**
_____ 1.	sphincter of Oddi *(1479)*	a. Biliary drainage tube
_____ 2.	T-tube *(1480)*	b. Hepatobiliary iminodiacetic acid scan
_____ 3.	cholangiography *(1461)*	c. Presence of gallstones
_____ 4.	HIDA scan *(1461)*	d. Stones in common bile duct
_____ 5.	laparoscopic cholecystectomy *(1480)*	e. Postoperative cholangiography
		f. Radiographic examination of bile ducts
_____ 6.	cholecystectomy *(1479)*	g. Radiographic examination of gallbladder
_____ 7.	cholecystitis *(1478)*	h. Removal of gallbladder
_____ 8.	cholecystography *(1460)*	i. Controls the flow of pancreatic juices and bile into the duodenum
_____ 9.	cholecystostomy *(1482)*	j. Laser or cautery is used to remove the gallbladder
_____ 10.	T-tube cholangiogram *(1461)*	k. Incision into the gallbladder (usually for drainage)
_____ 11.	choledocholithiasis *(1482)*	l. Biliary duct carcinomas
_____ 12.	cholangiomas *(1471)*	m. Inflammation of gallbladder
_____ 13.	lithotripsy *(1479)*	n. Series of shock waves through water or a cushion that breaks the stones into fragments
_____ 14.	cholelithiasis *(1478)*	

FILL-IN-THE-BLANK SENTENCES

15. Jaundice, the _____ of body tissues caused by abnormally high blood levels of bilirubin, is visible when the total serum bilirubin exceeds _____. *(1459)*

16. Chances for developing alcohol-related cirrhosis increase for women when they ingest more than _____ alcoholic drinks per day, and for men when they drink _____ drinks per day. *(1464)*

17. Cirrhosis of the liver and infection with hepatitis C or hepatitis B are factors in increased risk for primary _____ cancer. *(1471)*

18. There are approximately _____ people waiting for liver transplants; currently, only approximately 6000 transplants are performed annually. *(1475)*

19. More than 90% of cholecystitis cases are caused by _____. *(1478)*

20. The most common lifestyle risk factor for pancreatic cancer is _____. *(1485)*

MULTIPLE CHOICE

Directions: Select the best answer(s) for each of the following questions.

21. The nurse is providing teaching to a patient scheduled to undergo a needle liver biopsy. During the examination, the patient should be advised to: *(1462)*
    1. deeply inhale and hold breath until told to exhale.
    2. cough forcefully as the needle is withdrawn.
    3. inhale and exhale slowly and evenly as the needle is inserted.
    4. exhale and not breathe as the needle is inserted.

22. A T-tube was inserted during a cholecystectomy. What does the nurse expect to observe when assessing the patient? *(1480)*
    1. Greenish-yellow drainage from the tube
    2. Localized inflammation around the tube site
    3. Significant postoperative pain until the tube is removed
    4. Moderate amount of light-red bleeding from the tube

23. After a laparoscopic cholecystectomy, the patient reports shoulder pain. What should the nurse do? *(1481)*
    1. Perform gentle range-of-motion exercises to reduce shoulder discomfort.
    2. Assist the patient to ambulate to clear the residual carbon dioxide.
    3. Explain that the pain is a side effect of anesthesia.
    4. Reassure that the pain is expected and give an analgesic as ordered.

24. When caring for a patient with acute pancreatitis, which laboratory finding is the best indicator of the disorder? *(1463)*
    1. Low albumin
    2. Elevated lipase
    3. Increased blood glucose
    4. Elevated amylase

25. Which behavior places the patient at greatest risk to contract hepatitis E? *(1473)*
    1. Drinking water from a questionable source
    2. Engaging in unprotected anal and vaginal sex
    3. Sharing and reusing needles for illicit drug injection
    4. Traveling to Europe, Asia, or Australia

26. The nurse is talking to a patient who had an outpatient oral cholecystogram with poor visualization of the biliary tree. What question would the nurse ask to determine if the patient was compliant with the preparation for the test? *(1460)*
    1. "Did you take the laxative and the enema as directed by the health care provider?"
    2. "How many dye tablets did you take on the evening before the examination?"
    3. "When was the last time you had a meal that contained a lot of fiber?"
    4. "How much fluid did you consume on the morning of the examination?"

27. A young woman who is pregnant is having symptoms of cholecystitis and the health care provider has informed her that diagnostic testing is required. Which information brochure will the nurse prepare for this patient? *(1461)*
    1. "What You Need to Know About Ultrasonography for the Gallbladder"
    2. "Frequently Asked Questions About Oral Cholecystography"
    3. "Intravenous Cholangiography: A Patient's Guide for Decision-making"
    4. "Computed Tomography of the Abdomen as a Diagnostic Tool"

28. The patient had a hepatobiliary iminodiacetic acid (HIDA) scan. What instructions should the nurse give to the UAP who is assisting the patient with hygiene? *(1461)*
    1. Immediately flush all urine and stool.
    2. Wear your personal dosimeter at all times.
    3. Give care as usual; there are no special considerations.
    4. Watch for and report any bleeding at the puncture site.

29. The nurse hears in report that several patients are scheduled for diagnostic testing. The nurse must plan to take vital signs every 15 minutes (two times), then every 30 minutes (four times), and then every hour (four times) after which test? *(1462)*
    1. Serum ammonia test
    2. Needle liver biopsy
    3. Oral cholecystography
    4. Radioisotope liver scan

30. The nurse is instructing the UAP about assisting several patients with morning hygiene. Which patient needs to use a soft toothbrush with very gentle brushing action? *(1470)*
    1. Recently diagnosed with hepatitis A
    2. Surgery pending for cholelithiasis
    3. In later stage of cirrhosis of the liver
    4. NPO for acute pancreatitis

31. A first-semester nursing student tells the nurse that she would like to teach and coach coughing and deep-breathing for several patients. Which patient(s) would be best for the nurse to recommend to the student? (Select all that apply.) *(1476, 1481)*
    1. Scheduled to have a cholecystectomy in two days
    2. Looks forward to having a liver transplant from a living donor
    3. Has cirrhosis of the liver and esophageal varices
    4. Prescribed several weeks of bedrest for chronic hepatitis
    5. Is on bedrest for acute pancreatitis with severe pain

32. The patient has symptoms of hepatic encephalopathy and the health care provider wants to be called about laboratory results. Which laboratory result should the nurse seek out to validate the suspected condition? *(1462)*
    1. Serum bilirubin
    2. Serum albumin
    3. Ammonia level
    4. Blood glucose

33. The health care provider orders an intramuscular immune serum globulin for a hospital employee who was exposed to hepatitis A. A dosage of 0.02 mL/kg of body weight is ordered. The employee weighs 155 lbs. How many mL should the nurse draw up? _____ *(1474)*

34. A patient with acute pancreatitis is refusing to have a nasogastric tube inserted and wants to leave the hospital. What can the nurse say to help the patient to accept the therapy? *(1483)*
    1. "I can give you pain medication before or after the procedure."
    2. "Let me call the health care provider so he can explain the therapy."
    3. "The tube will be inserted by our most experienced nurse, so don't worry."
    4. "The tube will decrease the nausea, vomiting, pain, and abdominal distention."

CRITICAL THINKING ACTIVITIES

Activity 1

35. A 34-year-old patient with a history of end-stage liver disease related to chronic hepatitis has been added to the waiting list to receive a liver transplant. During his preoperative education classes, he voices many questions and concerns. *(1475, 1476)*

   a.   What are the primary risks associated with the planned transplant? _____

   _____

   b.   What postoperative complications will the patient be at risk for? _____

   _____

   _____

   c.   How will the risk of organ rejection be handled? _____

   _____

   _____

   _____

   d.   Discuss the appropriate postoperative nursing care. _____

   _____

   _____

   _____

Activity 2

36. A 49-year-old patient comes to the emergency department complaining of right upper-quadrant pain. She reports that the pain began a few hours after eating at a local fast-food restaurant. Upon assessment, the abdomen is distended. The patient also has nausea and vomiting. *(1478, 1479)*

   a.   What does the nurse expect the patient to be diagnosed with? _____

   b.   What are some other signs and symptoms that may develop? _____

   _____

   c.   What diagnostic examinations may be used to help diagnose this patient? _____

   _____

   _____

   _____

Activity 3

37. a. Based on knowledge of the etiology and clinical course of pancreatic cancer, discuss some of the psychological challenges that a patient could face. *(1486)*

_____

_____

_____

_____

   b. What can the nurse do to assist the patient with these psychological challenges? _____

_____

_____

_____

_____

Care of the Patient with a Blood or Lymphatic Disorder

Answer Key: Textbook page references are provided as a guide for answering these questions. A complete Answer Key is provided in your Additional Learning Resources on Evolve.

SHORT ANSWER

Directions: Using your own words, answer each question in the space provided.

1. What are the three main functions of blood? *(1491)* _____

   _____

   _____

   _____

2. What are three functions of the lymphatic system? *(1495, 1496)* _____

   _____

   _____

   _____

3. What are two main functions of the lymph glands? *(1496)* _____

   _____

   _____

4. What are five functions of the spleen? *(1496, 1497)* _____

   _____

   _____

   _____

   _____

   _____

TRUE OR FALSE

Directions: Write T for true or F for false in the blanks provided.

_____ 5. Blood is slightly acidic, with a pH range of 7.05 to 7.25. *(1491)*

_____ 6. Body defense, such as the destruction of bacteria and viruses, is the primary function of the red blood cells. *(1493)*

_____ 7. Using the posterior superior iliac crest for bone marrow aspiration creates the greatest risk for penetrating the underlying structures during the procedure. *(1497)*

_____ 8. *Pancytopenia* means that all three major blood elements (red cells, white cells, and platelets) from the bone marrow are reduced or absent. *(1503)*

_____ 9. A patient with aplastic anemia could have symptoms related to infection, decreased oxygenation of tissues, and bleeding tendencies. *(1503)*

_____ 10. Hematopoietic stem cell transplant is the only available therapy with curative intent for sickle cell disease. *(1508)*

TABLE ACTIVITY

11. Directions: Complete the table below with the normal values for selected blood tests. *(1491)*

Blood Test	Normal Values
Red blood cells (RBCs)	Males: Females:
Hemoglobin	Males: Females:
Hematocrit	Males: Females:
Platelet count	
White blood cells (WBC) actual cell count	
Prothrombin time (PT)	
International Normalized Ratio (INR)	
Partial thromboplastin time (PTT)	

MULTIPLE CHOICE

Directions: Select the best answer(s) for each of the following questions.

12. The nurse is caring for a young patient who has had vomiting and diarrhea secondary to food poisoning, but he is usually very healthy. What would be an expected laboratory result for this patient? *(1491)*
    1. Elevated hemoglobin and hematocrit
    2. Normal hemoglobin and hematocrit
    3. Low platelet count
    4. Increased prothrombin time

13. The health care provider tells the nurse that the laboratory results show that the patient has bandemia. The nurse will plan to be extra vigilant for which condition? *(1493)*
    1. Deep vein thrombosis
    2. Thrombocytopenia
    3. Sepsis or septic shock
    4. Allergic response

14. Which patient is most likely to require testing for anti-D antibodies and/or an injection of RH immunoglobulin? *(1495)*
    1. An Rh-positive mother who is 28 weeks gestation
    2. Any woman who has an ectopic pregnancy
    3. An Rh-negative mother who had a miscarriage
    4. An Rh-positive mother impregnated by an Rh-negative father

15. When caring for patients who are Jehovah's Witnesses, which information applies for use of blood products? *(1499)*
    1. Some Jehovah's Witnesses may permit the use of certain blood volume expanders.
    2. It is not legal for this patient to refuse transfusions if the bleeding is truly life-threatening.
    3. Some Jehovah's Witnesses may consent to homologous blood transfusions.
    4. Jehovah's Witnesses believe that children are allowed to have blood in an emergency.

16. A patient with anemia has a nursing diagnosis of Activity Intolerance related to tissue hypoxia. Which task can be delegated to the UAP? *(1499)*
    1. Ask the patient how far he is able to ambulate and evaluate his abilities.
    2. Apply oxygen per nasal cannula if the patient reports shortness of breath.
    3. Explain the patient's limitations to visitors and encourage short visits.
    4. Assist the patient with self-care activities, such as hygiene and toileting.

17. The nurse is caring for a trauma patient who must be observed for signs and symptoms of occult bleeding and injury. Which sign/symptom is an early manifestation of hypovolemic shock? *(1500)*
    1. Orthostatic blood pressure
    2. Decreased red blood cell count
    3. Restlessness
    4. Decreased urine output

18. The patient had major abdominal surgery yesterday. He reported abdominal pain, and the nurse gave him an opioid pain medication as directed; 2 hours later, he reports that the pain is worse. What should the nurse do first? *(1500)*
    1. Check the medication administration record for other pain or adjunctive medications.
    2. Explain to the patient that pain medication can only be given as ordered every 4 to 6 hours.
    3. Reassess the abdomen and ask the patient to describe the pain to the best of his ability.
    4. Call the health care provider and obtain an order for laboratory studies or x-ray studies.

19. The nurse is caring for a postoperative patient who is demonstrating early symptoms of hypovolemic shock. The nurse is awaiting a return call from the health care provider. Which task can be delegated to the UAP? *(1501)*
    1. Take and report the blood pressure, pulse, and respirations every 15 minutes.
    2. Reinforce the dressings for saturation of blood or drainage.
    3. Apply oxygen and monitor the pulse oximetry readings every 5 minutes.
    4. Place the patient in a supine position and monitor respiratory effort.

20. The health care provider has recommended that the patient with sickle cell disease have a splenectomy. Which medication is likely to be discontinued for several days prior to the surgery? *(1504)*
    1. Diuretic medication
    2. Vitamin B$_{12}$
    3. Blood thinner
    4. Blood pressure medication

21. The nurse is caring for a patient experiencing an initial sickle cell crisis. What is the primary sign/symptom that the nurse should expect during the crisis? *(1507)*
    1. Jaundice
    2. Fever
    3. Fatigue
    4. Pain

22. What health promotion points should be emphasized for patients who have sickle cell disease? (Select all that apply.) *(1508)*
    1. Avoid high altitudes
    2. Drink large amounts of iced fluids
    3. Stay current with vaccinations
    4. Maintain very cold room temperatures
    5. Stop smoking and alcohol consumption
    6. Maintain vigorous exercise routine

23. The patient is diagnosed with primary polycythemia. Which assessments are of particular concern? *(1509)*
    1. Palpating for abdominal distention and checking bowel movements
    2. Checking for pain, warmth, swelling, redness, and pulses in arms or legs
    3. Monitoring temperature and watching for other signs of infection
    4. Frequently assessing for fatigue and activity intolerance

24. The laboratory calls to inform the nurse that the patient has a white cell count of 1000/mm^3 with a differential neutrophil count of less than 200/mm^3. Which action is the most important for the nurse to initiate while waiting for the health care provider to respond to the phone message? *(1511)*
    1. Review current medication list.
    2. Start protective isolation precautions.
    3. Check for signs/symptoms of infection.
    4. Teach the importance of hand hygiene.

25. A 6-year-old child is hospitalized for treatment of acute lymphocytic leukemia. Which activity would the nurse suggest to the child and parents? *(1514)*
    1. Drawing pictures that accompany storytelling
    2. Playing with and petting the pet therapy dog
    3. Walking in the garden courtyard
    4. Attending a party in the pediatric play area

26. The nurse is examining the patient and notices several areas of ecchymoses and petechiae. Which question(s) will the nurse ask to follow up on this observation? (Select all that apply.) *(1515, 1516)*
    1. What do you think is causing these bruises?
    2. Do you notice any bleeding when you brush your teeth?
    3. Have you had frequent nosebleeds?
    4. Are your stools a black or very dark red color?
    5. Are you using a hydrocortisone cream on these areas?
    6. How much meat and fresh produce do you consume per day?

27. The patient has a very low platelet count. Which instruction will the nurse give to the UAP about the care of this patient? *(1517)*
    1. Always wear a mask to prevent spreading respiratory droplets.
    2. Handle the patient very gently to avoid bruising and injury.
    3. Encourage the patient to take fluids to prevent dehydration.
    4. Assist the patient with hygiene to prevent undue fatigue.

28. An adolescent with hemophilia A wants to participate in a high school sports activity. In consultation with the health care provider, which sport would be the best? *(1519)*
    1. Football
    2. Soccer
    3. Wrestling
    4. Golf

29. The nurse reads in the record that the patient has a medical diagnosis of Hodgkin's disease Stage 1. Which sign/symptom would the nurse expect to see? *(1525)*
    1. Abnormal single lymph node
    2. Night sweats
    3. Weight loss
    4. Alcohol-induced pain

30. Based on the nurse's knowledge of non-Hodgkin's disease, what does the nurse consider when planning care for the patient who has recently started treatment? (Select all that apply.) *(1527)*
    1. Pain is likely to be localized in the spine and increased with movement.
    2. Disease is likely to be widespread and most body systems are affected.
    3. Patient could have side effects from chemotherapy.
    4. Patient and/or family may need support because prognosis is poor.
    5. Total assistance for ADLs is likely to be needed.

CRITICAL THINKING ACTIVITIES

Activity 1

31. A 63-year-old patient is seen with complaints of her "heart racing," nausea, sore tongue, and difficulty swallowing. Upon oral examination, her tongue is smooth and erythematous. *(1501, 1502)*

    a. What medical diagnosis would a nurse anticipate? _____

    b. What diagnostic tests will support this suspicion? _____

    _____

    c. What treatment options are available for this patient? _____

    _____

    d. After completing 2 months of treatment, the patient states she is feeling well and now plans to discontinue the treatments. How should the nurse respond to the patient?

    _____

    _____

Activity 2

32. A 32-year-old female patient comes for care with complaints of fatigue, dizziness, and pallor. Her history includes childbirth 3 months ago, a subgastrectomy 3 years ago, and hernia repair 18 months ago. Her Hgb level is 10 g/dL. *(1505, 1506)*

    a. Based on the nurse's knowledge, what is the anticipated medical diagnosis? _____

    _____

    b. What risk factors does this patient have that support development of this disorder? _____

    _____

    _____

c.   Identify other signs and symptoms that may accompany this disorder. _____

_____

_____

d.   Discuss six considerations for the administration of iron. _____

_____

_____

Activity 3

33. The nurse is caring for an older adult patient who reports bone pain that increases with movement. The medical diagnosis is multiple myeloma.

a.   Discuss the benefits of ambulation and fluid for this patient. *(1522, 1523)*_____

_____

_____

b.   What can the nurse do to encourage the patient to walk if he says that moving increases the pain? *(1522, 1523)*

_____

_____

_____

Activity 4

34. Use the nursing process and indicate general care for patients with disorders of the hematologic and lymphatic systems. *(1528, 1529)*

Assessment	
Nursing diagnoses	
Planning	
Implementation	
Evaluation	

Student Name_____ Date_____

Care of the Patient with a Cardiovascular or a Peripheral Vascular Disorder

Answer Key: Textbook page references are provided as a guide for answering these questions. A complete Answer Key is provided in your Additional Learning Resources on Evolve.

TRACING A DROP OF BLOOD

1. Directions: Trace a drop of blood around the systemic circulatory system. Start at the superior or inferior vena cava and identify the names of the blood vessels, the chambers of the heart, and the valves of the heart. End with the drop of blood at the aorta. *(1538)*

   Superior or inferior vena cava →

   _____ → _____ →

   _____ → _____ →

   _____ → _____ →

   _____ → _____ →

   _____ → _____ →

   _____ → Aorta.

2. Directions: Identify the impulse pattern of the electrical conduction system of the heart. Start at the SA node. *(1536)*

   SA node →

   _____ → _____ →

   _____ → _____

FIGURE LABELING

3. Directions: Label each of the coronary vessels that supply blood to the heart. *(1536)*

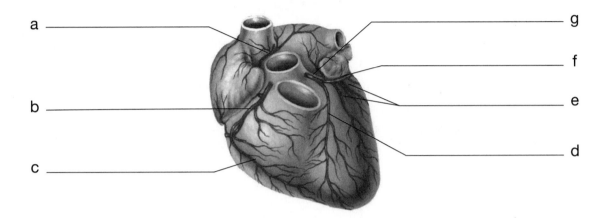

MATCHING

Directions: Match the term on the left with the explanation to the patient on the right. Record the letter of the correct choice in the space provided.

Term	**Explanation to the Patient**
_____ 4. Aneurysm *(1593)*	a. An electric shock to your chest; restores your regular heartbeat
_____ 5. Angina pectoris *(1553)*	b. Slow, steady heart rate
_____ 6. Arteriosclerosis *(1588)*	c. Part of the blood vessel is blocked
_____ 7. Atherosclerosis *(1588)*	d. The arteries are thicker and not as stretchy
_____ 8. Bradycardia *(1546)*	e. Chest pain and choking sensations that are relieved by nitroglycerin
_____ 9. Cardioversion *(1541)*	f. Bulging of an artery, like a tire with a bulge
_____ 10. Coronary artery disease *(1552)*	g. Removing the plaques from the inner part of arteries
_____ 11. Defibrillation *(1549)*	h. You do not have enough oxygen in your blood
_____ 12. Dysrhythmia *(1546)*	i. A blood clot or foreign matter travels in the bloodstream
_____ 13. Embolus *(1559)*	j. An abnormal heartbeat
_____ 14. Endarterectomy *(1591)*	k. A condition that causes the blood to stop going to the arteries around the heart
_____ 15. Heart failure *(1564)*	l. In order to breathe, you may have to sit or stand up
_____ 16. Hypoxemia *(1541)*	m. Shocking the heart to stop ventricular fibrillation, which prevents the heart from pumping blood
_____ 17. Intermittent claudication *(1582)*	n. Fluid is collecting in the lining around the lungs
_____ 18. Ischemia *(1553)*	o. You have too many red blood cells in your blood
_____ 19. Myocardial infarction *(1559)*	p. Your heart is not pumping effectively, causing fluid to settle in the lungs
_____ 20. Occlusion *(1559)*	q. The arteries are filling up with plaque and beginning to close
_____ 21. Orthopnea *(1572)*	r. The heart cannot pump correctly
_____ 22. Peripheral *(1581)*	s. Very fast heart rate that is steady
_____ 23. Pleural effusion *(1538)*	t. Cramps and weakness in your legs caused by decreased blood flow to your muscles
_____ 24. Polycythemia *(1541)*	u. A body part or organ is not getting enough blood, thus causin pain
_____ 25. Pulmonary edema *(1570)*	v. The heart is being damaged by the lack of blood
_____ 26. Tachycardia *(1546)*	w. Arms and legs

FILL-IN-THE-BLANK SENTENCES

Directions: Complete each sentence by filling in the blank with the correct word or phrase.

27. For many years, creatine phosphokinase (CK-MB) was the gold standard for the diagnosis of myocardial infarction, but now _____ are preferred. *(1542)*

28. Some researchers believe that elevated levels of homocysteine can be treated by administration of vitamins _____, _____, and _____. *(1543)*

29. Older Americans should have their cholesterol tested once every _____ years. *(1543)*

30. _____ and _____ have been identified as good forms of exercise to decrease the risk of developing cardiovascular disease. *(1545)*

31. _____ is pain (usually in the calves) brought on by exercise and relieved by rest. *(1582)*

32. For Buerger's disease, the most important patient behavior is _____. *(1595)*

MULTIPLE CHOICE

Directions: Select the best answer(s) for each of the following questions.

33. The nurse is caring for a patient who is on anticoagulant therapy. Which laboratory values are the most important to monitor? *(1541)*
    1. Prothrombin time, International Normalized Ratio, and partial thromboplastin time
    2. Blood glucose, potassium, sodium, calcium, and magnesium
    3. Enzyme creatine kinase, creatine phosphokinase, and myoglobin
    4. B-type natriuretic peptide and troponins 1 and 2

34. Laboratory results show a low hemoglobin for a patient diagnosed with myocardial infarction. What is the first therapy that the nurse would ensure to address this laboratory result? *(1563)*
    1. Obtain an order for an intramuscular iron supplement.
    2. Help the patient to order an iron-rich meal tray.
    3. Obtain an order for type and cross for blood transfusion.
    4. Check to see that oxygen is delivered as ordered.

35. The nurse is planning care for several patients who are scheduled to have diagnostic testing for cardiac disorders. Which patient will require postprocedural checks for peripheral pulses, color, and sensation of the extremity every 15 minutes for 1 hour? *(1538)*
    1. Needs cardiac catheterization to diagnose extent of atherosclerotic heart disease
    2. Is scheduled for electrocardiogram to identify specific cardiac dysrhythmias
    3. Requires chemically induced stress electrocardiogram for poor exercise tolerance
    4. Must have positron emission tomography because of coronary artery disease

36. The nurse is discussing modifiable risk factors for cardiovascular disease with a 23-year-old patient who is currently asymptomatic. What does the nurse recommend? *(1544)*
    1. Find out if any first-degree relatives had cardiovascular problems before 50 years of age.
    2. Stop smoking or consider greatly reducing the number of cigarettes smoked per day.
    3. Ask your health care provider for a cholesterol-lowering drug, such as simvastatin (Zocor).
    4. Monitor weight and calorie intake to maintain a body mass index of 30.

37. During a discharge teaching session, the patient voices concern about why her risk of heart disease is elevated simply because she has a history of diabetes mellitus. What is the best explanation to give to the patient? *(1545)*
    1. Fluctuating insulin levels cause vasoconstriction.
    2. Elevated blood glucose levels contribute to arterial damage.
    3. Diabetics are obese and thus at higher risk.
    4. Risk for heart disease is not higher for people with diabetes.

38. Which psychosocial behaviors are more likely to be associated with increased cardiovascular symptoms? *(1546)*
    1. Frequently in a hurry and easily irritated
    2. Easygoing and usually enjoys life
    3. Neat, organized, and pays attention to detail
    4. Pessimistic and generally expresses negativity

39. The patient's cardiac monitor shows a regular rhythm with a rate of 65 beats/min, P waves precede each QRS complex, QRS complexes are symmetrical and regularly spaced, and a normal T wave shows repolarization. What is the nurse's interpretation of monitor display? *(1546)*
    1. Vital signs should be immediately assessed.
    2. The monitor indicates a normal sinus rhythm.
    3. The monitor is showing a benign dysrhythmia.
    4. The patient should be assessed for chest pain.

40. The patient experiences dizziness and light-headedness while trying to pass a bowel movement. An immediate pulse check shows 45 beats/min that rapidly recovers to a regular rate of 70. What is the most probable cause of this episode of sinus bradycardia? *(1546)*
    1. Digitalis toxicity
    2. Endocrine disturbance
    3. Intracranial tumor
    4. Vagal stimulation

41. For which dysrhythmia would a pacemaker mostly likely be necessary? *(1552)*
    1. Sinus tachycardia
    2. Premature ventricular contractions
    3. Third-degree heart block
    4. Atrial fibrillation

42. The patient who had a myocardial infarction 2 weeks ago is now having frequent episodes of ventricular tachycardia. For this patient, what is the clinical significance of this dysrhythmia? *(1548)*
    1. Warning sign for ventricular fibrillation
    2. Expected finding at this stage
    3. Reaction to a beta-adrenergic blocker
    4. Treatment is given only for symptoms

43. The patient is on the cardiac monitor undergoing a diagnostic procedure. Suddenly, the health care provider says, "The patient is having ventricular fibrillation." Which piece of equipment is the most vital? *(1549)*
    1. Temporary pacemaker
    2. Defibrillator
    3. Bag-valve-mask
    4. Crash cart

44. A patient is being discharged after receiving a permanent pacemaker. What is the best rationale to give to the patient about refraining from sports such as tennis, swimming, golf, and weight-lifting for the first 6-8 weeks? *(1552)*
    1. "First, you have to be able to climb at least two flights of stairs."
    2. "Active sports will interfere with the pacemaker's fixed mode."
    3. "These sports are too strenuous and rapidly increase the heart rate."
    4. "The arm on the pacemaker side should not be lifted over the head."

45. The patient had a percutaneous transluminal coronary angioplasty with stent placement. What type of medication is the patient most likely to be prescribed for at least 3 months? *(1556)*
    1. Digitalis preparation
    2. Diuretic
    3. Opioid pain medication
    4. Anticoagulant

46. Which instruction would the nurse give to the patient for self-administration of nitrate medications? *(1557)*
    1. Refrigerate the oral tablets and nitroglycerin patches until use.
    2. Apply patches in the morning and remove them at bedtime.
    3. A burning sensation on the tongue indicates an allergic reaction.
    4. Pain relief should occur after a minimum of two doses.

47. For a patient with myocardial infarction, what symptom is the most important? *(1559)*
    1. Diaphoresis
    2. Palpitations
    3. Pain
    4. Shortness of breath

48. A 63-year-old patient presents with fever, increased pulse, epistaxis, and joint involvement. Heart murmurs are auscultated. The patient has a history of inadequately treated childhood group A β-hemolytic streptococci pharyngitis. These findings and history are consistent with which medical diagnosis? *(1575)*
    1. Cardiomyopathy
    2. Angina
    3. Left-sided heart block
    4. Rheumatic heart disease

49. A neighbor tells the nurse that he has indigestion that has lasted 60 minutes. He tried "taking nitroglycerin, but that didn't help." What should the nurse do first? *(1555)*
    1. Tell the neighbor to take an aspirin and then drive to the emergency department.
    2. Stay with the neighbor, assist him to remain calm, and call 911.
    3. Assess the neighbor's use of nitroglycerin and assess for other symptoms.
    4. Phone the neighbor's health care provider and ask for recommendations.

50. The health care provider is considering tissue plasminogen activator (TPA) for a patient who is having an acute myocardial infarction. The wife suddenly rushes to the nurse and says, "We forgot to tell you something." Which disclosure is a contraindication for TPA? *(1562)*
    1. "My husband is a Jehovah's Witness."
    2. "My husband recently had a head injury."
    3. "He forgot to take his insulin this morning."
    4. "He had a small heart attack last year."

51. The nurse is caring for a patient who is 40 hours post–myocardial infarction. Which instruction should be given to the UAP? *(1563)*
    1. Assist the patient to ambulate in the hall three times.
    2. Check to see if the patient is too tired to get up.
    3. Encourage the patient to independently get out of bed.
    4. Help the patient get to the commode chair.

52. What is the best method to help a patient comply with dietary restrictions associated with atherosclerotic heart disease? *(1565)*
    1. Tell him to avoid all foods that are high in fats.
    2. Remind him that total fat intake is 35-40% of total caloric intake.
    3. Tell him to eat 10-15 grams of soluble fiber every day.
    4. Teach him how to read the nutritional labels on food products.

53. The nurse is caring for a patient who has right ventricular heart failure. After therapy, the nurse sees that the patient has lost 5 pounds of weight. Assuming that all the weight represents fluid loss, how much fluid has the patient lost? _____ L *(1565)*

54. The patient with a history of heart failure tells the home health nurse, "Every night I sleep in this recliner chair. I feel better if I sleep with my head up." What will the nurse assess first? *(1566)*
    1. Check for dependent edema in the lower extremities.
    2. Look at accessibility to the bedroom and bathroom.
    3. Assess ability to independently move and ambulate.
    4. Ask about compliance with low-sodium, low-fat diet.

55. The nurse is supervising a nursing student who must administer digoxin to a patient. The nurse would intervene if the student performs which action? *(1570)*
    1. Stops to check the potassium level before administering the drug
    2. Asks the patient if he has any questions or concerns about the drug
    3. Tells the patient that his pulse is 55 beats/min and prepares to administer the drug
    4. Checks to see if the drug causes any interactions with other prescribed drugs

56. The patient arrives in the emergency department with severe dyspnea, agitation, cyanosis, audible wheezes, and a cough with blood-tinged sputum. What is the priority nursing action? *(1572, 1573)*
    1. Obtain a blood sample for arterial blood gases
    2. Administer oxygen
    3. Auscultate lung sounds
    4. Establish a peripheral IV

57. The nurse is caring for a patient with valvular heart disease. Which task could be assigned to the UAP? *(1574)*
    1. Identifying ADLs that cause fatigue
    2. Check meal trays for high-sodium foods
    3. Weigh the patient at the same time every day
    4. Explain the plan for rest periods

58. Which disorder of the cardiovascular system places the patient at highest risk for the potentially life-threatening condition of cardiac tamponade? *(1576)*
    1. Pericarditis
    2. Valvular heart disease
    3. Buerger's disease
    4. Endocarditis

59. Which sign/symptom indicates to the nurse that a patient with endocarditis is experiencing a serious and common complication of the disease? *(1578)*
    1. Fever and chills
    2. Joint pains and aches
    3. Sudden shortness of breath
    4. Petechiae on neck and chest

60. The nurse sees an elderly woman sitting in the waiting room and she is crying, "My granddaughter was just diagnosed with infective endocarditis. Those patients always die within a year." What should the nurse say first to comfort the grandmother? *(1579)*
    1. "Surgical procedures can repair the diseased valves."
    2. "These days, intensive antibiotic therapy cures 90% of patients."
    3. "If she is able to rest her heart, she will probably be okay."
    4. "We will do everything we can to take care of her."

61. Which patient should be counseled about the risk of cardiomyopathy related to lifestyle choices? *(1579)*
    1. High-risk sexual behavior
    2. Poor intake of dietary fiber
    3. Use of "crack" cocaine
    4. Social consumption of alcohol

62. The patient had a recent cardiac transplant. Which intervention is required for posttransplant care? *(1580)*
    1. Immunosuppressive therapy
    2. Pericardiocentesis
    3. Percutaneous transluminal angioplasty
    4. Contact isolation

63. What treatments and/or advice are given to patients who are prehypertensive? *(1585)*
    1. Diuretics and low-sodium diet
    2. Beta-adrenergic blockers and weight loss
    3. Angiotensin II receptor blockers and low-fat diet
    4. Lifestyle change and routine health appointments

64. The nurse is caring for a patient who has peripheral arterial disease with burning pain that occurs at rest in the right leg. For the nursing diagnosis of Ineffective Tissue Perfusion related to decreased arterial blood flow, which intervention will the nurse use? *(1590)*
    1. Elevate the leg on a pillow
    2. Use a covered ice compress
    3. Place the leg in a dependent position
    4. Encourage aerobic exercise for circulation

65. A patient receives a prescription for anticoagulant medication for treatment of arterial emboli. What dietary information should the nurse give? *(1592)*
    1. Do not increase intake of dark-green vegetables because of vitamin K.
    2. Take extra dairy products to ensure calcium intake and vitamin D.
    3. Eat fruits such as citrus and bananas that provide potassium.
    4. Avoid eating saturated fats by limiting use of butter, oils, and red meats.

66. The nurse is monitoring a patient who is waiting for diagnostic testing to determine if he has an aortic aneurysm. The patient suddenly reports severe chest pain. He becomes pale, weak, and confused. His pulse is 130 beats/min and blood pressure is 85/50 mm Hg. What should the nurse do first? *(1594)*
    1. Call the health care provider
    2. Put the patient in a supine position
    3. Assess pain and give opioid medication
    4. Establish a patent peripheral IV

67. The nurse is caring for a postsurgical patient. Which intervention is the most important in preventing deep vein thrombosis in the legs? *(1600)*
    1. Applying elastic compression stockings
    2. Elevating the lower extremities
    3. Ensuring early ambulation and mobility
    4. Measuring the calf circumference daily

CRITICAL THINKING ACTIVITIES

Activity 1

68. A 56-year-old man arrives in the emergency department seeking care. He is complaining of crushing chest pain. The pain is radiating down his left shoulder and arm. The patient, who has a history of angina, reports the pain is more severe and has lasted longer than a typical angina episode. *(1559-1563)*

 a. What does the nurse anticipate this patient's medical diagnosis will be? _____

 _____

 b. Discuss the pathology of this type of occurrence. _____

 _____

 c. During the medical diagnostic workup of this patient, what tests are likely to be ordered?

 _____

 _____

 d. What are the goals of the medical management of this patient? _____

 _____

 _____

 e. Identify four nursing interventions for this patient's care. _____

 _____

 _____

Activity 2

69. A 43-year-old Native American woman presents with complaints of "heaviness in her chest." She reports that it radiates down her left inner arm. Her medical history includes childbirth, pancreatitis, and hypertension. The medical diagnosis of angina is made. *(1553-1555)*

 a. What risk factors for heart disease does the patient have? _____

 _____

 _____

 b. What medications are used to treat angina? _____

 _____

 c. The patient asks the nurse, "What has caused this to happen?" How will the nurse respond to her inquiry?

 _____

Activity 3

70. A home health nurse is caring for a 73-year-old man who has heart failure. He has been hospitalized twice for exacerbations, but is currently stable and able to live independently in his own home.

   a. What changes related to aging would the nurse expect to find for this patient's cardiac system? *(1543, 1581)*

   _____

   _____

   b. What are common signs and symptoms of heart failure? *(1564, 1656)* _____

   _____

   _____

   c. Identify medication classes that are used in the medical management of heart failure. *(1567-1569)*

   _____

   _____

   d. Discuss patient teaching points for heart failure. *(1570)* _____

   _____

   _____

Activity 4

71. The nurse is working in an ambulatory walk-in clinic in an urban area. Many of the patients are homeless and the clinic staff sees many patients who have venous stasis ulcers.

   a. What is the pathophysiology of stasis ulcers and why are the homeless at particular risk for this disorder? *(1600)*

   _____

   b. Describe how the nurse would use PATCHES to assess venous disorders. *(1582)* _____

   _____

   _____

   _____

   c. Identify the signs and symptoms of venous stasis ulcers. *(1600)* _____

   _____

   _____

   d. Review the treatment options available for venous stasis ulcers and suggest how the nurse can assist homeless patients with these options. *(1601, 1602)*

   _____

   _____

Activity 5

72. Check the cupboards of an elderly relative or patient (or your own cupboards) and read nutritional labels on packages. Determine if a typical day's use of the products on the shelf would meet the nutritional restrictions for someone on a cardioprotective diet. (Don't forget to check condiments, if they are likely to be included in daily use.) Record your findings and the recommendations that you would make about the choice of food products. *(1565)*

_____

_____

_____

_____

_____

_____

_____

_____

_____

Care of the Patient with a Respiratory Disorder

chapter

48

Answer Key: Textbook page references are provided as a guide for answering these questions. A complete Answer Key is provided in your Additional Learning Resources on Evolve.

MATCHING

Medication Used for Respiratory Disorders

Directions: Match the medication used for a respiratory disorder on the left to the associated characteristic (action, side effect, or nursing implication) on the right. Indicate your answers in the spaces provided. (1637, 1638)

Medication	**Actions, Side Effects, or Nursing Implications**
_____ 1. Acetylcysteine (Mucomyst)	a. Vasoconstrictor, used for nasal congestion
_____ 2. Salmeterol (Serevent)	b. Beta$_1$- and beta$_2$-receptor agonist; could cause tachycardia, palpitations, angina, chest pain, myocardial infarction (MI), dysrhythmias, hypertension, restlessness, agitation, anxiety
_____ 3. Prednisone (Deltasone)	
_____ 4. Epinephrine (Adrenalin)	c. Bronchodilator; can cause anxiety, restlessness, insomnia, headache, seizures, tachycardia, dysrhythmias
_____ 5. Ethambutol (Myambutol)	d. Mucolytic agent; also used as antidote in acetaminophen overdose
_____ 6. Isoniazid (INH) (Nydrazid)	e. Used in prevention of exercise-induced asthma
_____ 7. Oxymetazoline (Afrin)	f. Antiinflammatory agent ; do not discontinue medication abruptly; dosage must be tapered slowly
_____ 8. Theophylline (Theo-Dur)	g. Antitubercular agent; requires baseline visual examination at start of therapy
_____ 9. Potassium iodide	h. Antitubercular agent; monitor liver function tests
_____ 10. Zafirlukast (Accolate)	i. For long-term treatment of asthma
	j. Expectorant, mucokinetic agent; could cause hyperkalemia

FILL-IN-THE-BLANK SENTENCES

Directions: Complete each sentence by filling in the blank with the correct word or phrase.

11. Carbon dioxide and oxygen diffuse between blood and lung _____ and alveolar air. *(1612)*

12. At rest, the normal inspiration lasts about _____ seconds and expiration about _____ seconds. *(1612)*

13. When stimulated by increasing levels of blood _____, decreasing levels of blood _____, or increasing blood acidity, the chemoreceptors send nerve impulses to the respiratory centers, which in turn modify respiratory rates. *(1612)*

14. The pco_2 level is _____ in primary respiratory acidosis and _____ in primary respiratory alkalosis. *(1617)*

15. _____ are tissue growths on the nasal tissues that are frequently caused by prolonged sinus inflammation. *(1620)*

TRUE OR FALSE

Directions: Write T for true or F for false in the blanks provided.

_____   16.   Aspirated foreign bodies are more likely to lodge in the left main stem bronchus. *(1610)*

_____   17.   Lung cancer is now the leading cause of death from cancer for men only. *(1650)*

_____   18.   Cigarette smoking is by far the most common cause of emphysema and chronic bronchitis. *(1659)*

_____   19.   In general, infants and young children with pulmonary tuberculosis (TB) do not require isolation precautions because they rarely cough and their bronchial secretions contain few acid-fast bacilli (AFB) compared with adults with pulmonary TB. *(1637)*

TABLE ACTIVITY

20. Directions: Complete the table by filling in the normal values for an arterial blood gas. *(1617)*

pH:	
$Paco_2$:	
Pao_2:	
HCO_3^-:	
Sao_2:	

MULTIPLE CHOICE

Directions: Select the best answer(s) for each of the following questions.

21. The patient had a permanent tracheostomy placed several months ago. The nurse will design interventions for the patient's inability to: *(1625)*
    1. breathe independently and safely.
    2. secrete adequate amounts of mucus.
    3. physiologically produce normal speech.
    4. swallow without choking or gagging.

22. A patient with a chronic lung disorder comes to the clinic and tells the nurse, "I feel like I am getting sick again." What questions would the nurse ask? (Select all that apply.) *(1612, 1613)*
    1. "How's your breathing? Can you describe it?"
    2. "Are you coughing? Can you describe the cough?"
    3. "When did you first notice the worsening of symptoms?"
    4. "What were your last arterial blood gas results?"
    5. "Do you use oxygen at home? If so, does it help?"
    6. "Have you noticed a change in your ability to do routine activities?"

23. The patient arrives at the emergency department and displays significant respiratory distress. Which objective finding is generally regarded as a late sign of respiratory distress? *(1613)*
    1. Shows increased respiratory rate
    2. Has adventitious breath sounds
    3. Assumes orthopneic position
    4. Demonstrates flaring of nostrils

24. A patient was brought to the emergency department because he was involved in a motor vehicle accident. The patient shows mild respiratory distress and expansion of the right side of the chest is decreased compared to the left. The history and data are indicative of which disorder? *(1649)*
    1. Pleural effusion
    2. Pneumothorax
    3. Empyema
    4. Pulmonary edema

25. Which patient has the greatest need for a helical computed tomography scan, which is considered a new and improved technology? *(1655)*
    1. A disoriented elderly man who may have a pulmonary embolus
    2. A toddler who might have swallowed a metallic foreign body
    3. A patient who requires a sample of lymph node tissue for biopsy
    4. A patient who was exposed to tuberculosis several decades ago

26. The nurse is caring for a patient who had a bronchoscopy. Which task can be delegated to the UAP? *(1615)*
    1. Give clear fluids after checking for the gag reflex.
    2. Assist the patient to a semi-Fowler's position.
    3. Report signs of laryngeal edema, such as stridor.
    4. Check sputum for signs of hemorrhage.

27. The patient needs a thoracentesis for therapeutic reasons. Which position should the nurse help the patient to assume for the procedure? *(1616)*
    1. Seated on the bed; head and arms resting on a pillow placed on an overbed table
    2. Placed in a supine position with the anterior-lateral chest draped for ready access
    3. Positioned in a recumbent prone position with head resting on forearms and hands
    4. Situated in a side-lying position on affected side and uncovered to the waist

28. The nurse hears in change of shift report that 1500 mL of fluid was removed during the therapeutic thoracentesis procedure. What is the most important intervention that the nurse will plan to do? *(1616)*
    1. Perform routine postprocedure assessments.
    2. Increase the fluid intake to compensate for the loss.
    3. Watch for signs and symptoms of pulmonary edema.
    4. Follow up to get the results of the fluid specimen.

29. What special consideration is needed for an arterial blood gas for a patient who is taking warfarin (Coumadin)? *(1655)*
    1. The dietary therapy associated with the drug is likely to alter the results.
    2. The drug increases fragility of the vessels, so the specimen is hard to obtain.
    3. The drug alters the amount of oxygen that hemoglobin can carry.
    4. The clotting times are longer than normal, so pressure is held for 20 minutes on the puncture site.

30. The nursing student uses an automatic blood pressure cuff to take vital signs. To be efficient, the student simultaneously attaches the pulse oximeter to the patient's same hand. The pulse oximeter reading is below 90%. What should the student do first? *(1618)*
    1. Report the findings to the nurse or instructor.
    2. Redo the pulse oximeter reading on the other hand.
    3. Assess the patient for shortness of breath.
    4. Document the finding in the patient's record.

31. A patient was treated for epistaxis with nasal packing saturated with 1:1000 epinephrine. During the postprocedure assessment, the nurse notices that the patient swallows frequently. Which question should the nurse ask? *(1619)*
    1. Does your throat feel swollen or painful?
    2. Would you like some cool fluids to drink?
    3. Is blood running down the back of your throat?
    4. Do you taste the epinephrine in the back of the throat?

32. What is likely to be included in the discharge instructions for a patient who was treated for epistaxis? (Select all that apply.) *(1620)*
    1. Use a vaporizer.
    2. Use saline nose drops.
    3. Apply nasal lubricants.
    4. Take aspirin for pain as needed.
    5. Vigorously blow to remove clots.
    6. Avoid inserting foreign objects into nose.

33. What is the nurse's role in allergy testing? *(1621)*
    1. Uses a lancet to prick the skin with different allergens
    2. Evaluates the response to different allergens
    3. Advises the patient about allergens to avoid
    4. Determines schedule for retesting questionable allergens

34. The nurse is eating in a restaurant. At a nearby table, several men are talking, laughing, drinking alcohol, and eating steak. Suddenly, the nurse hears, "Heh! Are you all right?" Which behavior signals a need to intervene for choking? *(1623)*
    1. Vigorous coughing
    2. Running from the room
    3. Hand over throat
    4. Waving hands frantically

35. A patient is diagnosed with viral laryngitis. Which discharge instruction is the most important to relieve the inflammation and edema of the vocal cords? *(1629)*
    1. Use a mild analgesic, such as acetaminophen for pain.
    2. Complete the full course of antibiotics.
    3. Rest the voice; communicate with gestures or by writing.
    4. Suck on throat lozenges to promote comfort.

36. The nurse is performing a rapid strep screen. What is the rationale for obtaining two throat swabs? *(1629)*
    1. The first swab is likely to be contaminated, so a backup swab is needed.
    2. If the rapid strep test is negative, the second swab is sent for culture.
    3. The second swab is given to the patient, in case the rapid strep is positive.
    4. The first and second swabs are grown in different types of culture media.

37. A patient comes to the clinic and reports decreased appetite, generalized malaise, and a decreased sense of smell. Gentle palpation over the sinus area elicits pain. Which piece of equipment should the nurse prepare so the health care provider can do some diagnostic testing during the physical examination? *(1630)*
    1. Tongue blade
    2. Percussion hammer
    3. Penlight
    4. Cotton-tipped applicator

38. A patient is diagnosed with acute bronchitis. Although the patient is instructed to increase fluids to 3000-4000 mL per day, which fluid is specifically not recommended because of the respiratory condition? *(1632)*
    1. Coffee
    2. Soda
    3. Orange juice
    4. Milk

39. What is the primary problem for the health care team in identifying respiratory disorders such as Legionnaires' disease, severe acute respiratory syndrome, and anthrax? *(1632-1634)*
    1. They are agents used in global germ warfare.
    2. The percentage of morbidity and mortality is high.
    3. They require isolation because transmission is airborne.
    4. At first, symptoms are similar to other respiratory disorders.

40. What is the biggest problem for patients who are being treated for tuberculosis? *(1640)*
    1. All the patient's contacts have to be identified and treated.
    2. Infection control measures are complex and expensive.
    3. Many have rapid disease progression with mortality rates up to 89%.
    4. Drug therapy lasts 6 to 9 months and about 50% are noncompliant.

41. A patient recently diagnosed with peripherally located lung cancer reports he is experiencing severe chest pain. Based on the nurse's knowledge of the pathophysiology of this pain, which therapy does the nurse anticipate? *(1645, 1651)*
    1. Bronchodilators
    2. Thoracentesis
    3. Mechanical ventilation
    4. Corticosteroids

42. The patient is diagnosed with pleurisy. During auscultation of the lungs, what is the nurse most likely to hear? *(1613)*
    1. Interrupted crackling or bubbling sounds more common on inspiration
    2. Deep, loud, low, coarse sound (like a snore) during inspiration or expiration
    3. Dry, creaking, grating, with a machinelike quality loudest over anterior chest
    4. High-pitched, musical, whistlelike sound during inspiration or expiration

43. A patient being treated for atelectasis has been prescribed acetylcysteine (Mucomyst). What is the purpose of this medication? *(1648)*
    1. Reduce the risk of infection
    2. Dilate the bronchioles
    3. Enhance the cough reflex
    4. Reduce viscosity of secretions

44. For a patient with a chest tube, which task could be delegated to the UAP? *(1646)*
    1. Assist to ambulate with water-seal below the level of the chest.
    2. Check to make sure that all connections are secure and intact.
    3. Observe for and report hypoventilation or increased dyspnea.
    4. Assess quantity and quality of drainage in the collection chamber.

45. The nurse is reviewing the admission orders for a patient who was stabilized in the emergency department and then admitted for a diagnosis of pulmonary edema. Which order is the nurse most likely to question? *(1653)*
    1. Oxygen 2 liters per nasal cannula
    2. Notify provider with all blood gas results
    3. IV normal saline at 250 mL per hour
    4. Place on telemetry monitor

46. A patient is admitted for a deep vein thrombosis in the left leg. He is in good spirits during the AM assessment, but later in day he reports feeling mildly short of breath with a sense of impending doom. What should the nurse do first? *(1655)*
    1. Obtain an order for an arterial blood gas.
    2. Check the vital signs and pulse oximeter reading.
    3. Assess the left leg for warmth, redness, or swelling.
    4. Alert the RN about possible pulmonary embolus.

47. Which patient is most likely to develop acute respiratory distress syndrome (ARDS)? *(1657, 1658)*
    1. Was diagnosed and treated for sepsis 5 days ago
    2. Had direct trauma to chest during a fight 10 days ago
    3. Has a history of chronic obstructive pulmonary disease
    4. Has been treated for asthma since early childhood

48. Which instruction would the nurse give to the UAP related to assisting the patient who has emphysema with ADLs? *(1660)*
    1. Divide hygienic care into short sessions with 90 minutes of rest between.
    2. Defer the hygienic care until the patient has better activity tolerance.
    3. Assess the patient's response to ambulating and shorten walks accordingly.
    4. Perform range-of-motion exercises, unless the patient declines them.

49. For a patient with chronic bronchitis, what is the physiologic cause of polycythemia? *(1660)*
    1. Medication side effect
    2. Dehydration and fluid shifting
    3. Nutritional deficiency
    4. Compensation for chronic hypoxemia

50. For a patient with newly diagnosed asthma, what is the rationale for conducting an assessment of the home environment? *(1666)*
    1. Determine if the patient will have activity intolerance related to design of house
    2. Assess the safety of the environment related to the use of home oxygen
    3. Identify stimulants or allergens that are triggering the asthma attacks
    4. Evaluate the need for home health care to accomplish activities of daily living

CRITICAL THINKING ACTIVITIES

Activity 1

51. A 34-year-old man comes to the health care provider's office seeking care. He is complaining of fatigue and headaches in the morning. The nurse's assessment reveals he is 5'9" and weighs 293 pounds. His blood pressure is 155/92 mm Hg. His health history reveals elevated blood pressure, hernia repair, appendectomy, and recent injuries suffered from a motor vehicle accident after falling asleep while driving. During the interview, his wife states he should never be tired because he snores so loudly at night that she is the one who is kept awake. *(1622, 1623)*

    a. Based on the nurse's knowledge, what medical diagnosis is anticipated?_____

    _____

    b. What risk factors and elements of the patient's personal history support this diagnosis? _____

    _____

    _____

    _____

    c. Discuss the medical management of this condition. _____

    _____

    _____

    _____

    _____

Activity 2

52. A 72-year-old man is transferred from the nursing home to the hospital with a diagnosis of viral pneumonia. *(1640-1644)*

   a. What signs and symptoms are associated with this type of pneumonia? _____

     _____

     _____

   b. What diagnostic tests can the nurse expect to be completed for this patient? _____

     _____

     _____

   c. What types of medications may be prescribed for this patient?_____

     _____

     _____

   d. Identify nursing assessments that should be performed for this patient._____

     _____

     _____

Activity 3

53. Discuss factors that may influence medication compliance for tuberculosis patients and suggest interventions to increase compliance. *(1637-1640)*

_____

_____

_____

_____

_____

_____

_____

_____

_____

_____

_____

Activity 4

54. The nurse has arrived on the nursing unit and found that the patient has a closed chest drainage system. *(1647)*

    a. What nursing assessments should be performed for this patient? _____

    _____

    _____

    b. How should the tubing and the chest drainage system be positioned? _____

    _____

    _____

    c. What is indicated if there is no tidaling (air bubbling) noted in the water seal chamber?_____

    _____

    _____

    d. What does constant bubbling in the water seal chamber indicate? _____

    _____

    _____

Care of the Patient with a Urinary Disorder

Answer Key: Textbook page references are provided as a guide for answering these questions. A complete Answer Key is provided in your Additional Learning Resources on Evolve.

WORD SCRAMBLE

Directions: Unscramble the words that are related to pathology of the urinary system and then match the term to the correct definition or characteristic listed below.

Scrambled Term	Unscrambled Term	Definition or Characteristic
1. riaanu *(1681)*		
2. aimetoza *(1694)*		
3. terbaciuria *(1690)*		
4. sislydiahemo *(1715)*		
5. suriady *(1679)*		
6. airutameh *(1690)*		
7. urianoct *(1690)*		
8. guriailo *(1702)*		
9. dyniaprostato *(1693)*		
10. thiasisuro *(1697)*		

Definition or characteristic of terms related to pathology of the urinary system
a. Retention of excessive amounts of nitrogenous compounds in the blood
b. Blood in the urine
c. Excessive urination at night
d. Urinary output of less than 100 mL/day
e. Painful or difficult urination
f. Requires access to the circulatory system to route blood through the artificial kidney
g. Formation of urinary calculi
h. Decreased urinary output, less than 500 mL in 24 hours
i. Bacteria in urine
j. Pain in the prostate gland

SHORT ANSWERS

Directions: Using your own words, answer each question in the space provided.

11. What are the three major functions of the nephron? *(1673)*

    a. _____

    b. _____

    c. _____

12. Summarize the three phases of urine formation. *(1674)*

    a. _____

    b. _____

    c. _____

13. Identify three life span considerations for older adults related to the urinary system. *(1676)*

    a. _____

    b. _____

    c. _____

TABLE ACTIVITY

Directions: Complete the table below by supplying the normal range for urinalysis results and identify at least one factor that could influence the results. The first constituent is completed for you. (1677)

14. Urinalysis

Constituent	Normal Range	Influencing Factors
Color	Pale yellow to amber	Diabetes insipidus, biliary obstruction, medications, diet
Turbidity		
Odor		
pH		
Specific gravity		
Glucose		
Protein		
Bilirubin		
Hemoglobin		
Ketones		
Red blood cells		
White blood cells		
Casts		
Bacteria		

FIGURE LABELING

15. Directions: Identify the ileal conduit, stoma, and anastomosis on the figure below. *(1720)*

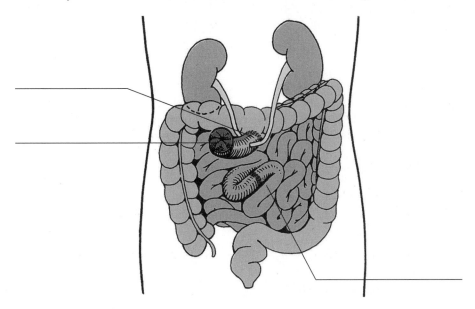

MULTIPLE CHOICE

Directions: Select the best answer(s) for each of the following questions.

16. A patient diagnosed with a urinary tract infection was directed to take sulfamethoxa-zole-trimethoprim (Bactrim) for 3 days and phenazopyridine (Pyridium) for 2 days. What abnormal finding would be expected to occur in the urine during treatment? *(1691)*
    1. An increase in pH
    2. Bright orange color
    3. Increase in leukocytes
    4. Presence of ketones

17. For patients with diabetes mellitus or starvation states, urinalysis will show the abnormal presences of ketones. What is the underlying physiology for this abnormality? *(1675)*
    1. Fatty acids are rapidly catabolized.
    2. Glucose is converted to ketones.
    3. Insulin levels are excessive.
    4. Glucose is transformed into fat.

18. Which patient condition is most likely to result in casts in the urine specimen? *(1677)*
    1. Type 1 diabetes mellitus
    2. Corticosteroid use
    3. Renal disease
    4. Urinary structure trauma

19. The nurse sees that the urine specific gravity results are 1.00o g/mL. Which patient condition is most likely to result in this abnormal finding? *(1678)*
    1. Diabetic ketoacidosis
    2. Hyperemesis gravidarum
    3. Water intoxication
    4. Febrile with poor skin turgor

20. Identify the renal disorders associated with an abnormal elevation in serum creatinine. (Select all that apply.) *(1678)*
    1. Prostatitis
    2. Glomerulonephritis
    3. Pyelonephritis
    4. Acute tubular necrosis
    5. Acute renal failure

21. A 49-year-old man's prostate-specific antigen (PSA) result is 9.5 ng/mL. Which condition(s) could be associated with this result? (Select all that apply.) *(1678)*
    1. Had a recent prostate biopsy
    2. Could be related to prostate cancer
    3. Suggests urinary tract infection
    4. Indicative of prostatitis
    5. Within normal limits

22. The nurse is planning care for several patients who will have diagnostic testing for urinary disorders. Which procedure is going to require the most time for postprocedural care? *(1679)*
    1. Kidney-ureter-bladder radiography
    2. Intravenous pyelogram
    3. Renal angiography
    4. Renal ultrasonography

23. During a urodynamic study, a patient is given bethanechol (Urecholine), a cholinergic drug. What is the expected effect of the medication? *(1680)*
    1. Relaxes the patient
    2. Reduces urine production
    3. Stimulates the atonic bladder
    4. Increases the uptake of dye

24. What instructions would the nurse give to the UAP for assisting a patient for the first 24 hours after a renal biopsy? *(1680)*
    1. Assist the patient to ambulate to the bathroom.
    2. Ask the patient about dizziness before ambulating.
    3. Withhold all foods and fluids for 24 hours.
    4. Remind the patient about bedrest for 24 hours.

25. The nurse is reviewing medication orders for a patient with advanced end-stage renal disease. The nurse would question the use of which type of medication? *(1682)*
    1. Antiemetic
    2. Antipruritic
    3. Vitamin supplement
    4. Osmotic diuretic

26. The nurse is caring for several elderly men who have problems with urinary disorders. Which patient is the best candidate for an external condom? *(1684)*
    1. Has Alzheimer's disease and recently pulled out an indwelling catheter
    2. Has urge incontinence and functional incontinence related to a hip fracture
    3. Has a urinary tract infection and is currently taking antibiotics
    4. Has an enlarged prostate and occasionally has trouble starting the stream

27. The UAP tells the nurse that the patient with a urinary catheter has urine output of less than 50 mL/hour. What should the nurse do first? *(1703)*
    1. Notify the RN and health care provider.
    2. Ask the UAP to recheck the amount.
    3. Assess the patient for renal failure.
    4. Check the function of the drainage system.

28. The nurse sees that the patient who is being discharged is prescribed spironolactone (Aldactone). Which laboratory result will the nurse verify before the patient goes home? *(1682)*
    1. Urinalysis
    2. Potassium level
    3. White cell count
    4. Blood urea nitrogen

29. A patient with benign prostatic hyperplasia (BPH) tells the nurse that he uses over-the-counter medications. Which medication is likely to create additional problems related to the BPH? *(1686)*
    1. Acetaminophen (Ibuprofen)
    2. Diphenhydramine (Benadryl)
    3. Vitamin K supplement
    4. Iron supplement

30. Which patient is most likely to benefit from learning about Kegel exercises? *(1686)*
    1. Experiences loss of urine during sneezing and lifting
    2. Has urinary retention secondary to chronic infection
    3. Has urge incontinence due to advanced Parkinson's disease
    4. Has a spastic bladder due to upper motor neuron lesion

31. The nurse and UAP are aware that no tension should be placed on urinary catheters; however the nurse should reinforce this principle for which patient? *(1707)*
    1. Has a suprapubic catheter for long-term management
    2. Has a three-way catheter for continuous bladder irrigation
    3. Has a Foley catheter after reconstruction of urethra
    4. Has a catheter and urometer for hourly measurements

32. For patients with nephrotic syndrome, which signs/symptoms is the nurse most likely to observe? *(1708)*
    1. Periorbital edema, pitting edema in legs, and crackles in lungs
    2. Sore throat or skin infection with fever and malaise
    3. Burning with urination, low back pain, hematuria, and fatigue
    4. Dysuria, weak stream, and increasing pain with bladder distention

33. The patient with acute glomerulonephritis is placed on bedrest. Which vital sign is of primary interest as an indicator of the success of the therapy? *(1709)*
    1. Temperature
    2. Pulse rate
    3. Respiratory rate
    4. Blood pressure

34. What is an early indicator of kidney failure that should be routinely checked for patients who are at high risk? *(1710)*
    1. Residual urine
    2. Albumin in the urine
    3. Ketones in the urine
    4. Prostate-specific antigen

35. What does the nurse do to assess the function of an arteriovenous fistula after a dialysis treatment? *(1715)*
    1. Flush with saline using strict aseptic technique.
    2. Palpate a thrill and auscultate for a bruit.
    3. Assess the distal pulses and check for sensation.
    4. Ask the patient about pain or discomfort at the site.

CRITICAL THINKING ACTIVITIES

Activity 1

36. A 42-year-old patient is admitted to the unit with a diagnosis of pyelonephritis. As the nurse collects data, she reveals a history of diabetes mellitus, and frequent urinary tract infections. *(1694, 1695)*

    a. What signs and symptoms would the nurse anticipate the patient to demonstrate? _____

    _____

    _____

    b. Discuss the diagnostic tests that may be used in the treatment of the patient and their probable results.

    _____

    _____

Activity 2

37. A patient reports to the emergency department complaining of severe flank pain, nausea, and vomiting. The patient reports that the pain starts in the flank area and radiates to the groin and inner thigh. A urinalysis reveals the presence of hematuria. *(1697, 1698)*

    a. What medical diagnosis can the nurse anticipate?_____

    _____

b. Discuss both the conservative and invasive techniques that may be used in the management of this condition.

_____

_____

c. After successful treatment, the nurse is preparing the patient for discharge. Discuss long-term preventive management options. Include diet and medications.

_____

_____

Activity 3

38. A 53-year-old man was in a motor vehicle accident 4 days ago. He sustained serious trauma with hypovolemia that was treated in the emergency department. He has been diagnosed with acute renal failure and is currently in the oliguric phase. *(1711, 1712)*

a. What potential clinical manifestations should the nurse be aware of when completing the nursing assessment?

_____

_____

b. Discuss the three phases of acute renal failure. _____

_____

_____

_____

c. The patient's wife asks if she can bring him a hamburger and fries from a local fast-food restaurant. How will the nurse respond?

_____

_____

Activity 4

39. A 22-year-old woman seeks care at the doctor's office complaining of burning with urination, perineal pain, and blood-tinged urine. She is diagnosed with a urinary tract infection. *(1690, 1691)*

a. Why are women more prone to urinary tract infections compared to men? _____

_____

b. What other signs and symptoms may be present?_____

_____

_____

c. What medical treatments can be anticipated in the management of this patient? _____

_____

_____

d. What self-care measures should the nurse suggest to the patient to prevent urinary tract infections?

_____

_____

_____

Student Name_____ Date_____

Care of the Patient with an Endocrine Disorder

Answer Key: Textbook page references are provided as a guide for answering these questions. A complete Answer Key is provided in your Additional Learning Resources on Evolve.

MATCHING

Directions: Match the hormone produced by the gland to the action on the target organ. Indicate your answer in the space provided.

Hormone (Endocrine Gland)

_____ 1. oxytocin (posterior pituitary) *(1726)*

_____ 2. antidiuretic (posterior pituitary) *(1726)*

_____ 3. thyroxine (thyroid) *(1728)*

_____ 4. calcitonin (thyroid) *(1728)*

_____ 5. parathormone (parathyroid) *(1728)*

_____ 6. mineralocorticoids (adrenal cortex) *(1728)*

_____ 7. glucocorticoids (adrenal cortex) *(1728)*

_____ 8. epinephrine (adrenal medulla) *(1729)*

_____ 9. norepinephrine (adrenal medulla) *(1730)*

_____ 10. insulin (pancreas) *(1729)*

_____ 11. glucagons (pancreas) *(1729)*

_____ 12. melatonin (pineal) *(1729)*

Action on Target Organ

a. Causes the kidneys to conserve water by decreasing the amount of urine produced

b. Promotes the release of milk and stimulates uterine contractions during labor

c. Decreases blood calcium levels by causing calcium to be stored in the bones

d. Growth and development; metabolism

e. Involved in glucose metabolism; provides extra reserve energy in times of stress; exhibits antiinflammatory properties

f. Causes the heart rate and blood pressure to increase

g. Increases the concentration of calcium in the blood and regulates phosphorus in the blood

h. Water and electrolyte balance; indirectly manages blood pressure

i. Secreted in response to decreased levels of glucose in the blood

j. Inhibits reproductive activities by inhibiting the gonadotropic hormones

k. Combines with epinephrine to produce "fight-or-flight" response

l. Secreted in response to increased levels of glucose in the blood

FIGURE LABELING

13. Directions: Label the figure below by indicating the position of the glands of the body. *(1726)*

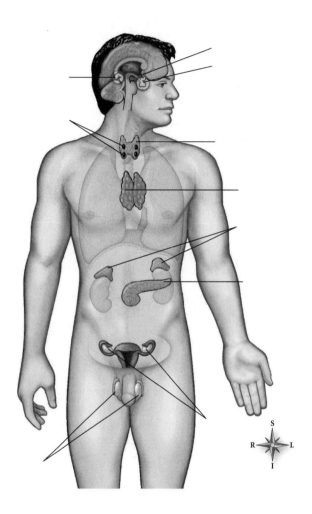

FILL-IN-THE-BLANK SENTENCES

Directions: Complete each sentence by filling in the blank with the correct word or phrase.

14. Diabetes insipidus is a metabolic disorder of the posterior pituitary in which _____ is deficient. *(1730)*

15. In nondiabetic patients, the beta cells are stimulated by increased blood glucose levels; insulin secretion reaches peak levels about _____ minutes after meals and returns to normal in _____ hours. *(1752)*

16. In type 2 diabetes, the main problem is an abnormal resistance to _____ action. *(1752)*

17. Patients should be educated that complications from diabetes can be greatly decreased by proper maintenance of the blood glucose levels of _____ and by appropriate HbA_{1c} levels of less than _____. *(1753)*

18. A patient with type 2 diabetes mellitus often has a history of _____, _____, _____, hypercholesterolemia, and cardiovascular risk (MI, stroke) before the disease is diagnosed. *(1753)*

19. _____ causes more cases of blindness in the United States than any other disease. *(1764)*

20. Approximately _____ of diabetic patients have to undergo either peritoneal dialysis or hemodialysis as a result of vascular changes that affect the kidney. *(1765)*

TABLE ACTIVITY

21. Directions: Complete the table below with the correct information about different types of insulin. *(1758)*

Type of Insulin	Injection Time (Before Meal)	Risk Time for Hypoglycemic Reaction	Peak Action	Duration
Lispro (Humalog)	5-15 min	No meal within 30 min		
Regular Humulin R Novolin R		Delayed meal or 3-4 hr after injection		2-4 hr
NPH/Regular Mix 70/30 Humulin Mix 70/30	30-60 min		30-60 min	6-12 hr
Lente		3-6 hr after injection		6-12 hr
Glargine (Lantus)	Usually take at 9 PM, once daily		1-2 hr	
Ultralente		6 hr after injection	4-6 hr	

MULTIPLE CHOICE

Directions: Select the best answer(s) for each of the following questions.

22. The nurse is talking to a 31-year-old woman who was recently diagnosed with acromegaly. The woman says, "My career is over. I'll become so hideous, I'm sure that I'll get fired." What is the most therapeutic response? *(1730)*
    1. "You have talents and abilities; surely those qualities will be considered."
    2. "Why don't you wait and cross that bridge when you come to it?"
    3. "You are thinking about how your life and career might change."
    4. "Let's talk about what you could do to enhance your appearance."

23. The school nurse is taking the height and weight measurements of all of the children at the beginning of the school year. Measurement for one of the students shows a deviation over two percentile levels from the median. What should the nurse do? *(1732)*
    1. Call the parents and ask about the child's birth weight and growth patterns.
    2. Contact the parents and suggest they take the child to the health care provider.
    3. Recheck the child's height and weight once a month for the next several months.
    4. Track the child's growth over time and compare findings to siblings and classmates.

24. Which nursing interventions should be employed for a patient with diabetes insipidus? (Select all that apply.) *(1734)*
    1. Assessment of skin turgor
    2. Daily weight measurement
    3. Fluid restriction
    4. Monitor intake and output
    5. Frequent ambulation

25. Which patient has the greatest risk for developing syndrome of inappropriate antidiuretic hormone (SIADH)? *(1735)*
    1. Has malignant cancer
    2. Has dormant tuberculosis
    3. Suffered head trauma
    4. Received opiate medication

26. The nurse is caring for a patient who is diagnosed with SIADH. Which assessment finding indicates that the disorder has progressed to neurologic involvement? *(1735)*
    1. An increased urge to drink fluids
    2. A decrease in serum sodium
    3. Progression to shock symptoms
    4. A change in mental status

27. For the patient with SIADH, the health care provider orders fluid restriction. Which finding best indicates that the therapy is working? *(1735)*
    1. Patient reports that he feels better.
    2. Vital signs are at patient's baseline.
    3. Serum sodium is gradually increased.
    4. Diuretics are gradually discontinued.

28. The nurse is caring for a patient who had a thyroidectomy. Which routine postoperative intervention would the nurse clarify with the health care provider? *(1739)*
    1. Inspect dressing for bleeding and drainage.
    2. Give clear liquids; progress to soft diet.
    3. Encourage coughing and deep-breathing.
    4. Observe surgical site for signs of infection.

29. The patient tells the nurse that the health care provider wants to test her for Graves' disease. What symptoms is the patient most likely to exhibit? *(1737)*
    1. Weight loss, increased appetite, and nervousness
    2. Intolerance to cold, constipation, and lethargy
    3. Skeletal pain, pain on weight-bearing, and paranoia
    4. Polyphagia, polydipsia, and polyuria

30. The nurse is reviewing the patient's medication orders and sees that the patient is prescribed levothyroxine (Synthroid). Which laboratory result will indicate efficacy of therapy? *(1741)*
    1. Blood glucose less than 250 mg/dL
    2. Normalization of urine specific gravity
    3. Gradual improvement of serum sodium level
    4. Normalization of thyroid-stimulating hormone level

31. The nurse is caring for a patient who had a thyroidectomy 6 hours ago. The patient now exhibits extreme anxiety and irritability with a severe elevation in pulse, blood pressure, and temperature. The nurse would initiate emergency measures for which postoperative complication? *(1739)*
    1. Hypovolemic shock
    2. Thyroid crisis
    3. Airway obstruction
    4. Septic shock

32. The nurse reads in the patient's chart that a firm, fixed, small, rounded, painless nodule was felt during palpation of the thyroid gland. The nurse prepares to support the patient when the health care provider informs about the need for diagnostic testing for: *(1743)*
    1. myxedema.
    2. colloid goiter.
    3. thyroid cancer.
    4. cretinism.

33. The nurse is caring for a patient who has a pathologic fracture secondary to hyperparathyroidism. Which food needs to be taken off the patient's breakfast tray? *(1745)*
    1. Glass of whole milk
    2. White toast with jam
    3. Sugared cereal flakes
    4. Fried egg with bacon

34. Why is the diuretic medication furosemide (Lasix) prescribed for a patient with hyperparathyroidism? *(1745)*
    1. Preserve existing kidney function
    2. Decrease fluid retention and edema
    3. Encourage the elimination of serum calcium
    4. Decrease blood pressure

35. The LPN is assisting an RN with a patient who needs emergency administration of calcium gluconate for hypoparathyroid tetany. The RN is preparing the medication. What task should the LPN/LVN perform under the supervision of the RN? *(1746)*
    1. Assess the patient for medication allergies.
    2. Place the patient on electrocardiographic monitoring.
    3. Assess the patency of the intravenous access.
    4. Verify the order for calcium gluconate.

36. For patients who have hypoparathyroidism, why is it important for the nurse to encourage foods such as soy milk, white rice, jam, honey, lemon-lime soda, cucumbers, lettuce, peppers, tomatoes, and non-organ meats? *(1746)*
    1. These foods supply extra calcium, which is needed to treat hypocalcemia.
    2. These foods are low in phosphorus, and serum phosphorus is elevated.
    3. These foods supply vitamin D, which improves the absorption of calcium.
    4. These foods are low in fat and will not be metabolized into ketones.

37. Urine excreted by a patient with diabetes insipidus will exhibit which characteristics? *(1733)*
    1. Dilute, with a specific gravity of 1.005–1.030 g/mL
    2. Dilute, with a specific gravity of 1.001–1.005 g/mL
    3. Concentrated, with a specific gravity of 1.005–1.030 g/mL
    4. Concentrated, with a specific gravity of 1.001–1.005 g/mL

38. A patient asks what causes his unsightly goiter. Based on knowledge of pathophysiology, what does the nurse tells the patient? *(1742)*
    1. The growth is harmless, like a fluid-filled cyst that can be drained.
    2. There is fluid retention in the face and neck because of a blockage.
    3. The gland usually enlarges because of lack of iodine in the diet.
    4. The surrounding tissue becomes inflamed and swollen because of infection.

39. Cortisol is responsible for what bodily function? *(1728)*
    1. Regulates sodium levels
    2. Regulates potassium levels
    3. Provides energy during stress
    4. Responds to decreased glucose levels

40. What type of insulin administration is indicated in the management of hyperglycemia related to diabetic ketoacidosis? *(1767)*
    1. Lente insulin given subcutaneously
    2. Ultralente insulin given subcutaneously
    3. NPH 70/30 given intravenously
    4. Regular insulin given intravenously

41. A patient is diagnosed with corticosteroid-induced Cushing's syndrome. Which statement by the patient indicates a need for additional patient teaching? *(1748)*
    1. "I would like to try a dose reduction."
    2. "I am going to stop taking the medication."
    3. "I prefer trying a gradual discontinuation."
    4. "I am changing to the alternate-day regimen."

42. The patient with Cushing's syndrome has high risk for impaired skin integrity. What instructions will the nurse give to the UAP to prevent skin impairment? *(1748)*
    1. Handle very gently to prevent bruising and ecchymosis.
    2. Assess for signs of erythema, edema, or infection.
    3. Frequently wash the skin to prevent irritation.
    4. Assist females to remove extra hair with a safety razor.

43. The nurse is caring for a patient who is admitted with Addison's disease. During the AM assessment, the nurse notes very high temperature and orthostatic hypotension. Laboratory results show hyponatremia and hyperkalemia. How does the nurse interpret these findings? *(1749)*
    1. These are expected findings for this disorder; continue routine assessment.
    2. The frequency of assessment should be increased; reassess status every 1-2 hours.
    3. These are signs of impending addisonian crisis; notify the health care provider.
    4. These should be documented as abnormal findings; compare data for trends.

44. The principal manifestation of pheochromocytoma is severe hypertension. What other symptoms are likely to accompany the excessive secretion of catecholamines (i.e., epinephrine and norepinephrine)? *(1751)*
    1. Lethargy, constipation, and depression
    2. Tachycardia, diaphoresis, and anxiety
    3. Kussmaul's respiration, hypotension, and drowsiness
    4. Excessive thirst, increased urine output, and lethargy

45. Which diagnostic test is the best for monitoring long-term compliance for patients with diabetes mellitus? *(1755)*
    1. Fasting blood glucose (FBG)
    2. Postprandial (after a meal) blood glucose (PPBG)
    3. Patient self-monitoring of blood glucose (SMBG)
    4. Glycosylated hemoglobin (HbA$_{1c}$)

46. Which patient needs to test the urine for ketones as part of their self-care management? *(1753)*
    1. Gestational diabetic who has started insulin
    2. Type 2 diabetic who is preparing to exercise
    3. Type 1 diabetic who has a febrile infection
    4. An older diabetic who cannot perform SMBG

47. The pharmacy delivers a bag of insulin to be delivered as a piggyback infusion. The label says that 100 units of regular insulin is mixed in 500 mL of normal saline. How many mL would be required to deliver 3 units per hour? _____ *(1767)*

48. A nurse hears in shift report that a diabetic patient has been NPO since midnight for a surgical procedure that should happen this morning. On assessment, the patient is irritable, and his skin is cool and clammy. His blood glucose is 45 mg/dL. What should the nurse do first? *(1766)*
    1. Give the patient some juice and a peanut butter sandwich.
    2. Administer 50% glucose per emergency protocol.
    3. Call the operating room and cancel the procedure.
    4. Call the health care provider and inform about findings.

CRITICAL THINKING ACTIVITIES

Activity 1

49. A 19-year-old woman seeks care because of excessive thirst, hunger, and fatigue. She reports she has not been able to sleep all night for the past few weeks because of needing to go to the bathroom. *(1754, 1762, 1764)*

    a. Based on the nurse's knowledge, what medical diagnosis is anticipated?_____

    _____

    b. What other clinical manifestations may occur in this patient?_____

    _____

    _____

    _____

    _____

c. Describe what the nurse will teach the patient about administering insulin. _____

_____

_____

_____

_____

d. Upon realizing this condition is not curable, the patient asks what acute and long-term complications are associated with diabetes. How will the nurse respond to this inquiry?

_____

_____

_____

_____

Activity 2

50. The parents of a 6-year-old boy report to the health care provider with concerns about their son's height. They report that he is the smallest child in the school. The parents are of normal stature. Assessment reveals that the child is indeed significantly small for his age. *(1733)*

a. What diagnostic tests can be anticipated? _____

_____

_____

b. What other clinical manifestations may be exhibited by a child with dwarfism? _____

_____

_____

c. Another question voiced by the parents concern future implications for their child. How will the nurse respond?

_____

_____

_____

d. What medical treatment will be prescribed for this patient? _____

_____

_____

Activity 3

51. Discuss considerations for older adults related to endocrine disorders. *(1764)* _____

_____

_____

_____

_____

Activity 4

52. Why should patients with endocrine disorders be advised to wear medical alert jewelry? *(1737, 1744, 1764)*

_____

_____

_____

_____

Care of the Patient with a Reproductive Disorder

Answer Key: Textbook page references are provided as a guide for answering these questions. A complete Answer Key is provided in your Additional Learning Resources on Evolve.

FIGURE LABELING

1. Directions: Label the parts of the female reproductive organs. *(1778)*

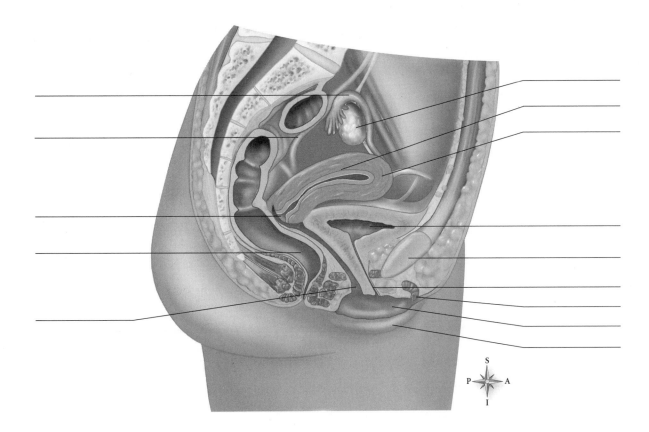

MATCHING

Directions: Match the birth control method with the description. Indicate your answers in the spaces provided. (1839-1841)

	Method		**Description**
_____	2. combination pill	a.	Take two within 72 hours of coitus; repeat if vomiting occurs; take second dose 12 hours later
_____	3. morning-after pill	b.	Consists of a thin flexible rod, which is inserted subdermally
_____	4. progestin-only pill	c.	Rubber thimble-shaped shield covering cervix, held in place by suction
_____	5. medroxyprogesterone (Depo-Provera)	d.	Device inserted into uterus; flexible object made of plastic or copper wire
_____	6. Implanon	e.	No pill-free days
_____	7. diaphragm	f.	Double-ring system fitted into vagina up to 8 hours before intercourse
_____	8. cervical cap	g.	Contains both estrogen and progesterone
_____	9. male condom	h.	Only drug given by injection every 3 months
_____	10. female condom	i.	Dome-shaped latex cap with flexible metal ring
_____	11. intrauterine device	j.	Thin rubber sheath fitting over erect penis
_____	12. rhythm method	k.	Bilateral surgical ligation and resection of ductus deferens
_____	13. tubal sterilization	l.	Crushing, ligating, clipping, or plugging of fallopian tubes
_____	14. hysterectomy	m.	Requires periodic abstinence during fertile portion of menstrual cycle
_____	15. vasectomy	n.	Surgical removal of uterus; 100% effective

FILL-IN-THE-BLANK SENTENCES

Directions: Complete each sentence by filling in the blank with the correct word or phrase.

16. Prostate enlargement is increasingly common with each decade after _____ years of age. *(1781)*

17. By _____ years of age, children are aware that they will remain boys or girls and that no outward change in their appearance will alter this. *(1781)*

18. It is believed that the average breast tumor is present for _____ years before it is palpable. *(1786)*

19. All pregnancy tests, regardless of method, are based on detection of _____, which is secreted in the urine after the fertilization of the ovum. *(1787)*

20. The appearance of the male climacteric phase is gradual and occurs between _____ and _____ years of age. *(1796)*

TRUE OR FALSE

Directions: Write T for true or F for false in the blanks provided.

_____ 21. The hymen can only be ruptured during sexual intercourse. *(1779)*

_____ 22. In giving patients information about sexuality, the implication is that the nurse agrees with specific beliefs. *(1782)*

_____ 23. CA-125 can detect primary ovarian cancer. *(1787)*

_____ 24. Delaying childbearing by women with endometriosis is not recommended as worsening of the condition may result in a loss of fertility. *(1805)*

SHORT ANSWER

Directions: Using your own words, answer each question in the space provided.

25. Identify three functions of the organs of the male reproductive system. *(1776)*

a. _____

b. _____

c. _____

26. Nurses may intervene in sexual problems among patient populations through what four strategies? *(1783)*

a. _____

b. _____

c. _____

d. _____

27. What are the most common disturbances related to menstruation? *(1788)*

a. _____

b. _____

c. _____

d. _____

e. _____

28. What are the major goals of treatment of vaginal infections? *(1801)*

a. _____

b. _____

c. _____

d. _____

29. What are the four main factors that contribute to STIs being among the world's most common communicable diseases? *(1832)*

a. _____

b. _____

c. _____

d. _____

FIGURE LABELING

30. Directions: Label the lymph nodes of the axilla. *(1817)*

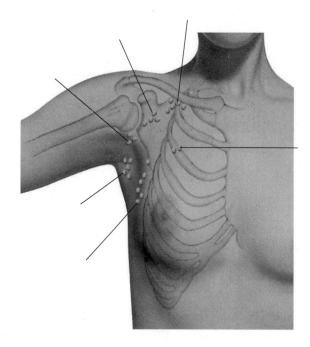

MULTIPLE CHOICE

Directions: Select the best answer(s) for each of the following questions.

31. Which illnesses can result in actual inabilities to function sexually? (Select all that apply.) *(1783)*
    1. Diabetes mellitus
    2. End-stage renal disease
    3. Primary syphilis
    4. Hypertension
    5. Spinal cord injuries

32. Which woman needs to be advised to have an annual Pap smear? *(1784)*
    1. A 17-year-old who has been sexually active since age 14
    2. A 19-year-old who has never been sexually active
    3. A 31-year-old who had three normal consecutive Pap smears
    4. A 25-year-old who had a hysterectomy for traumatic injury

33. In caring for men who have had diagnostic testing of the reproductive system, the nurse would provide the comfort measures of scrotal support and an ice application for which diagnostic test? *(1787)*
    1. Semen analysis
    2. Prostatic smear
    3. Testicular biopsy
    4. Prostate-specific antigen

34. Following a cystoscopy, which finding would be considered normal? *(1787)*
    1. Elevated temperature
    2. Decreased urinary output
    3. Pink-tinged urine
    4. Low-back pain

35. For which condition is the nurse most likely to use a heat application as a comfort measure? *(1790)*
    1. Amenorrhea
    2. Dysmenorrhea
    3. Menorrhagia
    4. Metrorrhagia

36. The nurse is interviewing a patient who reports that her menstrual periods seem heavier than usual. Which question(s) would the nurse ask? (Select all that apply.) *(1792)*
    1. "How many days have you had menstrual flow?"
    2. "How many days would your period typically last?"
    3. "How many pads or tampons are you saturating per day?"
    4. "How frequently would you normally change a pad/tampon?"
    5. "Do you take aspirin or other anticoagulant medications?"
    6. "Have you recently started a rigorous exercise program?"

37. Which disorder is most likely to be treated with an antidepressant medication? *(1793)*
    1. Premenstrual dysphoric disorder
    2. Premenstrual syndrome
    3. Pelvic inflammatory disease
    4. Polycystic ovarian syndrome

38. A 55-year-old woman reports that she went through menopause 3 years ago, but has started to have menstrual flow again and she wonders if she should start using birth control again. What should the nurse say? *(1812)*
    1. "Resuming birth control is a good idea if you don't want to get pregnant."
    2. "Pregnancy is probably not likely since you went through menopause three years ago."
    3. "Vaginal bleeding after menopause is not expected. See your health care provider."
    4. "Does your current flow look like it did before you went through menopause?"

39. What is the physiologic rationale that supports use of calcium and vitamin D supplements for postmenopausal women? *(1795)*
    1. These supplements are an alternative to hormone replacement therapy to relieve hot flashes.
    2. Decreased bone density occurs with menopause; calcium and vitamin D support bone health.
    3. Calcium and vitamin D mimic estrogen and progesterone in their structure and function in the body.
    4. Postmenopausal women are more likely to decrease active exercises that contribute to bone health.

40. For most menopausal women, which symptom/condition could be relieved by the use of a water-soluble lubricant, such as KY? *(1796)*
    1. Pruritus
    2. Phimosis
    3. Dyspareunia
    4. Procidentia

41. The woman is undergoing a tubal insufflation test. Which outcome suggests that the fallopian tubes are blocked? *(1787)*
    1. No pain or other symptoms are experienced during the test.
    2. The patient experiences shoulder pain during the test.
    3. A high-pitched bubbling is auscultated over the abdomen.
    4. A radiographic film shows free gas under the diaphragm.

42. A 57-year-old male patient confides in the nurse that he doesn't feel as productive or sexually powerful as he used to. What should the nurse say first? *(1797)*
    1. "I understand how you feel; aging makes us feel like time is slipping away."
    2. "You'll be okay. Look at all the things you have accomplished so far."
    3. "What factors are contributing to the changes that you see in yourself?"
    4. "Let's talk about ways that you can cope with your loss of sexual power."

43. The nurse is reviewing the medication lists for several patients. Which combination of medications must be immediately brought to the attention of the health care provider? *(1798)*
    1. Sildenafil citrate (Viagra) and nitrates (nitroglycerin tablets)
    2. Vitamin B_6 supplement and ibuprofen (Motrin)
    3. Cefoxitin (Mefoxin) and steroids (Prednisone)
    4. Danazol (Danocrine) and vitamin E supplement

44. The nurse places the patient with pelvic inflammatory disease in a Fowler's position. What is the rationale for using this position for this patient? *(1802)*
    1. Facilitate respiratory effort
    2. Prevent aspiration
    3. Facilitate vaginal drainage
    4. Decrease strain on the abdomen

45. What is an early manifestation of toxic shock syndrome? *(1803)*
    1. Decreased urine output
    2. Flulike symptoms
    3. Desquamation of palms
    4. Hypotension

46. What advice does the nurse give about tampon use in order to prevent toxic shock syndrome? *(1803)*
    1. Use an applicator to insert super-absorbent tampons.
    2. Wash hands thoroughly after inserting a tampon.
    3. Tampons should be changed every 8 hours.
    4. Alternate the use of tampons with use of pads.

47. Radiation has been scheduled for a patient diagnosed with breast cancer. When developing the plan of care, when should the nurse anticipate radiation will take place? *(1821)*
    1. Radiation will begin within 72 hours after surgery.
    2. Radiation will begin within 1 week after surgery.
    3. Radiation will begin 2 to 3 weeks after surgery.
    4. Radiation will begin 4 to 6 weeks after surgery.

48. An advantage of brachytherapy over traditional radiation therapy is that brachytherapy: *(1821)*
    1. is more cost-effective.
    2. will take less time to complete.
    3. is associated with fewer side effects.
    4. uses a lower dosage of radiation.

49. Anemia is a side effect associated with chemotherapy. Which medications may be ordered to manage this complication? *(1821)*
    1. Epoetin alfa (Procrit)
    2. Prochlorperazine (Compazine)
    3. Granisetron (Kytril)
    4. Ondansetron (Zofran)

50. Tamoxifen has been ordered to manage a patient diagnosed with breast cancer. Which characteristics are associated with tamoxifen? (Select all that apply.) *(1821)*
    1. Inhibits the growth-stimulating effects of estrogen
    2. Hormonal agent of choice for postmenopausal women
    3. Used to manage recurrent breast cancer
    4. Used to prevent breast cancer in high-risk individuals
    5. Used for women desiring continued fertility

51. An autologous bone marrow transplant is planned for a patient with breast cancer. Which statement is correct? *(1822)*
    1. Radiation is administered before the transplant to reduce the cancerous growth.
    2. Patient will donate bone marrow, from which stem cells will be harvested.
    3. Chemotherapy administration reduces success for the bone marrow transplant.
    4. Plasmapheresis is performed on the donor stem cells before transplantation.

52. A 22-year-old woman who has a history of cervical dysplasia is scheduled for a conization procedure to remove a small eroded area on her cervix. What nursing care is appropriate for this procedure? *(1784)*
    1. Assess for allergies to seafood or iodine.
    2. Monitor for bleeding after the procedure.
    3. Encourage fluids prior to the procedure.
    4. Remind to refrain from using deodorants.

53. When teaching a patient about the rationale for prescribing oral contraceptives to treat dysmenorrhea, the nurse's statement is based on the understanding that oral contraceptives will: *(1790)*
    1. suppress ovulation by increasing prostaglandin levels.
    2. suppress ovulation by increasing estrogen levels.
    3. suppress ovulation by inhibiting prostaglandin levels.
    4. promote ovulation by increasing estrogen levels.

54. What is the treatment of choice for primary syphilis? *(1834)*
    1. Penicillin
    2. Acyclovir
    3. Valtrex
    4. Tetracycline

55. A 22-year-old man comes to the clinic with complaints of urethritis, dysuria, and purulent penile discharge. What medical diagnosis should be anticipated? *(1835)*
    1. Genital herpes
    2. Syphilis
    3. Chlamydia
    4. Gonorrhea

56. A patient who has a pessary reports foul-smelling discharge, vaginal irritation, and difficulty with sexual intercourse. Which question should the nurse ask? *(1807)*
    1. Have you been using vaginal douching?
    2. Are you having burning with urination?
    3. How long has it been since it was cleaned?
    4. Do you use spermicidals for birth control?

CRITICAL THINKING ACTIVITIES

Activity 1

57. A 20-year-old patient reports to the family planning clinic for painful, erythematous vesicles on her genitals. She is scared and voices many questions and concerns about her condition. *(1832, 1833)*

    a. Based on the nurse's knowledge, what is anticipated to be her medical diagnosis? _____

    b. After being advised of her condition, the patient becomes tearful and asks what will be done to cure her. How should the nurse respond to her question?

    _____

    _____

    _____

    _____

    c. What treatment options and interventions are available to the patient? _____

    _____

    _____

    _____

d. What should be included in her patient education? _____

_____

_____

_____

_____

Activity 2

58. The nurse is preparing to discuss menstruation with a group of preteen girls. The nurse will include the following teaching points. *(1788)*

a. At what age do girls typically begin menstruation? _____

b. Approximately how much blood is lost during the average menstrual period?_____

c. List the hormones involved in the menstrual cycle._____

_____

d. What will the nurse tell the girls about personal hygiene? _____

_____

_____

_____

Activity 3

59. The nurse is originally from a very small farming town in the western United States, but after graduating, she decides to work in an urban clinic that serves an inner-city community in a very large city in the eastern part of the United States. *(1832)*

a. What are the risk factors for the clinic population that are likely to contribute to reproductive disorders?

_____

_____

_____

_____

b. What can the nurse do to prepare herself to help patients that may have gender identity beliefs or sexual practices that are different from her own?

_____

_____

_____

_____

Activity 4

60. Discuss the emotional impact for a couple who is undergoing diagnostic testing for infertility. *(1800)*

_____

_____

_____

_____

_____

_____

_____

_____

Care of the Patient with a Visual or Auditory Disorder

Answer Key: Textbook page references are provided as a guide for answering these questions. A complete Answer Key is provided in your Additional Learning Resources on Evolve.

FIGURE LABELING

1. Directions: Label the anatomy of the eye. *(1848)*

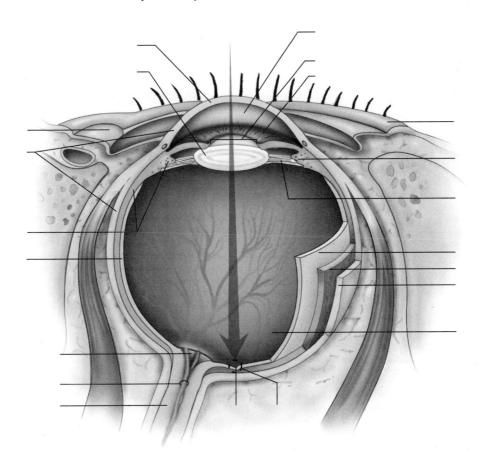

CROSSWORD PUZZLE

2. Use the clues to complete the crossword puzzle.

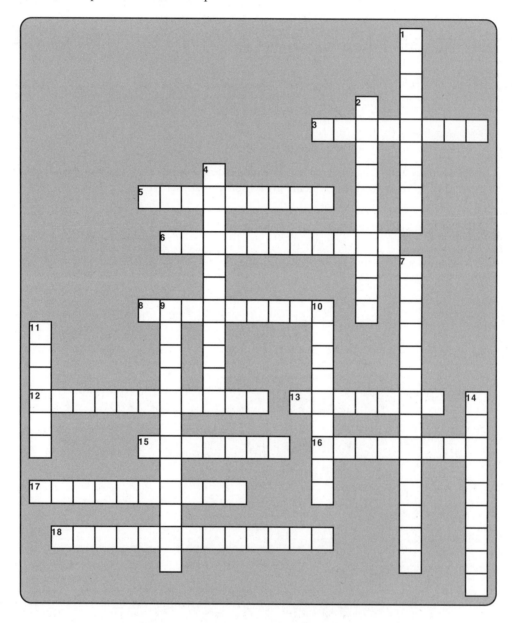

Across

3. Crystalline opacity or clouding of the lens *(1860)*
5. Inflammation of the cornea *(1858)*
6. Defect in curvature of eyeball surface *(1854)*
8. Infection of eyelid margin *(1856)*
12. A hearing deficit secondary to aging *(1891)*
13. Agents that cause the pupil to constrict *(1869)*
15. Sensation of moving or spinning *(1878)*
16. Ringing or tinkling sounds in the ear *(1882)*
17. A type of refractory error *(1851)*
18. Inflammation of the labyrinthine canals of the inner ear *(1884)*

Down

1. Farsightedness *(1854)*
2. Cross-eyed *(1854)*
4. Infection of one of the mastoid bones *(1884)*
7. Pinkeye *(1857)*
9. Chronic progressive deafness caused by the formation of spongy bone *(1886)*
10. Dilating drops *(1851)*
11. Nearsightedness *(1854)*
14. Involuntary, rhythmic movements of the eyes *(1878)*

TRUE OR FALSE

Directions: Write T for true or F for false in the blanks provided.

_____ 3. Most cataracts are caused by chronic eye infections. *(1860)*

_____ 4. The incidence of diabetic retinopathy greatly increases in relation to how long the patient has diabetes mellitus and how well their blood glucose levels are controlled. *(1862)*

_____ 5. Central vision damaged by macular degeneration can be restored by photocoagulation. *(1865)*

_____ 6. There is a direct relationship between vascular hypertension and ocular hypertension. *(1870)*

_____ 7. The deaf community believes that life without hearing is healthy and functional and that deafness is not a disease that needs to be cured. *(1891)*

FILL-IN-THE-BLANK SENTENCES

Directions: Complete each sentence by filling in the blank with the correct word or phrase.

8. The normal visual field range is _____ degrees. *(1852)*

9. A patient with glaucoma tests above the normal range of _____ mm Hg. *(1868)*

10. Primary open-angle glaucoma is medically treated by the use of beta blockers, _____, and carbonic anhydrase inhibitors. *(1869)*

11. The four taste sensations are _____, _____, _____, and _____. *(1890)*

SHORT ANSWER

Directions: Using your own words, answer each question in the space provided.

12. What four basic processes are necessary to form an image? *(1850)*

    a. _____

    b. _____

    c. _____

    d. _____

13. Define the following types of blindness. *(1852)*

    a. Total blindness: _____

    b. Functional blindness: _____

    c. Legal blindness: _____

14. What group of disorders characterizes glaucoma? *(1867)*

    a. _____

    b. _____

    c. _____

15. Briefly define the six types of hearing loss. *(1879)*

a. _____

b. _____

c. _____

d. _____

e. _____

f. _____

FIGURE LABELING

16. Directions: Label the anatomy of the external, middle, and inner ear. *(1875)*

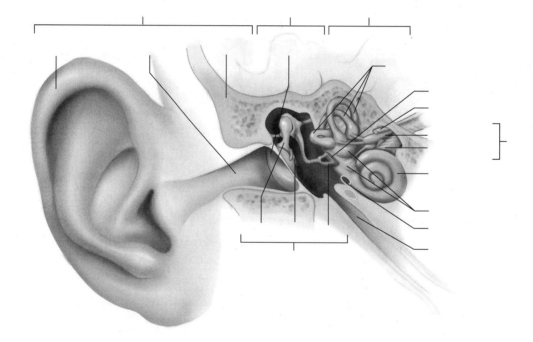

MULTIPLE CHOICE

Directions: select the best answer(s) for each of the following questions.

17. The patient shows loss and deterioration in the automated perimetry test. Which activity is the patient most likely to have difficulty with? *(1851)*
    1. Reading a newspaper or book
    2. Driving through the neighborhood
    3. Looking at a laptop computer screen
    4. Going on a moonlight stroll down the street

18. Which diagnostic test requires an assessment of allergies to seafood or iodine? *(1851)*
    1. Snellen's test
    2. Slit-lamp examination
    3. Fluorescein angiography
    4. Tonometry

19. The nurse hears in the shift report that the patient has diplopia. Which task will be the most difficult for the patient? *(1852)*
    1. Sitting upright in bed
    2. Reading an information brochure
    3. Listening to a radio broadcast
    4. Eating a sandwich with fries

20. The nurse is orienting the patient to the hospital environment. He is just learning to use a cane as an assistive device for partial blindness. Which interventions would the nurse use? (Select all that apply.) *(1852)*
    1. Walk silently beside the patient, so that he can hear environmental noises.
    2. Suggest that the cane be used to identify borders or objects in pathways.
    3. Walk behind the patient, so that the pathway is clear for him/her.
    4. Advise to walk slowly, especially since the environment is unfamiliar.
    5. Describe the general layout of the room and the adjacent hallway.

21. For which eye condition are patients most likely to report trying to first self-treat with over-the-counter eyewear? *(1855)*
    1. Astigmatism
    2. Strabismus
    3. Myopia
    4. Hyperopia

22. A patient with myopia is thinking about having refractory surgery to correct the problem. What should the patient do prior to the surgery? *(1855)*
    1. Arrange to take at least 2 weeks off from work for recuperation.
    2. Stop wearing contact lenses for 1 to 2 weeks before surgical evaluation.
    3. Stop taking any medications for at least 2 days before the surgery.
    4. Use sterile hydrating eyedrops for at least 2 weeks prior to surgery.

23. The nurse's teenage son tells her that his contact lens fell out while he was hanging out in the park with his friends, so he used saliva to clean it off. What should the nurse say? *(1856)*
    1. "Did you ask if anybody had contact lens solution or a lens case?"
    2. "You know you are not supposed to do that, don't you?"
    3. "So, what are you planning to do if that happens again?"
    4. "Do you think glasses would be a better option for you?"

24. The nurse has a 10-year-old daughter who wants to invite two friends for a sleepover. Part of the entertainment for the night is to do "glamour makeovers." What should the nurse do? *(1872)*
    1. Tell the daughter that sharing eye makeup contributes to eye infections.
    2. Call the other parents and see if the friends currently have eye infections.
    3. Purchase three makeup kits from the drugstore and supervise the activity.
    4. Teach the children how to use a fresh cotton-tip applicator for application.

25. The home health nurse is supervising a parent who is demonstrating care for her child's conjunctivitis. The nurse would intervene if the mother performed which action? *(1858)*
    1. Used a clean washcloth to wipe away the secretions
    2. Applied a warm compress with a clean cloth for comfort
    3. Instilled the eyedrops in the lower conjunctival sac
    4. Taped an eyepad loosely over the affected eye

26. For a patient who is diagnosed with keratitis, which common symptom differentiates this disease from other inflammatory eye diseases? *(1858)*
    1. Elevated body temperature
    2. Severe eye pain
    3. Presence of halos or flashes
    4. Low white cell count

27. A patient has recently been diagnosed with keratoconjunctivitis sicca and a dry mouth. Which immune disorder is likely to be associated with this diagnosis and symptom? *(1859)*
    1. Sjögren's syndrome
    2. Acquired immunodeficiency syndrome
    3. Rheumatoid arthritis
    4. Type 1 diabetes mellitus

28. Patients with Sjögren's syndrome typically report: *(1859)*
    1. seeing floaters in the field of vision.
    2. color blindness.
    3. feeling worse in the morning.
    4. feeling that their eyes are gritty.

29. Ectropion is often characterized by: (Select all that apply.) *(1860)*
    1. tearing.
    2. redness of sclera.
    3. thick eye discharge.
    4. corneal dryness.
    5. outward turning of eyelid margin.

30. What diagnostic tests are used to confirm the presence of entropion? *(1860)*
    1. Amsler's grid
    2. Snellen's examination
    3. Ophthalmologic examination
    4. Pneumatic retinopexy

31. The typical type of visual distortions associated with diabetic retinopathy will include: *(1864)*
    1. tunnel vision that worsens in low lighting.
    2. a loss of visual acuity accompanied by "floaters."
    3. a sudden onset of peripheral vision loss and eye discomfort.
    4. reddened eyes accompanied by a yellow discharge.

32. A 65-year-old patient reports to the office complaining of visual deficits, including disturbances in color vision and visual clarity, and a darkened area in the center of vision. What medical diagnosis does the nurse anticipate will be made? *(1865)*
    1. Macular degeneration
    2. Glaucoma
    3. Herpetic keratitis
    4. Cataracts

33. Tonometry is used in the diagnosis of what condition? *(1868)*
    1. Corneal abrasions
    2. Blepharitis
    3. Glaucoma
    4. Retinal detachment

34. The patient has been diagnosed with a visual disorder. Contact lenses have been prescribed. Which statement indicates the need for further instruction? *(1855)*
    1. "Photophobia, dryness, burning, or tearing are expected symptoms."
    2. "I will use proper lens care solutions and a clean lens case."
    3. "I will need to be careful not to mix up my left and right lenses."
    4. "Washing and drying my hands before handling my lenses is essential."

35. Following cataract surgery, which activity is the ophthalmologist most likely to discourage? *(1861)*
    1. Going to the movies
    2. Lifting a grandchild
    3. Walking on a sunny day
    4. Sleeping with a spouse

36. Based on research, supplemental zinc, beta-carotene, vitamins C and E, and a diet rich in fruits and dark-green leafy vegetables would be recommended for which eye disorder? *(1864)*
    1. Age-related macular degeneration
    2. Senile cataracts
    3. Retinal detachment
    4. Glaucoma

37. A patient reports seeing flashing lights and floaters and a dark area in the outer peripheral vision. What is the most important question to ask for suspicion of retinal detachment? *(1866)*
    1. "Are you having severe pain in the affected eye?"
    2. "Is the darkened area getting progressively larger?"
    3. "Do you have type 1 diabetes mellitus?"
    4. "Do you have a family history of eye problems?"

38. The nurse's neighbor is trying to remove an eyelash that has gotten in her eye. The nurse would intervene if the neighbor used which method? *(1872)*
    1. Flushed the eye gently with tap water
    2. Tried blinking and crying to stimulate tears
    3. Used a clean cotton-tipped swab to wipe the cornea
    4. Used a sterile pad to wipe the corner of the eye

39. The nurse is on a camping trip and one of the campers gets poked in the eye with a stick. The end of the stick is protruding from the eye. What should the nurse do first? *(1872)*
    1. Gently remove the stick and then flush the eye with water.
    2. Cover the eye and stick with a paper cup and secure with tape.
    3. Have the camper sit quietly in the car and drive him to the hospital.
    4. Remain calm and control the bleeding with direct pressure.

40. The health care provider informs the nurse that the patient had an abnormal Romberg test. Which safety precaution will the nurse initiate? *(1878)*
    1. Make sure the room has adequate natural lighting.
    2. Do a physical demonstration of how to use the call light.
    3. Announce self to avoid suddenly startling the patient.
    4. Assist the patient to stand and get balance before walking.

41. The nurse's toddler received a prescription for antibiotics to treat acute otitis media. The antibiotics and acetaminophen where given as recommended, but the toddler is still crying with pain. What should the nurse try first? *(1882)*
    1. Have the toddler swallow cool fluids.
    2. Place a warm compress over the affected ear.
    3. Use distraction until the acetaminophen works.
    4. Call the provider and ask for a sedative prescription.

42. The nurse is reviewing the patient's medication list and sees the patient takes meclizine (Antivert). What instructions should be given to the UAP? *(1883)*
    1. Face the patient directly when speaking to him.
    2. Assist the patient to ambulate because he gets dizzy.
    3. Keep the head of the bed elevated at least 30 degrees.
    4. Assist the patient to clean his eyes with a clean washcloth.

43. Which intervention applies to positioning the patient after a stapedectomy? *(1888)*
    1. Keep the operative side facing upward.
    2. Elevate the head of the bed to at least 90 degrees.
    3. Turn, cough, and deep-breathe every 2 hours.
    4. Use a neck brace for the first 2 hours.

CRITICAL THINKING ACTIVITIES

Activity 1

44. An 18-year-old patient has just returned from surgery for the enucleation of his right eye after injuries suffered in an automobile accident. *(1873)*

    a. Discuss the nursing interventions that will be required over the next 24 hours._____

    _____

    _____

    _____

    b. What findings are indicative of complications and warrant an immediate report to the health care provider?

    _____

    c. The patient expresses concerns about his appearance. How will the nurse address his concerns?

    _____

    _____

Activity 2

45. A 20-year-old patient reports worsening ear pain. After completing his history, it is determined he recently had an ear infection and he failed to take the full course of prescribed medications. His other signs and symptoms include fever, headache, malaise, and purulent exudates. *(1884)*

a. What should the nurse anticipate the patient's medical diagnosis will be? _____

_____

b. How did this condition occur? _____

_____

_____

c. Discuss the treatment and the prognosis of this condition. _____

_____

_____

_____

_____

Activity 3

46. The patient had a car accident and is returning to the nurse's unit from vitrectomy surgery of the right eye. List the appropriate nursing interventions for this patient. *(1875)*

_____

_____

_____

_____

_____

_____

_____

Activity 4

47. Refer to Box 52-2 on p. 1877 and identify behaviors that you have noticed for someone you know who may be demonstrating a hearing loss. Has the person you identified admitted that he or she has a hearing loss?

_____

_____

_____

_____

Activity 5

48. If you were to suddenly lose your vision or hearing, how would the loss affect your current lifestyle and future plans?

   _____

   _____

   _____

   _____

   _____

   _____

   _____

   _____

Care of the Patient with a Neurologic Disorder

chapter

53

Answer Key: Textbook page references are provided as a guide for answering these questions. A complete Answer Key is provided in your Additional Learning Resources on Evolve.

FIGURE LABELING

1. Directions: Label the parts of the brain on the figure below. *(1899)*

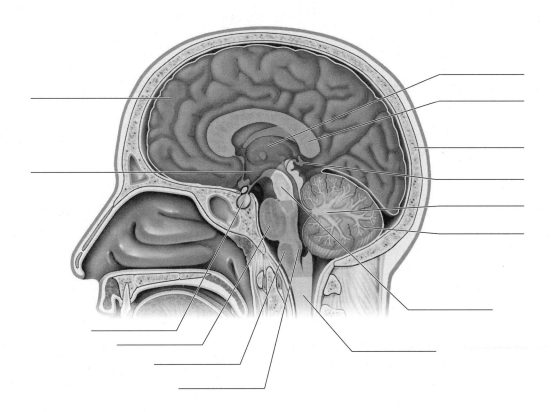

MATCHING

Directions: Match the cranial nerves to their functions. Indicate your answers in the spaces provided. (1902)

		Cranial Nerve		**Functions**

_____   2.   I—olfactory

_____   3.   II—optic

_____   4.   III—oculomotor

_____   5.   IV—trochlear

_____   6.   VI—abducens

_____   7.   VII—facial

_____   8.   VIII—acoustic (vestibulocochlear)

_____   9.   IX—glossopharyngeal

_____   10.   X—vagus

_____   11.   XI—spinal accessory

_____   12.   XII—hypoglossal

a. Eye movements, extraocular muscles, pupillary control (pupillary constriction)

b. Hearing; sense of balance (equilibrium)

c. Down and inward movement of eye

d. Shoulder movements (trapezius muscle) and turning movements of head (sternocleidomastoid muscles)

e. Sense of smell

f. Vision

g. Sense of taste on anterior two-thirds of tongue; contraction of muscles of facial expression

h. Sensations of throat, taste, swallowing movements, gag reflex, taste posterior one-third of tongue, secretion of saliva

i. Lateral movement of eye

j. Sensations of throat, larynx, and thoracic and abdominal organs; swallowing, voice production, slowing of heartbeat, acceleration of peristalsis

k. Tongue movements

FILL-IN-THE-BLANK SENTENCES

Directions: Complete each sentence by filling in the blank with the correct word or phrase.

13. The two main structural divisions of the nervous system are the _____ nervous system and the _____ nervous system. *(1959)*

14. The cerebrum is the largest part of the brain and contains five major areas: _____, _____, _____, _____, and _____. *(1959)*

15. _____ is a generalized impairment of intellect, awareness, and judgment. *(1951)*

16. _____ disease is characterized by abnormal and excessive involuntary writhing and twisting movements of the face, limbs, and body. *(1938)*

17. In untreated cases of brain abscess, the mortality rate approaches _____%. *(1950)*

TRUE OR FALSE

Directions: Write T for true or F for false in the blanks provided.

_____   18.   Pain receptors are not adaptable—they are specific for pain only—and pain impulses continue at the same rate as long as the stimulus is present. *(1912)*

_____   19.   Amyotrophic lateral sclerosis usually results in death 2 to 6 years after diagnosis. Respiratory tract infection secondary to compromised respiratory function is usually the cause. *(1937)*

_____   20.   Seventy to eighty percent of people who become infected with the West Nile virus develop encephalitis or meningitis. *(1949)*

_____   21.   Few patients with advanced HIV disease (AIDS) ever actually develop neurologic symptoms. *(1950)*

_____   22.   Most elderly people will eventually experience dementia. *(1903)*

FIGURE LABELING

23. Directions: In the figure below, identify decorticate and decerebrate responses and the flexion and extension characteristics of the upper and lower extremities. *(1915)*

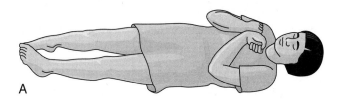

A

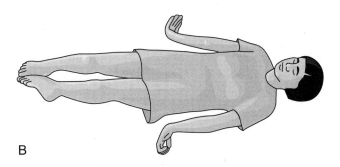

B

WORD SCRAMBLE

Levels of Consciousness

Directions: Unscramble the letters to reveal the correct spelling of terms related to level of consciousness and then match them to the correct definition or description. (1904)

Scrambled Term	Unscrambled Term	Definition or Characteristic
24. treal		
25. orientdisation		
26. porstu		
27. tosecomasemi		
28. esotamoc		

Description
a. Responds to verbal commands with moaning or groaning, if at all; seems unaware of surroundings
b. Is in impaired state of consciousness, characterized by obtundation and stupor, from which a patient can be aroused only by energetic stimulation
c. Unable to respond to painful stimuli; cornea and pupillary reflexes are absent; cannot swallow or cough; is incontinent of urine and feces; electroencephalogram pattern demonstrates decreased or absent neuronal activity
d. Unable to follow simple commands; thinking slowed; inattentive; flat affect
e. Responds appropriately to auditory, tactile, and visual stimuli

MULTIPLE CHOICE

Directions: Select the best answer(s) for each of the following questions.

29. What behavior(s) would be considered normal neurologic changes related to aging? (Select all that apply.) *(1903)*
    1. Drives slower to compensate for slowed reaction time
    2. Demonstrates slight tremor while holding teacup when tired
    3. Takes a foreign language class, but can't keep up with classmates
    4. Does needlework, but has more trouble with fine, small stitches
    5. Rearranges items on countertop, but action serves no purpose
    6. Frequently misplaces keys or eyeglasses, but can usually find them

30. The nurse is assessing the "fund of knowledge" component of the patient's awareness. Which question would the nurse use to assess this component? *(1904)*
    1. "What month is it? And what day of the week is it today?"
    2. "What did you have for dinner last night?"
    3. "If you had $3.00 and gave me half, what would you have?"
    4. "Who was president before Obama took office?"

31. The nurse is assessing a patient who had a serious head injury. During the assessment, the patient spontaneously opens his eyes; is oriented to person, place, and time; and can follow the nurse's commands. How would the nurse document his Glasgow coma score? *(1904)*
    1. GCS within normal limits
    2. GCS insufficient
    3. GCS 3
    4. GCS 15

32. The nurse is using the FOUR Score coma scale to assess a patient who suffered a stroke. Which assessment is an integral part of this scale? *(1905)*
    1. Checking the blood pressure and pulse
    2. Checking orientation to person, place, and time
    3. Assessing the respiratory rate and pattern
    4. Evaluating the ability to make good judgments

33. The nurse hears in report that the patient has motor aphasia. Which intervention will the nurse plan to use when communicating with this patient? *(1905)*
    1. Talk slower, be patient, and enunciate very clearly.
    2. Face the patient so that he can watch the lips move.
    3. Obtain a set of picture cards and encourage gestures.
    4. Be kind and caring, but limit verbal communication.

34. The nurse is checking the gag reflex prior to giving liquids to a patient who had a bronchoscopy earlier in the day. Which cranial nerve is the nurse testing? *(1905, 1906)*
    1. Trochlear
    2. Abducens
    3. Trigeminal
    4. Glossopharyngeal

35. The nurse is caring for a patient who has unilateral neglect that includes the nondominant hand. For which task is the patient most likely to require assistance? *(1906)*
    1. Putting on her blouse
    2. Brushing her hair
    3. Using the remote control
    4. Writing a letter

36. The patient is scheduled to return from having a lumbar puncture. What instructions will the nurse give to the UAP about the care of this patient? *(1907)*
    1. Help the patient ambulate in the halls.
    2. Keep the head of the bed at 30 degrees.
    3. Patient needs to be NPO for several hours.
    4. Report if the patient has numbness or tingling.

37. The nurse is caring for a patient who had cerebral angiography and the vascular system was accessed through the carotid artery. In the immediate postprocedure assessment, what is the priority? *(1909)*
    1. Watching for infection at the puncture site
    2. Assessing for reaction to contrast media
    3. Observing for respiratory difficulties
    4. Assessing for nausea and vomiting

38. A 35-year-old man who suffers from tension headaches requests opioid medications for the debilitating pain. Why is the health care provider unlikely to grant the patient's request? *(1911)*
    1. Opioids are avoided because of the risk of abuse.
    2. Tension headache pain does not warrant opioid use.
    3. Pain receptor sites will not respond to opioids.
    4. Tension headaches are controlled by reducing stress.

39. Which food may cause or worsen a migraine headache? *(1910)*
    1. Italian foods
    2. Apples
    3. Dairy products
    4. Ripened cheese

40. In caring for a patient with a headache, which instruction will the nurse give to the UAP? *(1911)*
    1. Assist the patient to turn every 2 hours.
    2. Keep the room quiet and dark.
    3. Refresh warm compress as needed.
    4. Maintain NPO status for nausea.

41. The nurse is reviewing the medication list for a patient who is diabetic and sees that gabapentin (Neurontin) is prescribed. Which pain assessment will the nurse make? *(1913)*
    1. Low-back pain with movement
    2. Dull or throbbing headache
    3. Burning or tingling in lower legs
    4. Stiffness in joints in the morning

42. What is an early sign of increased intracranial pressure? *(1914)*
    1. Change in level of consciousness
    2. Decreased or abnormal respirations
    3. Increased systolic blood pressure
    4. Increased or widening pulse pressure

43. The nurse is checking the pupils of a patient who sustained a serious head injury. Which pupil response is the most ominous? *(1914)*
    1. Pupil reacts, but is sluggish.
    2. Pupil is fixed and dilated.
    3. Pupil is dilated, but will slowly constrict.
    4. Pupil on affected side is larger.

44. Select the measures that may be implemented to reduce venous volume in a patient experiencing increased intracranial pressure. (Select all that apply.) *(1916)*
    1. Restrict fluid intake.
    2. Place head in flexed position.
    3. Avoid flexion of the hips.
    4. Administer enemas as needed.
    5. Administer oxygen.

45. The patient has residual hemiplegia following a stroke. Which instructions will the nurse give to the UAP? *(1917)*
    1. Assist the patient to ambulate to the bathroom.
    2. Put the unaffected arm through range of motion.
    3. Place in a prone position if the patient can tolerate it.
    4. Use pillows to keep the upper arm in abduction.

46. The nurse hears in report that the 33-year-old patient with multiple sclerosis (MS) is withdrawn, depressed, and emotionally labile. The nurse knows that emotional changes are part of the disease. What other aspect(s) of the disease is/are likely to be contributing to the patient's emotional state? (Select all that apply.) *(1925, 1926)*
    1. Exacerbations and remissions are continuous; deterioration progresses.
    2. The symptoms are vague, insidious, and widely distributed.
    3. No specific treatments exist, although many treatments have been tried.
    4. Multiple body systems are affected and function is lost in every area.
    5. If cured in the early stages, patient can maintain independence and self-care.

47. A resident with Parkinson's disease lives at a long-term care facility. The patient has a flat facial expression, hand tremors, and bradykinesia. Which instruction will the nurse give to the UAP to address the bradykinesia? *(1929)*
    1. He has a shuffling gait and needs assistance to prevent bumping into objects.
    2. He has trouble bending to tie his shoes because of muscle soreness and aches.
    3. He has trouble eating soup or drinking coffee because of fine hand tremors.
    4. He has resistance to motion, so he may seem stiff when you put on his shirt.

48. What is an early subjective symptom that the patient may report that would be characteristic of myasthenia gravis? *(1936)*
    1. Muscle weakness in the extremities
    2. Eyelid drooping and double vision
    3. Trouble swallowing
    4. Weak, nasal-sounding voice

49. What is the single most important modifiable risk factor for stroke? *(1938)*
    1. Cigarette smoking
    2. Sedentary lifestyle
    3. Hypertension
    4. Obesity

50. The patient who had a stroke exhibits dysphagia. Which intervention will the nurse use? *(1918)*
    1. Mix solid and liquid foods together to facilitate swallowing.
    2. Assist the patient to drink water after every bite of food.
    3. Offer the patient a drinking straw or a covered plastic cup.
    4. Check mouth on the affected side for accumulation of food.

51. The patient comes to the clinic and is exhibiting stroke symptoms. The health care provider believes that the patient is a possible candidate for thrombolytic therapy. What are the most important actions for the clinic staff to perform? *(1942)*
    1. Rapid triage and transport to a stroke center
    2. Draw blood for coagulation tests and establish IV
    3. Obtain a CT or MRI to rule out hemorrhagic stroke
    4. Explain the risks and benefits of therapy to the patient

52. In caring for a patient with trigeminal neuralgia, what instructions would the nurse give to the UAP about assisting with hygiene and meals? *(1945)*
    1. Use gentle touch when assisting with shaving.
    2. Encourage the patient to drink cold liquids.
    3. Ask the patient if he prefers to do his own care.
    4. Offer to cut the patient's food into bite-sized pieces.

53. A patient who is diagnosed with Bell's palsy will need to know how to use which device? *(1946)*
    1. Eating utensil with a universal cuff
    2. Eyeshield to be applied at night
    3. Footboard for the end of the bed
    4. A volar wrist splint for extension

54. In caring for a patient who is diagnosed with Guillain-Barré syndrome (GBS), what is the priority assessment? *(1948)*
    1. Paralysis in the legs
    2. Respiratory function
    3. Change of mental status
    4. Loss of bowel control

55. The nurse is caring for a patient who is diagnosed with bacterial meningitis. For this patient, what is the rationale for keeping the room quiet and dark? *(1949)*
    1. Light and noise increase the subjective experience of pain.
    2. Patient needs extra rest and sleep to facilitate recovery.
    3. Any increased sensory stimulation may cause a seizure.
    4. Critically ill patients do better in quiet environments.

56. What is considered a prominent early sign of a brain tumor? *(1951)*
    1. Speech impairment
    2. Morning headache
    3. Change in personality
    4. Memory loss

57. A young man who sustained a serious head injury several years ago is a resident in a long-term care facility. After the injury, he demonstrated intermittent poor judgment and occasional physical aggression. Today, he is trying to leave the facility. What should the nurse do first? *(1954)*
    1. Speak calmly and redirect him to another activity.
    2. Obtain an order for a PRN antianxiety medication.
    3. Allow him to wander around, but keep an eye on him.
    4. Instruct a UAP to perform one-on-one observation.

58. The UAP tells the nurse that a patient with a spinal cord injury has a systolic blood pressure of 190/100 mm Hg. The nurse observes that the patient is diaphoretic, restless, and has "gooseflesh" and a headache. What should the nurse do first? *(1955)*
    1. Recheck the blood pressure.
    2. Check the bladder for distention.
    3. Check the rectum for impaction.
    4. Put the patient in a sitting position.

CRITICAL THINKING ACTIVITIES

Activity 1

59. The school nurse is accompanying a group of children on a field trip. One of children suddenly reports feeling odd and then sits down on the ground. As the nurse eases her to a supine position, the child demonstrates tonic-clonic jerking movements of the body. The nurse notes secretions and drooling from the child's mouth and the lips are slightly cyanotic. The child is unable to respond to her name and her eyes are rolled back and upwards. *(1921, 1924)*

    a. Describe what the nurse should do. _____

    _____

    _____

    b. What information should the nurse record and report to the health care provider? _____

    _____

    _____

Activity 2

60. A 58-year-old man reports he experienced numbness in his legs, a loss of sensation in his arms, and an inability to speak. Upon questioning, he reported that the entire event lasted only about 15 minutes. *(1940)*

    a. What condition/disorder has the patient experienced? _____

    b. Since this event was short in duration, is it of any long-term significance? Why or why not?

    _____

    _____

    _____

    c. What is the most frequently prescribed antiplatelet agent for this condition? _____

    _____

Activity 3

61. a. It is likely that you know or will know someone who has Alzheimer's disease. What are the warning signs? *(1934, 1935)*

_____

_____

_____

_____

    b. Discuss the effect that Alzheimer's disease has on family and society. *(1934, 1935)* _____

_____

_____

_____

_____

    c. What are things you can do and teach your patients to do that will help prevent Alzheimer's disease? *(1934, 1935)*

_____

_____

_____

_____

Care of the Patient with an Immune Disorder

Answer Key: Textbook page references are provided as a guide for answering these questions. A complete Answer Key is provided in your Additional Learning Resources on Evolve.

FIGURE LABELING

1. Directions: Label the figure below with the correct names of the organs of the immune system. *(1965)*

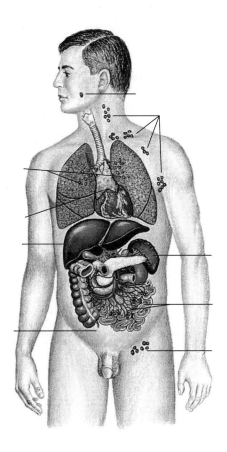

MATCHING

Directions: Match the term related to the immune system with the defining characteristics.

	Term		**Defining Characteristics**
_____	2. autoimmune disorders *(1964)*	a.	Provides a specific reaction to each invading antigen and has the unique ability to remember the antigen that caused the attack
_____	3. innate system *(1964)*		
_____	4. immunoincompetence *(1963)*	b.	Immune response is too weak or too vigorous and system malfunctions
_____	5. adaptive immunity *(1965)*	c.	Systemic lupus erythematosus, celiac disease, thyroid disease, inflammatory bowel disease, type I diabetes, multiple sclerosis, myasthenia gravis, psoriasis, rheumatoid arthritis
_____	6. allergen *(1966)*		
_____	7. immunization *(1966)*		
_____	8. active immunity *(1966)*	d.	Includes intact skin and mucous membranes, cilia, stomach acid, tears, saliva, sebaceous glands, and secretions and flora of the intestines and vagina
_____	9. cellular immunity *(1966)*		
_____	10. complement system *(1967)*	e.	Process by which resistance to an infectious disease is induced or increased
_____	11. allergies *(1964)*	f.	Substance that can produce a hypersensitive reaction in the body, but may not be inherently harmful
		g.	Caused by hyperactive responses against environmental antigens
		h.	Antibodies produced by one's own body
		i.	Negative effects include rejection of transplanted tissues, contact hypersensitivity reactions, and certain autoimmune diseases
		j.	Functions in a "step-by-step" series

SHORT ANSWER

Directions: Using your own words, answer each question in the space provided.

12. What are the three main functions of the immune system? *(1963)*

    a. _____

    b. _____

    c. _____

13. What are the four Rs of the immune response? *(1966)*

    a. _____

    b. _____

    c. _____

    d. _____

14. Identify the five factors influencing hypersensitivity. *(1976)*

    a. _____

    b. _____

    c. _____

    d. _____

    e. _____

15. List 14 items in the health care environment that could contain latex. *(1972)* _____

    _____

    _____

    _____

    _____

MULTIPLE CHOICE

Directions: Select the best answer(s) for each of the following questions.

16. In caring for an older adult, what instructions would the nurse give to the UAP that address changes related to aging for the immune system? (Select all that apply.) *(1967, 1968)*
    1. Promptly assist with toileting to prevent urinary stasis.
    2. Increase fluids (unless contraindicated) to thin secretions.
    3. Apply a thin layer of lotion after bathing to prevent dry skin.
    4. Watch for elevated temperature associated with serious infection.
    5. Perform scrupulous hand hygiene and don clean gloves.
    6. Offer frequent oral hygiene because of decreased saliva production.

17. What is the theory behind progressively increasing the doses of the allergens during perennial immunotherapy? *(1968)*
    1. Inhibits the release of leukotrienes and reduces allergic symptoms
    2. Allows the individual to build up a tolerance without having symptoms
    3. Competes with histamine by attaching to the cell surface receptors
    4. Inhibits further release of chemical mediators from mast cells

18. If medications are administered in error to a patient who is hypersensitive, which route will produce the most rapid allergic reaction? *(1969)*
    1. Oral
    2. Transdermal
    3. Intravenous
    4. Topical

19. The nurse and a friend are ordering lunch. The friend takes 50 mg of diphenhydramine (Benadryl) and then orders oysters, saying, "I'm allergic to oysters, but I just love them, so I take Benadryl." What should the nurse say? *(1969)*
    1. "Do you have your cell phone, so we can call 911?"
    2. "Every time you eat oysters, the reaction will get worse."
    3. "You are an adult and you can make your own choices."
    4. "If I have to resuscitate you, I am not going to be happy."

20. The nurse is trying to do an environmental assessment for an elderly patient who is having continuous allergic reactions, but the patient vaguely rambles on about pets, dust, a broken vacuum cleaner, and mold. What is the best intervention to use for this patient? *(1969)*
    1. Use simplified and focused yes-or-no questions.
    2. Make an environmental checklist for the patient.
    3. Obtain information from a close relative.
    4. Obtain an order for a home health nurse visit.

21. Within 15 minutes of initiating a blood transfusion, the patient reports shortness of breath, chills, and urticaria. After stopping the transfusion and notifying the health care provider, which laboratory test must be completed? *(1974)*
    1. Urinalysis
    2. Electrolytes
    3. Platelet count
    4. White blood cell count

22. The suppressed humoral immune response in older adults is associated with: *(1975)*
    1. degeneration of the spleen.
    2. decreased production of white blood cells.
    3. reduction in effectiveness of white blood cells.
    4. decreased immunoglobulin levels.

23. During plasmapheresis, the plasma may be replaced with which of the following? (Select all that apply.) *(1975, 1976)*
    1. Normal saline
    2. Lactated Ringer's solution
    3. Albumin
    4. 10% dextrose
    5. Fresh-frozen plasma
    6. Dextrose 5% and half normal saline

24. The nurse gives a patient his immunotherapy injection and immediately he demonstrates wheezes, impaired breathing, and hypotension. The nurse initiates the anaphylaxis protocol. What is the nurse's first action? *(1971)*
    1. Establish an IV to administer 1:10,000 epinephrine hydrochloride.
    2. Adminster 1:1000 epinephrine hydrochloride subcutaneously.
    3. Prepare the equipment and assist the provider to intubate the patient.
    4. Administer a 50-mg oral dose of diphenhydramine (Benadryl).

25. What are examples of passive immunity? (Select all that apply.) *(1966)*
    1. Mother breastfeeds her baby
    2. Antivenom given after a snakebite
    3. Immunoglobulin administered postexposure
    4. Child gets hepatitis B vaccine
    5. Patient reports having measles during childhood

26. In caring for a patient who recently had an organ transplant, which instructions would the nurse give to the UAP to protect this immunosuppressed patient? *(1974)*
    1. The most dangerous period is 7 to 10 days after the transplant.
    2. Remind visitors to check at the nurses' station before entering.
    3. If you are pregnant, the patient's chemotherapy may harm the baby.
    4. If you have a cough or skin infection, don a mask and gown.

27. The nurse is caring for a patient who underwent plasmapheresis. What is the most important assessment to make after the procedure? *(1976)*
    1. Monitor intake and output.
    2. Check blood pressure.
    3. Assess mental status.
    4. Evaluate pain.

CRITICAL THINKING ACTIVITIES

Activity 1

28. A 22-year-old patient has just completed allergy testing. Her health care provider has prescribed a regimen of weekly allergy shots. *(1968)*

   a. What special precautions should be taken with the patient after the injection? _____

   _____

   _____

   b. What teaching should be provided for a patient who is receiving allergy shots at home? _____

   _____

   _____

   _____

   c. After administering the shots at home for more than a month, the patient calls and reports she has been ill and unable to take the medications for the past 2 weeks. How should the nurse advise the patient?

   _____

   _____

Activity 2

29. A 67-year-old patient voices concern about his health status. He reports he never used to "get sick," but now has been hospitalized three times in the last month with a variety of illnesses. *(1968)*

   a. Discuss how aging affects the immune system. _____

   _____

   _____

   _____

   b. What should the nurse recommend for measures related to preventing immune disorders in an older patient?

   _____

   _____

   _____

Activity 3

30. Design actual questions that the nurse could use to take a detailed history about a rash to help the health care provider diagnose the patient's allergies. Include: (1) onset, nature, and progression of signs and symptoms; (2) aggravating and alleviating factors; and (3) frequency and duration of signs and symptoms. Assess environmental, household, and occupational factors. *(1969)*

_____

_____

_____

_____

_____

_____

_____

_____

_____

_____

_____

_____

Care of the Patient with HIV/AIDS

Answer Key: Textbook page references are provided as a guide for answering these questions. A complete Answer Key is provided in your Additional Learning Resources on Evolve.

MATCHING

Nutritional Management: HIV Infection

Directions: Match the condition associated with HIV infection with the recommended dietary therapy. Indicate your answers in the spaces provided. (2005)

	Condition		Dietary Recommendation
_____	1. fatigue	a.	High-calorie, high-protein foods
_____	2. anemia	b.	Soft or puréed foods
		c.	High-calorie foods
_____	3. altered taste	d.	Diet as tolerated
_____	4. fever	e.	High-iron foods
		f.	High-fiber foods
_____	5. candidiasis	g.	Lactose-free, low-fat, low-fiber, and high-potassium foods
_____	6. nausea and vomiting	h.	Low-fat foods
_____	7. diarrhea		
_____	8. constipation		

TRUE OR FALSE

Directions: Write T for true or F for false in the blanks provided.

_____ 9. Studies have shown that in communities where needle-exchange programs have been established, drug use does not increase and rates of HIV infection are controlled. *(2012)*

_____ 10. HIV can only be transmitted via contaminated equipment used for illicit drugs such as heroin or cocaine. *(2010)*

_____ 11. It is impossible to contract HIV by receiving a blood product due to current testing used to detect HIV in donated blood. *(1983)*

_____ 12. HIV is classified as "slow" retrovirus or a lentevirus. After infection with these types of viruses, a long time passes before specific signs and symptoms appear. *(1985)*

_____   13.   For patients with end-stage HIV disease who undergo palliative care, the focus will be to relieve pain and give emotional support; intravenous therapy, blood transfusions, and antibiotic usage would not be considered. *(2000)*

_____   14.   The CDC's recommendations state that informed consent is not needed for HIV testing, but nurses should be aware that state law may require informed consent before drawing blood to test for HIV. *(2009)*

TABLE ACTIVITY

15.   Directions: In the table below, add the signs and symptoms that the nurse will see in primary HIV infection (acute illness) and signs and symptoms that appear in early HIV disease (symptomatic infection). *(1988)*

Primary HIV infection (acute illness)	Early HIV disease (symptomatic infection)

MULTIPLE CHOICE

Directions: Select the best answer(s) for each of the following questions.

16.   Which behavior combined with viral load status creates the highest risk for contracting HIV? *(2010)*
   1.   Infected partner in mid-stage HIV performs insertive oral intercourse.
   2.   Uninfected partner receives anal intercourse from infected partner in primary stage.
   3.   Infected partner in mid-stage receives vaginal intercourse from uninfected partner.
   4.   Uninfected partner performs insertive oral intercourse on infected partner in late stage.

17.   What factors increase the risk of HIV for intravenous drug users? (Select all that apply.) *(1983)*
   1.   Poor nutritional status and poor hygiene
   2.   Exchanges sexual activity for drugs
   3.   Impaired judgment due to illicit drug use
   4.   Less likely to use condoms during sex
   5.   Has ready access to sterile equipment
   6.   Routinely uses "booting" during injection

18.   Which health care worker has sustained the greatest risk for HIV after being exposed to body fluids from patients who are HIV-positive? *(1984)*
   1.   Deep puncture with a hollow-bore needle filled with blood from a patient's vein
   2.   Splashed in the face with saliva and mucus during oral suctioning and hygiene
   3.   Glove tears while cleaning the perianal area of a patient who has postpartum bleeding
   4.   Patient vomits copious amounts of bloody fluid over the front of the worker's uniform

19. For a health care worker who must take post-exposure antiviral therapy, which signs/symptoms suggest that the worker is developing the most likely adverse effect of the drug therapy? *(1984)*
    1. Fatigue, activity intolerance, and a low red blood cell count
    2. Decreased urine output and elevated blood urea nitrogen
    3. Jaundice, malaise, and abnormal liver function tests
    4. Chest pain, arrhythmias, and elevated troponin levels

20. Perinatal or vertical transmission has been reduced by initiating which combination of interventions? *(1985)*
    1. Breastfeeding, enhanced maternal nutrition, and voluntary HIV testing
    2. Bottle-feeding, antiretroviral therapy for HIV-infected mothers, and cesarean birth
    3. Early prenatal care, natural childbirth, and antiretroviral therapy for HIV-infected babies
    4. Inducing labor during mid-stage HIV, and giving zidovudine syrup to neonate at birth

21. For a CD_4^+ lymphocyte level of 200 cells/mm³, which clinical manifestations are most likely to be observed? *(1988)*
    1. Generally asymptomatic
    2. Mild flulike symptoms
    3. Opportunistic infections
    4. Fatal respiratory complications

22. What differentiates typical progressors from long-term nonprogressors and rapid progressors? *(1988)*
    1. Their physiologic response to standard antiviral therapy
    2. The age of the patient (i.e., rapid progressors are usually older)
    3. The length of time between seroconversion and symptom onset
    4. The number and combination of risk factors at time of exposure

23. The patient is advised to be tested for viral load 4 to 6 months after exposure. What is the clinical significance of having a lower viral set point at this stage? *(1988)*
    1. Used to determine the risk for exposing partner to HIV
    2. Predicts minor transient respiratory or skin infections
    3. Helps to determine the type and timing of therapy
    4. Used as a predictor for long-term survival

24. A 32-year-old patient diagnosed with HIV reports she is looking into some alternative and complementary therapies to treat her disease. What is the best response? *(1995)*
    1. "You should only rely on prescribed medications. "
    2. "Those therapies can be costly and ineffective."
    3. "What kind of therapies are you considering?"
    4. "Let me know how they work for you."

25. While caring for a known HIV-positive patient in the emergency department, the nurse notices the phlebotomist preparing to draw blood. Which nursing action is correct? *(2001)*
    1. Do nothing, because all patients should be treated with Standard Precautions.
    2. Ask the technician if the nurse can see him before he starts the procedure.
    3. Flag the chart to let all health care professionals know the patient's status.
    4. Discretely hand a second pair of gloves to the technician as a signal.

26. An HIV-positive patient voices concern about his recurring bouts of diarrhea, because he is making every effort to follow the treatment plan. What factors contribute to the diarrhea? (Select all that apply.) *(2002)*
    1. Side effects of the medications
    2. Infections of the gastrointestinal tract
    3. Damage to the intestinal villi
    4. Malabsorption in the intestinal tract
    5. Insufficient personal hygiene

27. A 34-year-old patient has recently been diagnosed with HIV-associated cognitive motor complex. Which assessment will the nurse initiate? *(2006)*
    1. Presence of numbness or tingling in hands or feet
    2. Level of consciousness based on Glasgow coma scale
    3. Home safety assessment to identify obstacles in hallways
    4. Pain in the extremities when ambulating or bending

28. The nurse is talking to a 17-year-old sexually active adolescent who is reluctant to use condoms because "It just doesn't feel as good." Which barrier to prevention is the adolescent demonstrating? *(2009, 2010)*
    1. Denial of risk
    2. Fear of alienation
    3. Lack of access
    4. Anxiety about sex

29. Which sexual activity would be considered the safest? *(2010)*
    1. Mutual monogamy
    2. Mutual masturbation
    3. Vaginal sex with condom
    4. Serial monogamy

CRITICAL THINKING ACTIVITIES

Activity 1

30. A nursing student has just been stuck by a needle while providing care for a patient whose lifestyle has placed him at high risk for HIV infection. After reporting to the clinic, she has questions. *(2012)*

    a. What course of action should be taken initially? _____

    _____

    _____

    _____

    _____

    b. What patient-based factors will affect her level of susceptibility?_____

    _____

    _____

    _____

    _____

    c. Upon hearing the recommendation for her to begin prophylactic drug therapy, she asks to wait a few days before beginning the medication regimen. How would you advise her?

    _____

    _____

    _____

    _____

    _____

d. After a discussion of the need to begin the medications as soon as possible, she asks for an explanation concerning the pros and cons of taking the drugs.

_____

_____

_____

_____

e. The student voices concerns about having contact with her husband and child. How will the nurse respond to her concerns?

_____

_____

_____

_____

Activity 2

31. A commercial sex worker has used the clinic for treatment for sexually transmitted diseases over the past 3 years, but had always declined testing for HIV. Recently, the worker came in more frequently for a variety of infections that never seemed to fully resolve. Several nurses and health care providers talked to this patient about HIV testing and the benefits of early detection, but the patient said she assumes a "don't know, don't tell" position and that she tries to get all of her customers to use condoms. Several months later, the worker is admitted to the hospital for treatment of opportunistic infection secondary to HIV disease. Discuss the legal and ethical dilemmas for the clinic staff. *(2012, 2013)*

_____

_____

_____

_____

_____

_____

_____

_____

_____

_____

_____

Activity 3

32. Think about your personal feelings and concerns about taking care of a patient with HIV or AIDS. If possible, interview a nurse (or a patient) who experienced the early days of the HIV epidemic. Compare and contrast your own personal feelings to those of people who experienced the early days of HIV disease.

_____

_____

_____

_____

_____

_____

_____

_____

_____

_____

Care of the Patient with Cancer

chapter
56

Answer Key: Textbook page references are provided as a guide for answering these questions. A complete Answer Key is provided in your Additional Learning Resources on Evolve.

MATCHING

Directions: Match the terms to the correct definition. Indicate your answers in the spaces provided.

	Terms		Definition
_____	1. alopecia *(2032)*	a.	Malignant tumors
_____	2. autologous *(2035)*	b.	Malnutrition, marked by weakness and emaciation
_____	3. benign *(2022)*	c.	Loss of hair due to the destruction of hair follicles
_____	4. biopsy *(2023)*	d.	Removal of a small piece of living tissue
_____	5. cachexia *(2036)*	e.	Origin within an individual
_____	6. carcinogen *(2017)*	f.	Change in taste
_____	7. carcinoma *(2022)*	g.	Not recurrent or progressive; nonmalignant
_____	8. immunosurveillance *(2022)*	h.	Substances known to increase the risk for developing cancer
_____	9. dysgeusia *(2037)*	i.	Immune system's recognition and destruction of newly developed abnormal cells
_____	10. leukopenia *(2029)*	j.	Process by which tumor cells spread
_____	11. malignant *(2022)*	k.	Reduction in the number of circulating white blood cells
_____	12. metastasis *(2022)*	l.	Therapy to relieve uncomfortable symptoms, but does not produce a cure
_____	13. neoplasm *(2026)*	m.	Abnormal cell growth with a loss of normal role and function and ability to spread to other body sites
_____	14. palliative *(2026)*	n.	Reduction in the number of circulating platelets
_____	15. stomatitis *(2032)*	o.	Uncontrolled or abnormal growth of cells
_____	16. sarcoma *(2022)*	p.	Malignant tumors of connective tissues
_____	17. thrombocytopenia *(2031)*	q.	Inflamed, sore, ulcerated areas developing within the patient's mouth

SHORT ANSWER

18. What are four quality-of-life factors that affect cancer patients and their families? *(2038)*

   a. _____

   b. _____

   c. _____

   d. _____

19. Name five common concerns voiced by cancer patients. *(2038)*

   a. _____

   b. _____

   c. _____

   d. _____

   e. _____

20. What are the leading primary cancer sites for men? *(2016)*

   a. _____

   b. _____

   c. _____

   d. _____

21. What are the leading primary cancer sites for women? *(2016)*

   a. _____

   b. _____

   c. _____

   d. _____

22. What are cancer's seven warning signals? *(2021)*

   a. _____

   b. _____

   c. _____

   d. _____

   e. _____

   f. _____

   g. _____

TRUE OR FALSE

Directions: Write T for true or F for false in the blanks provided.

_____ 23. The American Cancer Society indicates that in the United States, one out of every two men will develop cancer in their lifetime. *(2016)*

_____ 24. Cancer incidence is higher in African Americans than in any other race. *(2017)*

_____ 25. If a female has genes *BRCA1* or *BRCA2*, she has a 25% risk of having breast cancer during her lifetime. *(2019)*

_____ 26. Cancer cells are not subject to the usual restrictions placed on cell proliferation by the host. *(2022)*

FIGURE LABELING

27. Directions: On the figure below, identify the four types of biopsy depicted. *(2024)*

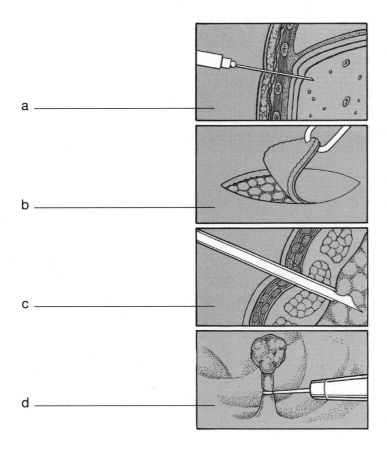

a _____

b _____

c _____

d _____

CLINICAL APPLICATION OF MATH

28. The American Cancer Society recommends adults engage in at least 150 minutes of moderate physical activity each week or 75 minutes of vigorous activity each week. *(2021)*
    a. Patient A desires to exercise five times a week doing moderate physical exercise. How many minutes per day will the patient have to spend for each session? _____ min
    b. Patient B desires to exercise six times a week doing moderate physical exercise. How many minutes per day will the patient have to spend for each session? _____ min
    c. Patient C desires to exercise three times a week doing vigorous physical exercise. How many minutes per day will the patient have to spend for each session?_____ min
    d. Patient D desires to exercise seven times a week doing vigorous physical exercise. How many minutes per day will the patient have to spend for each session?_____ min

29. The nurse knows that a 5% weight loss places the patient at risk for malnutrition and the health care provider should be notified. If the patient weighs 140 pounds, how many pounds would be considered a 5% loss? _____ pounds *(2037)*

TABLE ACTIVITY

30. Directions: Fill in the normal values in the table below. *(2031)*

	Male	**Female**
Erythrocytes (RBCs)	million/mm³	million/mm³
Hemoglobin	g/dL	g/dL
Hematocrit	%	%

MULTIPLE CHOICE

Directions: Select the best answer(s) for each of the following questions.

31. What is the single most important lifestyle modification that can reduce risk for cancer? *(2017)*
    1. Eat a low-fat, high-fiber diet.
    2. Stop smoking.
    3. Avoid excessive sun exposure.
    4. Limit alcohol consumption.

32. Which dietary recommendation to decrease risk for cancer comes from the National Cancer Institute? *(2018)*
    1. Eat four to five servings of lean protein each day.
    2. Eat at least two servings of yellow cheese each day.
    3. Add several types of beans to your diet every week.
    4. Eat at least five servings of fruit and vegetables each day.

33. The patient states that she knows vitamin C is an important nutrient in the prevention of cancer, but she really dislikes citrus fruits. What is the best alternative source that the nurse could suggest? *(2018)*
    1. Taking a vitamin C supplement
    2. Trying citrus juice in place of fruit
    3. Eating strawberries or tomatoes
    4. Eating carrots or cauliflower

34. The nurse is talking to a 23-year-old woman about breast self-examination (BSE). What does the nurse tell the patient about timing and frequency of doing BSE? *(2021)*
    1. Perform the examination monthly on the first day of your menses.
    2. Perform the examination on the first day of every month.
    3. Perform the examination if you notice a discharge from the nipple.
    4. Perform the examination 2 to 3 days after your period ends.

35. A prostate-specific antigen (PSA) test is usually recommended at age 50. Beginning at age 40, members of which ethnic group need to be advised to get the test? *(2026)*
    1. Asian American
    2. African American
    3. Native American
    4. Caucasian American

36. According to clinical staging classification, which stage indicates the most extensive cancer with the poorest prognosis? *(2023)*
    1. Stage 0
    2. Stage I
    3. Stage III
    4. Stage IV

37. According to the TNM classification system, which set of parameters suggests the best prognosis? *(2023)*
    1. $T_0; N_0; M_0$
    2. $T_x; N_x; M_x$
    3. $T_{is}; N_1; M_1$
    4. $T_4; N_4; M_4$

38. The patient is having a radioisotope bone scan. He has had the radioactive material injected into his arm and the nurse encourages him to drink water for the next several hours. What is the purpose of encouraging fluids? *(2024)*
    1. Radioisotope that is not picked up by the bone will be flushed through the kidneys.
    2. The radioactive material could be harmful to the kidneys if not diluted and voided.
    3. The fluid enhances the contrast media and facilitates visualization of tumor areas.
    4. Extra fluid thins secretions and improves the visualization of the lung fields.

39. The health care provider is considering magnetic resonance imaging (MRI) for a patient who might have a spinal tumor. Prior to the MRI, the nurse would notify the provider if the patient disclosed which information? *(2025)*
    1. History of depression
    2. Family history of breast cancer
    3. History of hip fracture
    4. History of deep vein thrombosis

40. The health care provider informs the nurse that the patient may have metastasis to the bone. The provider requests that the nurse notify him immediately with the relevant results. Which test will the nurse be watching for? *(2025)*
    1. Serum calcitonin
    2. Alkaline phosphatase
    3. Carcinomaembryonic antigen
    4. CA-125

41. The patient has a positive guaiac test, but he tells the nurse that he may have not followed the dietary instructions correctly. Which food substance is most likely to cause a false positive? *(2026)*
    1. A rare hamburger
    2. A double fudge sundae
    3. French fries with catsup
    4. Caffeinated soda

42. The nurse is present when the health care provider tells the patient that a combination of surgery, radiation, and chemotherapy are needed to treat his cancer. Afterwards, the patient angrily says, "I'm not going to spend my last days getting poked by that doctor. I'm leaving the hospital!" What should the nurse say? *(2037)*
    1. "I respect your decision, but is there anything I can do to help?"
    2. "Don't be hasty, you have just had bad news; wait for a while."
    3. "Please don't leave. The doctor is just trying to help you."
    4. "You are upset; that's understandable. Let me call your doctor."

43. The nurse is giving instructions to the UAP on how to assist with hygiene for a patient who is currently undergoing external radiation over a large portion of the trunk. What will the nurse say? *(2028)*
    1. Gently clean the skin with a mild soap and flush with warm water.
    2. Do not put lotion, cream, or body powder over the marked areas.
    3. Help the patient take a shower, but use tepid water and a soft cloth.
    4. Shower according to usual procedure, but don't scrub the skin.

44. In caring for the patient who is being treated with internal radiation, what is the most important part of the nursing process for the nurse to prevent self-exposure? *(2028)*
    1. Assessment
    2. Planning
    3. Implementation
    4. Evaluation

45. The nurse is instructing the UAP on how to assist the patient who received an applicator of radioactive material in the vagina. What instructions should the nurse give? *(2028)*
    1. Spend a maximum of 10 minutes to help with a bed bath from the waist up.
    2. Assist the patient with perineal care because vaginal discharge is likely.
    3. Help the patient ambulate to the shower if she is feeling well enough to walk.
    4. Turn the patient every 2 hours and remind her to do range-of-motion for her arms.

46. The patient is placed on neutropenic precautions for a neutrophil count of fewer than 1000/mm³. Which order would the nurse question? *(2030)*
    1. Take vital signs every 4 hours.
    2. Report temperature > 100.4° F (38° C).
    3. Catheterize for urine specimen.
    4. Administer filgrastim (Neupogen).

47. The patient has stomatitis secondary to chemotherapy. Which intervention will the nurse use? *(2030)*
    1. Suggest that the patient suck hard candy or chew gum.
    2. Help the patient rinse with mouthwash every 2 to 4 hours.
    3. Use a sponge-tipped applicator to perform frequent mouth care.
    4. Suggest drinking warm soup, tea, or other hot liquids.

48. The patient is receiving epoetin alfa (Epogen). Which laboratory finding indicates that the therapy is helping? *(2031)*
    1. Normalization of the white cell count
    2. Improvement of the red cell count
    3. Increase in the platelet count
    4. Normalization of the electrolytes

49. Which observation would be consistent with a platelet count of fewer than 20,000/mm³? *(2031)*
    1. Extreme fatigue
    2. Decreased urine output
    3. High fever
    4. Bleeding gums

50. While caring for a 23-year-old patient undergoing chemotherapy, the patient voices concerns about her hair loss. The nurse advises her that: *(2032)*
    1. the loss of her hair will not be permanent.
    2. hair loss will only affect facial areas.
    3. the hair just stops growing temporarily.
    4. when the hair grows back, it will be thicker.

51. During meal planning for a cancer patient, the patient reports that things have a "strange" taste, which is affecting her appetite. Select those possible responses that accurately pertain to her concern. (Select all that apply.) *(2037)*
    1. This is a common occurrence and will get better after her treatments end.
    2. This phenomenon is a permanent and unfortunate consequence associated with cancer.
    3. Onion and ham may help to improve the taste of her vegetables.
    4. Lemon juice is frequently used with success to mask these taste alterations.
    5. Eat anything that you feel like, just to keep up your caloric intake.

52. Select those factors shown to have an impact on the determination of how well a patient will cope with a diagnosis of cancer. (Select all that apply.) *(2038)*
    1. Age at the time of the diagnosis
    2. Availability of significant others
    3. Presence of symptoms
    4. Socioeconomic status
    5. Gender
    6. Ability to express feelings

53. The nurse is reviewing the patient's medication list and sees that the patient is taking ondansetron (Zofran). What additional intervention will the nurse plan to use? *(2032)*
    1. Minimize food odors or noxious smells.
    2. Help the patient dangle before walking.
    3. Check the pulse before giving the drug.
    4. Place a sign on the door to limit visitors.

54. What is an early sign/symptom of tumor lysis syndrome? *(2034)*
    1. Anuria
    2. Muscle weakness
    3. Paresthesias
    4. Tetany

55. What is the most effective regimen to manage the patient's cancer pain? *(2036)*
    1. Patient-controlled analgesia
    2. Bolus dose for breakthrough pain
    3. Round-the-clock, fixed dose
    4. PRN, based on assessment

CRITICAL THINKING ACTIVITIES

Activity 1

56. During a routine checkup, a 40-year-old man voices questions about his potential for developing colon cancer. He relates his concerns about the recent death of his maternal grandfather from colon cancer. *(2018, 2019, 2026)*

    a. Discuss how a family history of colon cancer affects the recommendations for screening examinations for this patient.

    _____

    _____

    _____

    _____

    b. What preventive behaviors should be included in discussions with this patient? _____

    _____

    _____

    _____

    _____

Activity 2

57. A 32-year-old patient is undergoing radiation therapy for treatment of cervical cancer. *(2027-2029)*

    a. The patient's mother asks for clarification concerning the differences between radiation therapy and chemotherapy.

    _____

    _____

    _____

    _____

b. After returning to her room after the first treatment, the patient asks if she can shower. Discuss this patient's request.

_____

_____

_____

_____

c. What precautions should be observed with this patient? _____

_____

_____

_____

_____

d. The patient's husband asks about the visitation policy for the couple's 2-year-old daughter. How should the nurse respond?

_____

_____

_____

_____

e. Identify nursing interventions for the care of this patient. _____

_____

_____

_____

_____

_____

_____

Professional Roles and Leadership

chapter

57

Answer Key: Textbook page references are provided as a guide for answering these questions. A complete Answer Key is provided in your Additional Learning Resources on Evolve.

SHORT ANSWER

Directions: Using your own words, answer each question in the space provided.

1. What are the key components of a cover letter? *(2042, 2043)* _____

   _____

   _____

2. What are the advantages of membership in professional organizations? *(2048)* _____

   _____

   _____

3. Discuss certification programs, continuing education opportunities, and furthering education programs that are available for the LPN/LVN. *(2048-2050)*

   _____

   _____

   _____

4. For the NCLEX-RN® and NCLEX-PN® examinations, identify the following. *(2051)*

   a. Minimum number of questions: _____

   b. Maximum number of questions: _____

   c. Maximum time allowed:_____

   d. Goal of CAT testing: _____

   e. Average time to receive results:_____

   f. Approval for candidate to take the test given by:_____

   g. Examples of alternate-item format questions:_____

5. Why is it important for the LPN/LVN to be familiar with the nurse practice act of the state where he/she decides to work? *(2053)*

_____

_____

_____

6. List all of the possible job settings for an LPN/LVN. *(2053-2057)*_____

_____

_____

_____

_____

FILL-IN-THE-BLANK SENTENCES

Directions: Complete each sentence by filling in the blank with the correct word or phrase.

7. A(n) _____ is a nurse with more experience and knowledge who is willing to assist a novice to learn the skills of the profession through counseling, role modeling, and teaching. *(2053)*

8. _____ is a specialty that "integrates nursing science, computer science, and information science to manage and communicate data, information, knowledge, and wisdom in nursing practice." *(2058)*

9. _____ for nurses is becoming increasingly important in a society that has become lawsuit-conscious. *(2061)*

10. If a nurse or a coworker becomes addicted to drugs or alcohol, the only option is _____. *(2064)*

MULTIPLE CHOICE

Directions: Select the best answer(s) for each of the following questions.

11. There has been an earthquake in the area, and disaster victims are being brought into the emergency department. In this situation, the type of leadership that is the most effective for the nurse manager is: *(2057)*
    1. democratic.
    2. autocratic.
    3. situational.
    4. laissez-faire.

12. The nursing student will be in a position to take the NCLEX-PN® within a few months. However, her fiancé is likely to be transferred to another state within the next year. What should the student do? *(2052)*
    1. Wait until the fiancé has moved and then apply to that state board of nursing to take NCLEX-PN®.
    2. Wait until after legally married to take the NCLEX-PN® so that the license will be issued under her married name.
    3. Apply to take the NCLEX-PN® in the current state of residency and investigate reciprocity or endorsement with other states.
    4. Apply to take the NCLEX-PN® in the current state of residency and then retake the NCLEX-PN® in the permanent state of residency.

13. A new nurse is unsure of the order that is written, but believes that it is appropriate. What should the nurse do first? *(2059)*
    1. Transcribe it to the medication administration record.
    2. Report the problem to the nursing supervisor.
    3. Wait until the health care provider returns to the unit and ask for clarification.
    4. Ask a charge nurse or senior nurse to look at the order.

14. The patient had surgery in the morning, and during the evening requests medication for pain. The nurse administers a preoperative dose of an opioid medication. One hour later, the patient reports that the pain is unrelieved and the nurse realizes that she made an error. What should the nurse do first? *(2060-2061)*
    1. Check the postoperative orders and give the correct dose.
    2. Inform the patient that additional medication cannot be given at this time.
    3. Report the error to the provider and ask for a one-time order for pain medication.
    4. Make out an incident report and document actions in the patient record.

15. The nurse is caring for several patients. Which task(s) can be delegated to the UAP? (Select all that apply.) *(2058)*
    1. Taking the morning vital signs
    2. Changing the linens for isolation patients
    3. Restocking the medications and intravenous solutions
    4. Ambulating patients in the hallway
    5. Assessing skin condition while bathing
    6. Transcribing orders during the night shift

16. Which action could be considered negligence by the nurse and could potentially result in the loss of the nursing license? *(2053)*
    1. Fails to check patient allergies prior to administering medication, but patient suffers no harm
    2. Fails to report change of patient status to provider and later the patient has to be taken for emergency surgery
    3. Fails to give medication within the time limit established by the facility's policies and procedures
    4. Fails to come to work on time and so off-going nurse has to stay later to cover patient care

17. The nurse overhears another nurse, who is a friend, discussing patient information in the cafeteria. There are several visitors nearby and it appears that they are also overhearing the conversation. What should the nurse do first? *(2046, 2061)*
    1. Take the nurse aside and tell her that others are listening.
    2. Report the nurse to risk management.
    3. Walk over to the nurse and quickly change the subject.
    4. Write an incident report and submit it anonymously.

18. The nurse is assigned to be the chairman of a patient satisfaction committee. The committee will include nurses, UAPs, and unit secretaries from other units in the hospital. Which style of leadership would be most useful? *(2056)*
    1. Autocratic
    2. Democratic
    3. Laissez-faire
    4. Situational

19. The nurse is working in a long-term care facility and instructs the UAP to assist several patients with morning hygiene and report back if anyone is having any problems. What delegation error has the nurse made? *(2058)*
    1. Has assigned the UAP too many patients
    2. Has given the UAP a task that is not within scope of practice
    3. Has given broad and generalized instructions to the UAP
    4. Has failed to give feedback on the UAP's performance

20. The new nurse is having difficulty with time management. She feels very frustrated and ends up staying late every day to complete her work. What should be the first step to improve time management? *(2058, 2059)*
    1. Ask for help if falling behind schedule.
    2. Stop socializing with colleagues.
    3. Reflect on how the time is being spent.
    4. Set goals every day and stick to them.

CRITICAL THINKING ACTIVITIES

21. Identify a job or a practice setting that you would like to apply for. Describe what you will need to do in order to increase your chances of getting your first choice of position. *(2042, 2043)*

_____

_____

_____

_____

_____

22. The nurse has just started a new job, but has never worked the night shift before. Identify self-care behaviors that the nurse could use for each of the following. *(2047)*

    a. Staying alert at work: _____

    _____

    b. Getting to sleep: _____

    _____

    c. Balancing life with work: _____

    _____

    d. While there are many disadvantages to working the night shift, the nurse is looking forward to the new job and decides to focus on some of the advantages. Identify several things that could be considered a benefit of being on this shift. (Hint: Interview several night-shift nurses to get a variety of opinions.) *(2045-2047)*

    _____

    _____

    _____

    _____

23. a. Listen to several different nurses give change-of-shift report. Describe the strong points of the reports and describe parts of the reports that could have been improved. *(2061)*

    _____

    _____

    _____

    _____

    _____

    _____

b. Compare and contrast different styles of report that you have seen on clinical units (e.g., tape recordings, rounding on patients, etc.). If you have only seen one method, interview nurses and discuss with classmates or senior students. *(2061)*

_____

_____

_____

_____

_____

24. A nurse has been working at the same job for several years. She has always worked hard and tried to give good care to the patients, even when conditions at the hospital were less than ideal. Lately, she feels exhausted and depressed and often she finds herself complaining to other nurses about working conditions and the lack of gratitude that seems to come from patients, families, and nursing administration.

a. What factors can contribute to burnout among nurses? *(2061, 2062)* _____

_____

_____

_____

_____

_____

b. What are the signs and symptoms of burnout? *(2062)* _____

_____

_____

_____

_____

_____

c. What are strategies to prevent burnout? *(2062, 2063)* _____

_____

_____

_____

_____

_____

Notes

Notes